CURRENT THERAPY IN FOOT AND ANKLE SURGERY

CURRENT THERAPY SERIES

CURRENT THERAPY IN
FOOT AND
ANKLE SURGERY

MARK MYERSON, M.D.

Director
Foot and Ankle Services
The Union Memorial Hospital
Assistant Professor of Orthopedic Surgery
The Johns Hopkins University School of Medicine
Baltimore, Maryland

B.C. Decker
An Imprint of Mosby–Year Book, Inc.

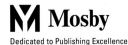

Dedicated to Publishing Excellence

Executive Editor: Susan M. Gay
Senior Managing Editor: Lynne Gery
Project Editor: Ross Goldberg

Copyright © 1993 by Mosby–Year Book, Inc.
A B.C. Decker imprint of Mosby–Year Book, Inc.

All rights reserved. No part of this publication may be reproduced,
stored in a retrieval system, or transmitted, in any form or by any
means, electronic, mechanical, photocopying, recording, or otherwise,
without prior written permission from the publisher.

Permission to photocopy or reproduce solely for internal or personal use is
permitted for libraries or other users registered with the Copyright Clearance
Center, provided that the base fee of $4.00 per chapter plus $.10 per page is
paid directly to the Copyright Clearance Center, 27 Congress Street, Salem, MA
01970. This consent does not extend to other kinds of copying, such as copying for
general distribution, for advertising or promotional purposes, for creating new collected
works, or for resale.

Printed in the United States of America

Mosby–Year Book, Inc.
11830 Westline Industrial Drive
St. Louis, MO 63146

NOTICE: The authors and publisher have made every effort to ensure
that the patient care recommended herein, including choice of drugs
and drug dosages, is in accord with the accepted standards and
practice at the time of publication. However, since research and
regulation constantly change clinical standards, the reader is
urged to check the product information sheet included in the
package of each drug, which includes recommended doses, warnings,
and contraindications. This is particularly important with new or
infrequently used drugs.

Library of Congress Cataloging in Publication Data

Current therapy in foot and ankle surgery / [edited by] Mark Myerson.
    p.   cm. — (Current therapy series)
   Includes bibliographical references and index.
   ISBN 1-55664-389-6
    1. Foot—Abnormalities—Surgery. 2. Foot—Wounds and injuries
—Surgery. 3. Ankle—Abnormalities—Surgery. 4. Ankle—Wounds and
injuries—Surgery. I. Myerson, Mark. II. Series.
    [DNLM: 1. Ankle—surgery. 2. Ankle Injuries—surgery. 3. Foot—
surgery. 4. Foot Diseases—surgery. WE 880 C9758]
RD781.C877 1993
617.5'85059—dc20
DNLM/DLC
for Library of Congress

92-48292
CIP

93 94 95 96 97 GW/MY 9 8 7 6 5 4 3 2 1

WE
880
C9758
1993

REID A. ABRAMS, M.D.

Assistant Professor of Orthopaedics, and Chief, Hand and Microvascular Surgery Service, University of California, San Diego, School of Medicine, San Diego, California

IAN J. ALEXANDER, M.D., FRCSC

Associate Professor of Orthopedics, Northeastern Ohio University College of Medicine, Rootstown; Staff, Orthopaedic Surgeons, Inc., Crystal Clinic, Akron, Ohio

RICHARD G. ALVAREZ, M.D.

Director, Southern Orthopaedic Foot and Ankle Center, Chattanooga, Tennessee

JUDITH FORD BAUMHAUER, M.D.

Orthopedic Surgery Resident, University of Vermont College of Medicine, Burlington, Vermont

JAMES L. BESKIN, M.D.

Clinical Assistant Professor of Orthopedics, Tulane University School of Medicine, New Orleans, Louisiana; Peachtree Orthopedic Clinic, Atlanta, Georgia

SUE C. BODINE-FOWLER, Ph.D.

Assistant Professor of Orthopaedics, University of California, San Diego, School of Medicine, San Diego, and Veterans Administration Medical Center, La Jolla, California

R. LUKE BORDELON, M.D.

Clinical Professor of Orthopaedics, Louisiana State University School of Medicine, New Orleans; Director, Foot Clinic, Doctors Hospital of Opelousas, Opelousas, Louisiana

MICHAEL J. BOTTE, M.D.

Associate Professor of Surgery, and Chief, Foot and Ankle Surgery, Department of Orthopaedic Surgery, University of California, San Diego, School of Medicine; Chief, Rehabilitation Medicine, Veterans Administration Medical Center, San Diego, California

JAMES W. BRODSKY, M.D.

Clinical Assistant Professor of Orthopaedic Surgery, University of Texas Southwestern Medical School at Dallas; Director, Orthopedic and Diabetic Foot Clinic, Veterans Administration Medical Center, Dallas, Texas

JASON H. CALHOUN, M.D., M.Eng.

Associate Professor of Orthopedics, University of Texas Medical Branch at Galveston, Galveston, Texas

CECIL A. CASS, F.R.C.S.

Clinical Lecturer, Orthopaedic Surgery, University of New South Wales; Senior Orthopaedic Surgeon, St. Vincent's General Hospital, Sydney, Australia

MICHAEL J. COUGHLIN, M.D.

Clinical Associate Professor of Surgery, Division of Orthopedics, Department of Surgery, Oregon Health Sciences University School of Medicine, Portland, Oregon; Private Practice, St. Alphonsus Regional Medical Center, Boise, Idaho

RICHARD S. DAVIDSON, M.D.

Clinical Assistant Professor of Orthopaedic Surgery, University of Pennsylvania School of Medicine, and Children's Hospital of Philadelphia, Philadelphia, Pennsylvania

FIONA L. DULBECCO, B.A.

Medical Student, University of California, San Diego, School of Medicine; Laboratory Technician, Neuromuscular and Microsurgical Research Laboratory, Veterans Administration Medical Center, San Diego, California

PETER EDWARDS, M.D.

Resident, Department of Orthopedics, West Virginia University School of Medicine, Morgantown, West Virginia

CAROL FREY, M.D.

Associate Clinical Professor of Orthopaedic Surgery, University of Southern California School of Medicine; Director, Orthopaedic Foot and Ankle Center, Orthopaedic Hospital, Los Angeles, California

3 0001 00259 4598

2717 3006

STANLEY C. GRAVES, M.D.

Associate Professor, University of Tennessee, Memphis, College of Medicine; Instructor and Staff, Campbell Clinic, Memphis, Tennessee

WILLIAM G. HAMILTON, M.D.

Assistant Clinical Professor of Orthopedic Surgery, Columbia University College of Physicians and Surgeons; Senior Attending, Orthopedic Surgery, St. Luke's–Roosevelt Hospital Center, New York, New York

JOHN D. HSU, M.D., C.M., F.A.C.S.

Clinical Professor of Orthopaedics, University of Southern California School of Medicine, Los Angeles; Chief of Orthopaedics, and Chairman, Department of Surgery, Rancho Los Amigos Medical Center, Downey, California

SHEPARD HURWITZ, M.D.

Associate Professor of Orthopaedics, University of Rochester School of Medicine; Director, Foot Surgery Service, University of Rochester Medical Center, Rochester, New York

MELVIN H. JAHSS, M.D.

Clinical Professor of Orthopaedic Surgery, Mount Sinai School of Medicine of the City University of New York; Attending and Chief, Orthopaedic Foot Service, Hospital for Joint Diseases Orthopaedic Institute, New York, New York

CARROLL A. LAURIN, M.D., FRCSC

Professor of Surgery, Maurice and Marthe Muller Chair of Orthopaedic Surgery, McGill University Faculty of Medicine; Surgeon-in-Charge, Division of Orthopaedic Surgery, Royal Victoria Hospital, Montreal, Quebec, Canada

GEORGE J. LIAN, M.D.

Assistant Clinical Professor of Orthopaedic Surgery, and Head, Foot and Ankle Service, University of California, Davis, School of Medicine, Davis, California

JON T. MADER, M.D.

Professor, Division of Infectious Diseases, and Chief, Division of Hyperbaric Medicine, Department of Marine Medicine, University of Texas Medical Branch at Galveston, Galveston, Texas

BERT MANDELBAUM, M.D.

Adjunct Assistant Professor of Orthopaedics, University of California, Los Angeles, School of Medicine, Los Angeles; Team Physician, Pepperdine University Hospital, Malibu, California

ROGER A. MANN, M.D.

Director, Foot Fellowship Program, Oakland; Associate Clinical Professor of Orthopaedic Surgery, University of California, San Francisco, School of Medicine, San Francisco, California

WILLIAM C. McGARVEY, M.D.

Orthopaedic Resident, Union Memorial Hospital, Baltimore, Maryland

HEIDI MULTHOPP-STEPHENS, M.D.

Foot and Ankle Fellow, Tampa Orthopedic Program, Tampa, Florida

MARK MYERSON, M.D.

Director, Foot and Ankle Services, The Union Memorial Hospital; Assistant Professor of Orthopedic Surgery, The Johns Hopkins University School of Medicine, Baltimore, Maryland

TYE J. OUZOUNIAN, M.D.

Clinical Instructor of Surgery and Orthopaedics, University of California, Los Angeles, School of Medicine; Attending Physician, Wadsworth Veterans Administration Medical Center, Los Angeles; and Active Staff, Tarzana Regional Medical Center, Tarzana, California

JOHN A. PAPA, M.D.

Attending, Orthopaedic Surgery, Orlando Regional Medical Center, and Orthopaedic Foot and Ankle Surgery, Matthews Orthopaedic Clinic, Orlando, Florida

GLENN B. PFEFFER, M.D.

Assistant Clinical Professor, and Chief, Orthopaedic Foot and Ankle Clinic, University of California, San Francisco, School of Medicine; Chief, Orthopaedic Foot and Ankle Surgery, California Pacific Medical Center, Pacific Campus, San Francisco, California

GEORGE E. QUILL, Jr., M.D.

Clinical Instructor of Orthopedic Surgery, University of Louisville School of Medicine; Director, Orthopedic Foot and Ankle Surgery, Louisville Orthopedic Clinic and The Foot and Ankle Center at Humana Hospital–Suburban, Louisville, Kentucky

RONALD QUIRK, F.R.C.S., F.R.A.C.S.

Consultant Orthopaedic Surgeon, The Australian Ballet, The Australian Ballet School, The Victorian College of the Arts, and The Australian Institute of Sport, Melbourne, Australia

E. GREER RICHARDSON, M.D.

Associate Professor of Orthopaedic Surgery, University of Tennessee, Memphis, College of Medicine; Director, Foot and Ankle Fellowship, and Staff, Campbell Clinic, Memphis, Tennessee

G. JAMES SAMMARCO, M.D.

Volunteer Professor of Orthopedics, University of Cincinnati School of Medicine, Cincinnati, Ohio

BRUCE J. SANGEORZAN, M.D.

Associate Professor of Orthopaedic Surgery, University of Washington School of Medicine, Seattle, Washington

TERENCE SAXBY, F.R.A.C.S.

Brisbane Orthopaedic and Sports Medicine Centre, Brisbane, Australia

MARK E. SCHAKEL II, M.D.

Private Practice, Santa Rosa Orthopaedic Medical Group, Santa Rosa, California

LEW C. SCHON, M.D.

Clinical Instructor of Family Medicine, University of Texas Health Science Center at Houston, Houston, Texas; Associate Director, Foot and Ankle Center, and Attending Orthopaedic Surgeon, The Union Memorial Hospital, Baltimore, Maryland

MICHAEL J. SHEREFF, M.D.

Associate Professor of Orthopaedic Surgery, Medical College of Wisconsin; Director, Division of Foot and Ankle Surgery, Milwaukee Regional Medical Center, Milwaukee, Wisconsin

FRANCESCA M. THOMPSON, M.D.

Assistant Clinical Professor of Orthopedic Surgery, Columbia University College of Physicians and Surgeons; Chief, Adult Orthopedic Foot Clinic, St. Luke's–Roosevelt Hospital Center, New York, New York

SAUL G. TREVINO, M.D.

Clinical Associate Professor of Orthopaedics, Baylor College of Medicine; Chief, Foot and Ankle Services, Veterans Administration Medical Center, Houston, Texas

To Melvin Jahss,

my mentor and friend,

whose insight and encouragement

have nurtured and inspired my

commitment to excellence

PREFACE

This text is an exciting amalgamation of current concepts of surgical techniques in foot and ankle surgery. The contributors are all internationally recognized experts in their field, who present their step-by-step approaches in their individual styles.

The emphasis in this text is on surgery and surgical technique. Yet this is not a "how to" text, which I think loses some value in too simplistic a format. The chapters present surgical techniques in a logical and focused manner, and highlight the pathophysiology and biomechanics of deformity. The surgical approaches are enhanced by numerous illustrations, most of which are published for the first time.

My goal in editing this text was to provide the reader with a comprehensive but succinct source for operative techniques in foot and ankle surgery. Although this is a multi-author text, I have included my own philosophy of treatment wherever possible. The result is a text that is easy to read and that I hope will be invaluable to anyone with an interest in foot and ankle surgery.

Mark Myerson, M.D.

CONTENTS

THE FOREFOOT

TOENAIL DEFORMITIES

GEORGE E. QUILL, JR., M.D.

The two most common, and often the most disabling, toenail deformities requiring surgical management are the ingrown toenail and the onychomycosis arising from deformity and infection of the nail bed of the great toe. The less common maladies afflicting the toenail may be treated expeditiously once one understands the principles involved in managing the ingrown or onychomycotic nail.

The basic mechanism in the pathogenesis of the ingrown toenail (Fig. 1) is improper nail trimming. When the entire nail plate is not allowed to passively grow out beyond the fleshy end of the toe before it is trimmed transversely, a spike of nail remains untrimmed at the lateral margin and is covered by soft tissue. Further nail growth, more "bathroom surgery," and local irritation

result in an infected, ingrown toenail. This self-inflicted mechanism is a much more common etiology of ingrown toenail than are congenital deformity, systemic disease, hallux valgus, trauma, or constrictive shoe wear.

Onychomycosis of the toes results most commonly from *Trichophyton rubrum* and *T. interdigitale* invasion from the lateral nail bed or under the proximal nail fold and cuticle (Fig. 2). As the integrity of the nail is damaged, dirt and air may enter the separated layers of the nail plate, resulting in a variety of deformities. Onychogryphosis is an abnormal thickening of the nail caused by a disordered growth of the germinal matrix or a thickening of the sterile matrix by cornification of the hyponychium (Fig. 3). A combined thickening of both the nail and the sterile matrix occurs. Onychogryphosis may be caused by fungal infection.

The literature is replete with attempts to stage or classify the type of ingrown toenail. Once the patient has symptoms significant enough to warrant an office visit, only two real types of clinical relevance exist: those ingrown nails associated with pus and those not associated with pus.

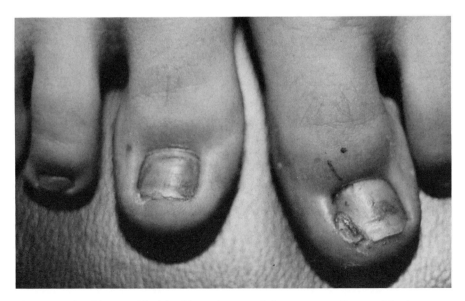

Figure 1 An 11-year-old girl with an ingrown left great toenail caused by improper trimming of the nail.

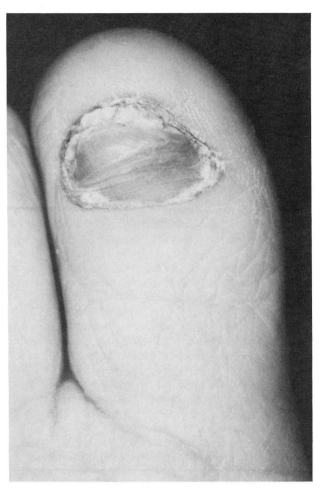

Figure 2 A 62-year-old female with steroid-dependent pulmonary disease and onychomycosis.

THERAPEUTIC ALTERNATIVES

Cases of onychomycosis and onychogryphosis presenting without significant pain or drainage should be left alone. I encourage women with this clinical entity to paint their nails and ignore the underlying deformity. Painful, nondraining cases of onychomycosis and onychogryphosis caused by fungus may be managed with oral griseofulvin therapy, but the patient must be willing to accept prolonged compliance with this method of therapy until the infecting organism is completely eradicated, a period usually no less than 6 months for toenail infection. The patient also must understand that there is a significant risk of hepatotoxicity, photosensitivity, and cross-sensitivity with penicillin. Other drug interactions have been reported. The patient also must be made aware that a high incidence of recrudescence of fungal infection occurs once the medication is discontinued.

Topical antifungal therapy alone has provided less than satisfactory long-term results.

In the past a score of nonoperative therapeutic alternatives for ingrown nails consisting of shoe wear modifications, the tedious application of subungual cotton wicks, silver nitrate therapy, chemical or thermal ablation, and laser therapy have not yielded uniformly positive results. Oral antibiotics and appropriate soaking of ingrown toenails in bactericidal solutions are most useful when employed as a prelude to surgical management of the significantly involved nail.

The most practical surgical options for management of the ingrown or fungally infected nail include the following:

1. Nail plate avulsion
2. Partial matrixectomy

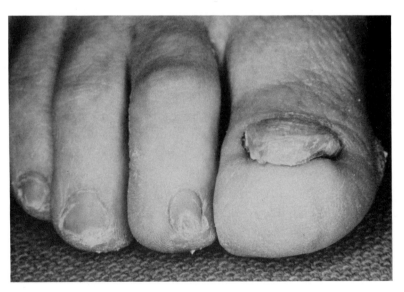

Figure 3 A 58-year-old female with insulin-dependent diabetes mellitus exhibiting significant onychogryphosis.

3. Obliteration of the nail bed without shortening of the terminal phalanx (Zadik's procedure)
4. A terminal Syme amputation and obliteration of the nail bed

The optimal operation achieves a cosmetic result by retaining the majority of the nail, is technically simple, has a low rate of morbidity and a low rate of nail deformity recurrence. In my experience nearly all toenail deformities can be managed by one or a combination of these four techniques, and all four should be incorporated in the surgeon's therapeutic approach.

PREFERRED APPROACH

Onychomycosis, Onychogryphosis, and Purulent Infection of the Entire Nail Bed

The significantly infected or enlarged nail that also causes difficulty with shoe wear should be managed with warm water and povidone-iodine soaks and oral antibiotic therapy until the earliest elective surgical date. I recommend that all these nail procedures are done in the outpatient operative suite where the patient can be made comfortable, the environment is sterile, and the lighting and instrumentation are optimal.

With the patient supine on the operating room table, digital block anesthesia is achieved with usually no more than 7 to 8 ml of an equal mixture of 1 percent lidocaine and 0.5 percent bupivacaine without epinephrine. A 10 minute povidone-iodine and surgical soap preparation is performed, and the patient's affected foot draped in the usual sterile, free fashion.

A disposable exsanguinating digit tourniquet (Tourni-cot) is applied to the level of the base of the involved digit. The patient who desires the least morbid procedure possible, and who is willing to comply with postoperative topical antifungal therapy, may be managed with avulsion of the nail plate.

Subungual dissection with a blunt-tipped tenotomy scissor or Freer elevator is done to the level of the lunula and the nail plate elevated from the sterile nail matrix. The Freer elevator is used to "peel" back the eponychium atraumatically, as well as the medial and lateral nail folds. The nail is delivered with a forceps or Kocher clamp. The underlying sterile matrix is superficially debrided, leaving the hyponychium flush with the nail bed to avoid premature arrest of the new nail's migration over the end of the fleshy part of the toe. No attempt at nail bed ablation is made. The nail bed is irrigated, the Tourni-cot removed, and manual compression applied to the bleeding nail bed for 3 to 5 minutes. A nonadherent, bulky, compressive dressing is applied and left in place for 48 hours, after which the patient may remove the dressing and soak the foot twice daily in warm water and povidone-iodine. The patient usually can wear soft shoes or tennis shoes within 3 to 4 days after the procedure. Fungoid tincture may be applied twice daily to the affected nail bed postoperatively.

The patient with clinically significant onychomycosis, onychogryphosis, or purulent subungual infection of the entire nail plate (most often the result of a traumatic subungual hematoma or neglect), and who desires the most expedient one-step management of the problem, may be managed with either Zadik's procedure or a terminal Syme amputation of the digit. Zadik recommends that if infection is observed under the lateral border of the nail, the nail should be avulsed as a first stage and excision deferred for 2 weeks.

Patient selection and timing of the surgery, as well as preoperative preparation, are similar to that described for nail plate avulsion. Zadik's procedure for obliteration of the nail bed without shortening the terminal phalanx is based on the tenet that the nail bed distal to the lunula makes no contribution to nail growth. The purpose of this procedure is to remove the nail-forming part of the nail bed and provide adequate skin coverage without shortening the distal phalanx.

Under digital block and Tourni-cot control, the skin over the base of the nail bed is raised as a flap, and the nail is avulsed. The part of the nail bed that lies proximal to the border of the lunula is excised sharply with a #15 blade. The skin flap is advanced and sutured without tension to the cut edge of the distal part of the nail bed. When the patient presents with deep lateral nail furrows, the lateral nail folds are excised and the skin edges are sutured to the edge of the nail bed, resulting in an H-shaped incision.

In my opinion the patient may be better managed with a terminal Syme amputation if these flaps appear to be under too much tension, or there is an underlying subungual exostosis or an exaggerated dorsal and upward curvature of the terminal phalanx. If the patient is willing to accept the cosmetic deformity of a terminal Syme procedure, the following procedure should be carried out after the appropriate timing and preoperative preparation.

After the appropriate preparation and draping and using Tourni-cot hemostasis and digital block anesthesia, the first step of the Syme procedure is avulsion of the nail, as described earlier. A sterile skin marker then is used to design a dorsal ellipse of skin and nail matrix (both sterile and germinal) for excision. This ellipse to be excised should be designed so that its closure as the distal skin is brought dorsally may be made appropriately without tension on the skin edges and without the formation of dog-ear flaps.

A #15 blade is used to sharply dissect down to bone well proximal to the proximal most extension of the germinal nail matrix, remaining distal to the interphalangeal joint, extensor hallucis longus, and flexor hallucis longus insertions. This is an extraperiosteal resection of skin, subcutaneous tissue, nail matrix, periosteum, and bone. A bone cutter is used to transect the distal tuft of the terminal phalanx, beveling the cut dorsally and smoothing it appropriately. The surgeon should take care not to fragment the phalangeal bone. Irrigation is performed, the dog-ears are trimmed, and the distal plantar flap is brought up to approximate the proximal dorsal wound margin. Absorbable deep sutures may be used to keep tension off the skin edges, which are closed with nonabsorbable sutures placed in a mattress fashion after removal of the Tourni-cot. Approximately one-fourth of the circumference of a ¼ inch Penrose drain is inserted and allowed to extend out the corner of the wound. This drain site should be kept as small as possible and yet still allow egress of fluid because it must close by secondary intention after the drain is removed 48 hours after the procedure (Fig. 4).

Medial, Lateral, or Simultaneous Medial and Lateral Ingrown Toenail

The patient with this toenail deformity and enough pain to warrant orthopedic referral is best managed with partial matrixectomy in a fashion similar to that described by Winograd or Heifetz. Preoperative preparation is as described earlier. The patient with pus need not be treated emergently, but if he or she comes to surgical management on an urgent basis, one carries out the

procedures in conjunction with prudent irrigation and debridement, and leaves the distal wound open as one might in the draining of an abscess found elsewhere. Ideally a week of oral antibiotics and twice-daily soaks in a dilute solution of warm water and povidone-iodine better prepare the patient for surgery. The following procedure may be carried out on either the medial or lateral nail margin, or in a combined fashion on both sides of the nail plate as clinically indicated, and still leave a cosmetically acceptable result.

Digital block anesthesia in the operating room is achieved. Povidone-iodine and surgical soap preparation is done, and the procedure is done under Tourni-cot hemostasis. A #15 blade is used to incise the eponychium longitudinally, beginning at a level of about 5 to 7 mm proximal to the base of the eponychium and at a distance of about 5 mm from the parallel ingrown nail fold. The incision is carried onto the nail plate, scoring the length of it and, if the hyponychium is thick and

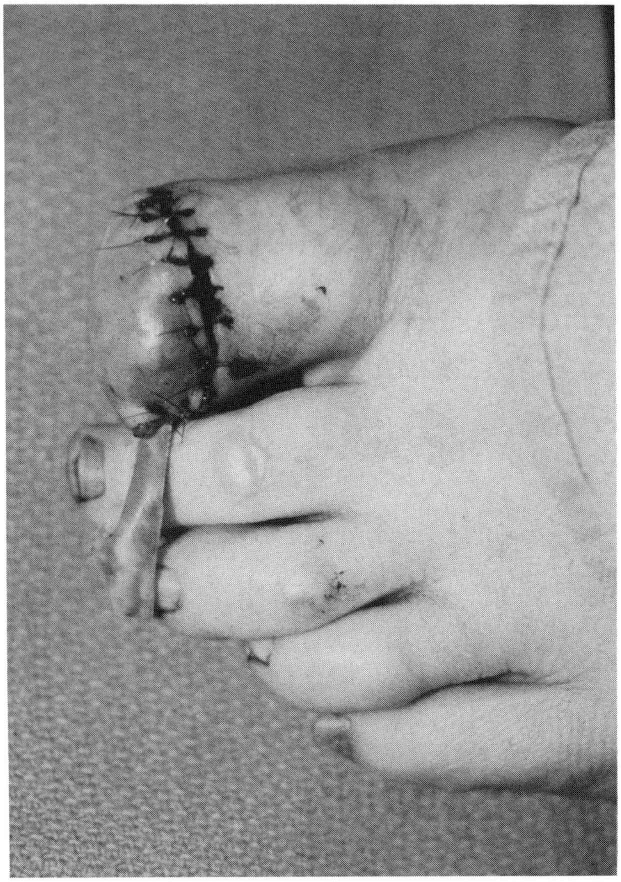

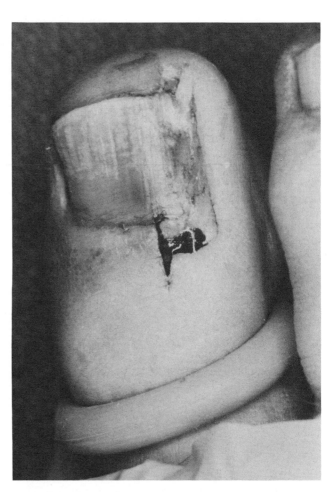

Figure 4 A 45-year-old female underwent a terminal Syme amputation of the hallux for painful nail bed deformity, resulting from a subungual glomus tumor. The residual flaps are contoured to accommodate the medial last of most women's shoes.

Figure 5 A 63-year-old diabetic male undergoing lateral partial matrixectomy. Note the lateral and distal "spike" of nail plate that had gone untrimmed and had become embedded in the lateral nail fold.

protuberant, the incision is carried into the distal 3 to 5 mm of hyponychium. A subungual Freer elevator is inserted distally to proximally, flipping the affected sterile nail plate margin (usually about one-fifth the entire width of the nail plate) up over the lateral nail fold. This maneuver usually exposes the typical self-inflicted spike of distal nail (Fig. 5). A straight Iris scissor is used to transect the nail plate along the line previously scored by the #15 blade. A single skin hook is used to reflect the eponychial flap, and a #15 blade is used to complete the germinal matrixectomy out to the level of the lunular matrix. This excision includes periosteum, but need not resect the entire length of the gutter as originally described by Winograd because this maneuver causes too much perioperative bleeding. A curette is used to ensure matrixectomy. If the lateral nail fold is extremely enlarged and inflamed, one may resect a small wedge of hyponychium distally, allowing the nail fold to more readily approximate the new margin of nail plate. Irrigation is done, one or two simple nonabsorbable sutures of 5.0 Prolene are placed in the eponychial fold, the Tourni-cot is removed, and manual pressure is

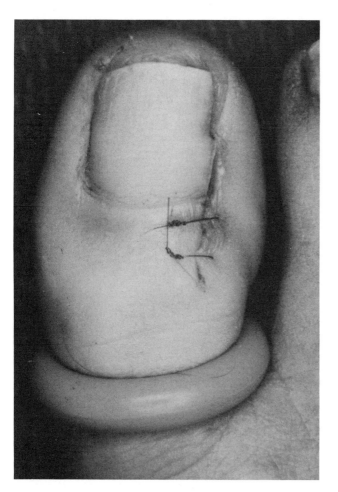

Figure 6 Hallux of 60-year-old female at completion of a lateral partial matrixectomy.

applied to the digit for 5 minutes before applying a nonadherent, bulky, slightly compressive dressing. The patient is told to expect some blood saturating the dressing, but is instructed not to remove the dressing until the second postoperative morning, when an eschar has formed. Twice-daily soaks in warm water and povidone-iodine are instituted, and the patient returns in 1 week for suture removal. If this is an elective partial matrixectomy and there is no pus, the hyponychium may be sutured and approximated as well. (The hyponychium becomes infected if it is closed in the face of pus.) If the appropriate width and margin of nail plate are resected, the lateral nail fold nicely approximates the margin of the nail plate without a suture once the edema and paronychial infection have resolved (Fig. 6).

PROS AND CONS OF SURGICAL TREATMENT OF TOENAIL DEFORMITIES

Avulsion

Advantages of avulsion are that it is an expedient procedure with little morbidity, and when it is combined with perioperative topical antifungal therapy, the patient is encouraged to take charge and play a major role in therapy. The major disadvantage of this procedure is its relatively high rate of recurrence of deformity.

Zadik's Procedure

The advantages of Zadik's procedure are that it is theoretically a one-step approach to nail ablation and preserves the terminal phalanx. The disadvantage of this procedure is the potential for partial recurrence of nail growth and deformity if one does not apply the appropriate knowledge of germinal nail matrix anatomy. Swelling, immobility, and the potentially dysvascular nature of the flaps also may lead to failure.

Winograd Partial Matrixectomy

The advantages of partial matrixectomy are that it is simple and expedient and in my clinical series has afforded permanent relief with a 0 percent recurrence rate of deformity and infection. This procedure may be applied to both sides of the nail and still leave an acceptable cosmetic result. Like incision and drainage of any abscess found elsewhere in the body, this operation may be performed even in the presence of a purulent infection. The disadvantage of the Winograd procedure is that the patient still must be educated in the appropriate trimming of the residual nail. In addition, bleeding is a nuisance.

Terminal Syme Procedure

The advantage of the terminal Syme procedure is that it usually affords a permanent correction of many toenail deformities and infections. The obvious disadvantage is that it involves amputating the distal portion of the terminal phalanx; many women feel it provides an unsatisfactory cosmetic result. A potential for recurrence exists after this procedure, but most recurrences actually represent inclusion cysts and not regrowth of nail.

SUGGESTED READING

Beaven DW, Brooks SE. Color atlas of the nail in clinical diagnosis. Chicago: Year Book Medical Publishers, 1988.
Heifetz CJ. Ingrown toe-nail: A clinical study. Am J Surg 1937; 38:298–315.
Winograd AM. A modification in the technic of operation for ingrown toenail. JAMA 1929; 92:229–230.
Zadik FR. Obliteration of the nail bed of the great toe without shortening of the terminal phalanx. J Bone Joint Surg 1950; 32B:66–67.

DISORDERS OF THE GREAT TOE SESAMOIDS

JAMES W. BRODSKY, M.D.

The great toe sesamoids have two basic functions. First, they provide the weight-bearing points for the first metatarsal, distributing its plantar forces over two points (i.e., twice that of each lesser metatarsal head). The medial sesamoid is usually, but not always, larger than the lateral, bears more weight, and is symptomatic somewhat more frequently. Second, the sesamoids increase the mechanical advantage of the flexor hallucis brevis (FHB) muscle, in whose tendon they are embedded, in a fashion analogous to the function of the patella relative to the quadriceps mechanism. Most presenting clinical problems are related to weight bearing, and most problems and complications of sesamoid surgery are related to loss of function of the surrounding tendinous apparatus.

PRESSURE LESIONS OF THE SESAMOIDS: PLANTAR ULCERATIONS AND PAINFUL, INTRACTABLE PLANTAR KERATOSIS

Painful calluses beneath the first metatarsal head usually are situated under the medial sesamoid. These are further accentuated by other accompanying deformities, especially the plantarflexed first ray of a cavus or cavovarus foot. This is true also for neurotrophic plantar ulcerations beneath the first metatarsophalangeal (MP) joint in patients, such as diabetics, with peripheral neuropathy. When either of these two types of plantar lesion fail to respond to conservative measures, the most commonly indicated procedure is partial medial sesa-

moidectomy, as outlined in the following section. Complete sesamoid excision also can be considered for these indications, but it has a somewhat higher complication rate. If insufficient pressure relief is obtained by partial sesamoidectomy alone, the surgeon can consider concomitant dorsiflexion osteotomy of the metatarsal by taking a basilar dorsally based closing wedge. Complete sesamoidectomy can be done if further pressure relief is necessary.

Partial Sesamoid Excision

Partial sesamoid excision almost always is performed on the medial sesamoid. The lateral sesamoid is seldom in a position to exert the pressure that indicates the need for this operation. Partial excision of the lateral sesamoid is technically difficult.

A horizontal incision is made, parallel to the plantar surface of the foot, but below the midline of the first ray, corresponding to a plane that is plantar to the metatarsal-sesamoid joint. The subcutaneous dissection is done with scissors, avoiding the plantar medial proper sensory nerve to the hallux. Neither the MP joint nor the metatarsal sesamoid joint is entered (Fig. 1).

The plantar surface of the fibers of the medial tendon of the FHB are identified. These are sharply incised in a longitudinal direction with a #15 blade in line with the fibers and peeled off the plantar surface of the medial sesamoid with the sharp end of a Freer elevator. Care is taken not to extend the incision in the fibers more than a few millimeters past either pole of the sesamoid so as not to disrupt the mechanism of the FHB tendon. The dissection is carried over to the lateral side of the bone, separating the fibers from the intersesamoid ligament and the tendon of the flexor hallucis longus (FHL), so that these structures are not bound to the bone at the time of bone resection (Fig. 2).

The plantar half of the sesamoid bone is then resected using a narrow blade on a micro-oscillating saw. Care is taken not to section the soft tissue structures,

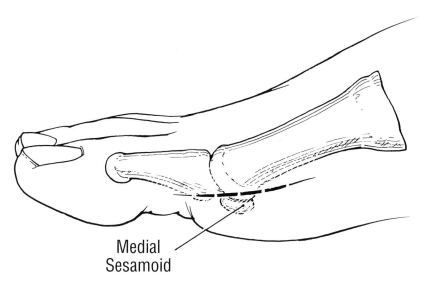

Figure 1 Incision for partial excision of the sesamoid.

Medial
Sesamoid

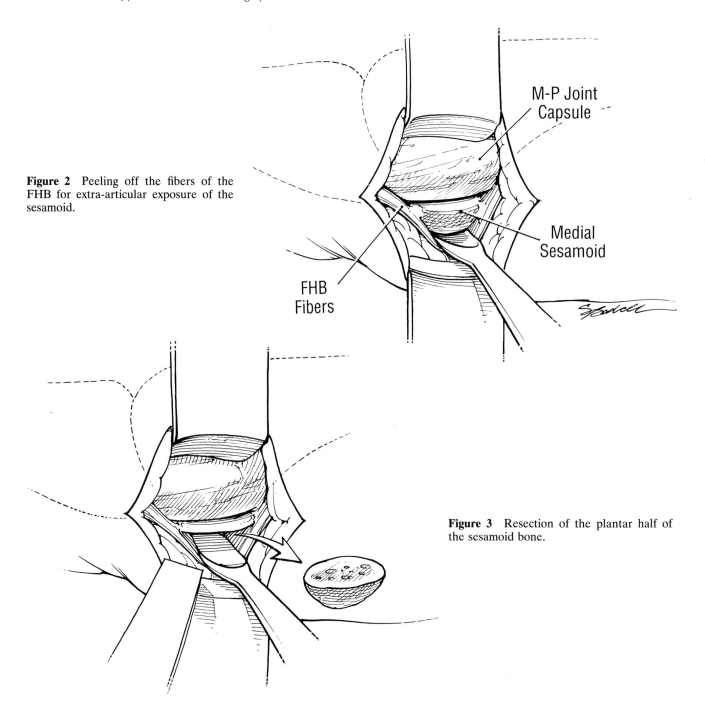

Figure 2 Peeling off the fibers of the FHB for extra-articular exposure of the sesamoid.

Figure 3 Resection of the plantar half of the sesamoid bone.

which *can* be cut if inadvertently held taut against the saw blade (Fig. 3).

The piece of bone is then removed by prying it loose with a small osteotome. Any remaining soft tissue attachments are divided with the #15 blade while rotating the piece into the wound. Avoid cutting blindly in the depth of this small incision to prevent injury to the FHL tendon.

The sharp edges of the remaining dorsal half of the bone are smoothed with a small rasp and the wound irrigated to remove all bony particles. The edges of the plantar fibers of the FHB are reapproximated with 3-0 or 2-0 absorbable sutures. The subcutaneous layer is not sutured to avoid injuring the superficial sensory nerves, and the skin is closed with a running subcuticular suture of 3-0 Prolene.

Pitfalls and Complications

Three problems may result from partial sesamoid excision. The first is incomplete relief of pressure, which may occur even if there has been resection of a sufficient amount of bone. In the patient with pain and a plantar keratosis, it may result in partial or incomplete pain relief and callus formation. In the patient with neuropathic ulceration, the ulcer may recur or fail to heal. Treatment is by excision of the remnant or occasionally by another more proximal technique to elevate the metatarsal head.

The opposing complication is fracture of the residual sesamoid, which has been thinned and does not withstand the pressure of weight bearing. Treatment is with immobilization, and if unsuccessful, excision of the remnant with reconstruction of the FHB tendon (see subsequent section).

Injury to the plantar medial sensory nerve is the third complication. Treatment is by resection of the incisional neuroma if unrelieved by injection.

SESAMOIDITIS VERSUS SESAMOID FRACTURE AND NONUNION

Pain under the sesamoids frequently is attributable to chronic inflammation, called *sesamoiditis.* This usually is distinguished from acute or chronic (or stress) fractures by negative radiographs. Diagnosis of a fractured sesamoid can be subtle, requiring both medial and lateral oblique views, as well as a special tangential sesamoid view. Fractures produce intensely positive technetium-99m bone scans, which should be performed with plantar views to best visualize the sesamoids. Occasionally sesamoiditis also can produce a strongly positive scan. This usually is not a problem if the radiographs are negative, but occasionally, in the case of a congenitally bipartite sesamoid (occuring in approximately 10 percent of the population), the distinction between sesamoiditis and fracture can be difficult. This distinction is important because surgery seldom is indicated for sesamoiditis. Many fractures likewise respond to nonoperative treatment as well, although healing usually occurs through fibrous rather than osseous ankylosis at the fracture site.

Surgical treatment should follow failure of conservative therapy including rest, anti-inflammatory medications, immobilization in walking casts, shoe modification, and molded shoe insoles. The most common operative procedure for symptomatic chronic fracture or nonunion is excision of the entire sesamoid *and* reconstruction of the FHB tendon, described later. For selected early cases, especially in athletes, bone grafting of the fractured sesamoid is a new alternative.

Complete Sesamoid Excision and Flexor Brevis Reconstruction

Medial sesamoid excision is done through a medial approach with an incision parallel to the sole and plantar to the midaxis of the MP joint, which enters the joint between the metatarsal and the sesamoid (Fig. 4). The incision is extended proximally and distally to improve the exposure, while taking care not to transect the FHB tendon. Adequate exposure is gained once the surgeon can visualize both sesamoids and the intersesamoid ligament, beneath which lies the FHL tendon. The sesamoid complex comprises a network of tendons merged around the sesamoid bones to form a sling under the first metatarsal head (Fig. 5A). Conceptualization of the cross-sectional anatomy of the sesmoid complex aids in understanding the surgical dissection (Fig. 5B).

The medial sesamoid then is painstakingly peeled out of the fibers of the flexor brevis, making maximal effort to preserve the fibers on the medial and lateral sides. Dissection is done alternating between a scalpel and a small elevator. Saving the plantar fibers is more difficult, because they are thinner and more easily torn in the process of removing the sesamoid. Loupe magnification is helpful. The intersesamoid ligament is the most important structure to preserve, because it is the key to successful reconstruction of the flexor brevis mechanism (Fig. 6).

Even if there is a painful fibrous nonunion, often it

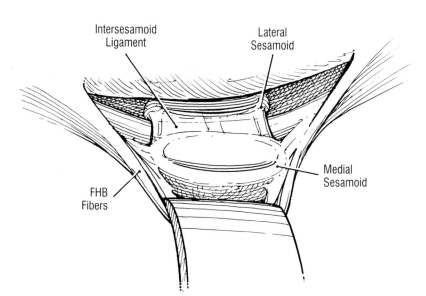

Figure 4 Exposure of the metatarsal-sesamoid joint for complete excision of sesamoid: visualization of both sesamoids and the intersesamoid ligament.

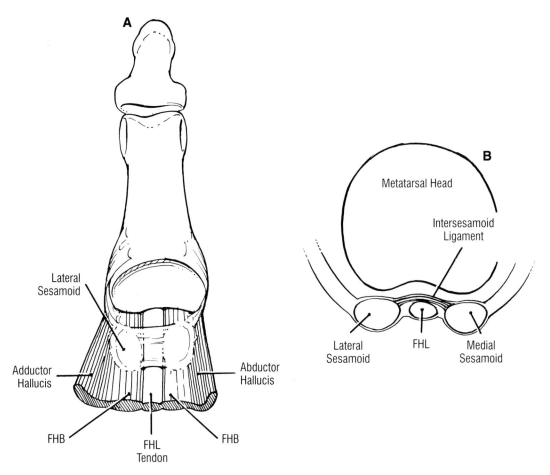

Figure 5 *A,* Cross-sectional view of the sesamoid complex. *B,* Dorsal view of the anatomy of the sesamoid complex (with the metatarsal head removed).

Figure 6 Dissecting out the medial sesamoid and preserving the intersesamoid ligament.

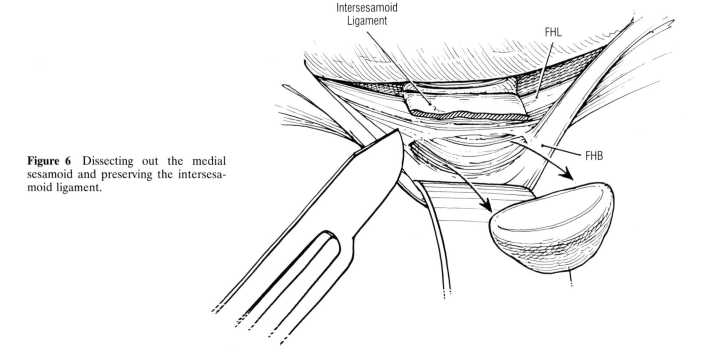

is possible to remove the sesamoid in one piece. A small hook on the bone helps to rotate it out while severing the remaining strands of tendon. At the same time, the hook is less likely than a clamp to crush or separate the specimen. The principles are the same even if the bone must be excised piecemeal. I attempt to remove it as a single specimen for pathologic section and examination in a longitudinal plane; the results are used for histologic confirmation of the fracture or nonunion.

The second, and equally technically challenging half of the operation, is the tendon reconstruction. Once the sesamoid has been removed, inspect the defect (Fig. 7). The intersesamoid ligament should be in reasonable condition, and the FHL tendon, which lies between the defect and the other sesamoid, usually is at least partially visible. The goal of the reconstruction is to achieve the best reapproximation of the combined FHB and medial capsular fibers to the intersesamoid ligament, taking care not to suture the FHL tendon. This tethers the remaining sesamoid with its tendon complex, preventing lateral drift of the lateral sesamoid, which would lead to a postoperative hallux valgus deformity. The converse is true when a lateral sesamoid is excised—namely, the risk of failing to reconstruct the FHB mechanism is a postoperative hallux varus, as documented in the literature on the classic McBride bunionectomy.

The reconstruction usually is done with three or four sutures of 0 absorbable suture, usually rethreaded on a small round needle such as a #6 Mayo needle. This is the most difficult and frustrating part of the procedure. The sutures first must be passed from the intersesamoid ligament and remaining lateral fibers of the FHB; the suture is pulled through and regrabbed with the needle

holder, then passed through the medial FHB fibers (Fig. 8). Each of the sutures is placed and tagged with a small mosquito hemostat. Once all the sutures have been placed, all are tied at the same time. Position of the great toe is checked and, if necessary, held in a corrected alignment while the sutures are tied.

The capsule of the MP joint then is sutured with interrupted 2-0 absorbable sutures, and the skin then is closed with interrupted or running subcuticular mono-filament sutures. The foot is dressed with a soft bulky bandage, and the patient is placed in a walking cast or prefabricated walking orthosis for 3 weeks. Active range-of-motion and strengthening exercises are started thereafter in progressive fashion. A cushioning, custom-molded shoe insert is employed after 1 month as needed for symptomatic relief of plantar tenderness.

Lateral Sesamoid Excision

Although some series suggest that lateral sesamoid injuries are relatively rare, in my series of 23 sesamoids excised for histologically documented fracture and/or

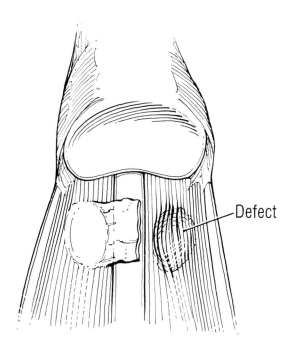

Figure 7 Defect after sesamoid has been removed.

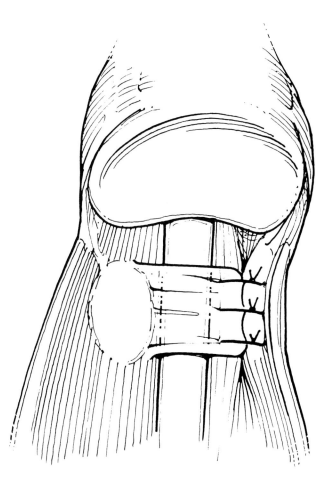

Figure 8 Placement of sutures from the intersesamoid ligament to the FHB remnant to reconstruct the FHB and sesamoid complex.

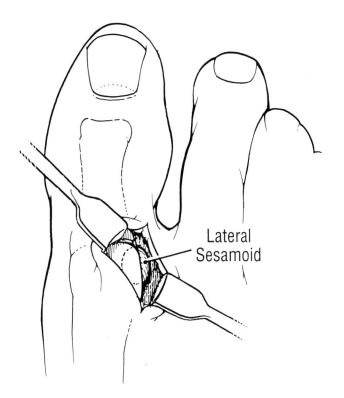

Figure 9 Incision for excision of lateral sesamoid.

nonunion, the number of medial and lateral sesamoids were about equal.

The technical difficulty of excising a lateral sesamoid is an order of magnitude greater than that of operating a medial sesamoid because the exposure frequently is difficult. The principles of FHB fiber preservation and the method of FHB reconstruction to the intersesamoid ligament are the same, except they are technically exasperating at times.

The first incision must be made dorsally, in the first metatarsal interspace, to approach the lateral side of the metatarsal-sesamoid joint (Fig. 9). If the tissues are lax, which is seldom the case in a young patient, the lateral sesamoid can be displaced into the web space, facilitat-

ing the dissection. Almost always, a second incision is required. A plantar incision has the advantage of proximity but the disadvantage of potential injury to the lateral plantar sensory nerve to the hallux, as well as the relative difficulty of retraction of the fat pad for visualization. A medial incision also has its disadvantages. It is somewhat difficult to pass the sutures for the flexor brevis reconstruction back and forth from medial to lateral sides of the joint. A medial incision still is preferable because it affords better exposure, allows good access to the medial side of the lateral sesamoid for the dissection from the intersesamoid ligament, and the medial capsulotomy is repaired easily with low risk of sensory nerve injury. Dissection and repair are done alternating back and forth between the two incisions, making this somewhat tedious. Once the sutures for the reconstruction all have been placed, the ends are passed out through the lateral incision to be tied (see Fig. 9).

Bone Grafting of the Sesamoid

A medial-plantar incision is utilized, placed over the medial sesamoid with the nonunion. The medial approach is used to prevent the possibility of a painful plantar scar. The joint is inspected and the procedure aborted if a smooth cartilage surface is not present. The approach to the nonunion itself is extra-articular. A trough is cut across the nonunion and it is curretted out, preferably with nonpower instruments so as not to burn the bone. Bone graft from the distal tibia or metatarsal is then packed across the nonunion. The fibers of the FHB are repaired and the patient is immobilized non–weight bearing in a slipper cast, followed by a walking cast or brace for a total of 6 to 8 weeks (the Anderson-McBryde technique).

SUGGESTED READING

Coughlin MJ. Sesamoid pain: Causes and surgical treatment. In: Instructional course lectures. American Academy of Orthopaedic Surgeons, 1990:23.

Van Hal ME, Keene JS, Lange TA, et al. Stress fractures of the great toe sesamoids. Am J Sports Med 1982; 10:122–128.

DISORDERS OF THE SECOND METATARSOPHALANGEAL JOINT

FRANCESCA M. THOMPSON, M.D.

This chapter describes the surgical management of a group of problems presenting at the second metatarsophalangeal (MP) joint: Freiberg's infraction, synovitis, and instability of the second MP joint ranging from subluxation to crossover toe to dislocation. Subluxation and instability are further discussed in the chapter *Claw Toes, Crossover Toe Deformity, and Instability of the Second Metatarsophalangeal Joint.*

FREIBERG'S INFRACTION

Usually first presenting in the adolescent, and sometimes erroneously diagnosed as interdigital neuroma, Freiberg's infraction is thought to result from an avascular necrosis of the lesser metatarsal head with resultant pain (type I stage). If it does not heal spontaneously, it can progress to the type II stage in which the articular cartilage is preserved, but osteophytes are present in the periarticular area. A later stage, type III, involves articular destruction and severe degenerative joint changes. These changes in types II and III are best visualized in an oblique radiograph of the forefoot.

Initially, conservative methods may suffice: relative rest, flat shoes, metatarsal pads, soft soles, rocker-bottom shoes. If pain persists in patients who have advanced to type II and type III disease, surgical debridement is indicated.

Under ankle block anesthesia with an ankle tourniquet, a longitudinal curvilinear incision is made around the extensor tendon, which is retracted to one side. The capsule is opened and the synovectomy performed. Dorsal osteophytes are debrided. If the articular surface is loose, it too is debrided, and the metatarsal head is reshaped to its former size. It may be necessary to remove the plantar condyles as in a DuVries arthroplasty. If extensive bone must be removed from both aspects of the joint, it may be necessary to stabilize the soft tissues by placing a purse-string suture through the volar plate structures. For type III disease an osteotomy of the metatarsal head as described by Gauthier is extremely useful. The plantar half of the articular surface of the MP joint usually is preserved, and is tilted dorsally to reconstitute the joint.

The patient is placed in a firm dressing and allowed to walk in a wood-soled shoe. After 3 to 4 weeks, passive motion at the MP joint is begun and closely monitored by the surgeon to promote optimal dorsiflexion without allowing dorsal subluxation to occur. Soon thereafter, the patient is allowed to return to any comfortable shoe wear. After 3 months, competitive sports may be resumed.

SYNOVITIS

Pain, swelling, and tenderness around the second MP joint indicate a synovitis that can be unrelated to systemic disease, and may result from mechanical factors. While the joint is stable, the synovitis may resolve with conservative methods, but if the pain and swelling persist, a synovectomy may be required. This is performed as described earlier. In many patients with intractable synovitis attributed to mechanical causes, mild asymptomatic hallux valgus may be present. In these patients the synovitis may be resolved only after surgical correction of the hallux.

SUBLUXATION OF THE METATARSOPHALANGEAL JOINT

Subluxation of the MP joint must be suspected whenever a patient presents with a complaint of forefoot pain. Every physical examination should check the stability of all the lesser MP joints to vertical stress. This is performed by grasping the metatarsal head with one hand, and the base of the proximal phalanx with the other, and applying a straight, *vertical* force to the proximal phalanx (Fig. 1). A normal MP joint cannot be displaced dorsally by this maneuver. An unstable MP joint can be displaced vertically, and with practice, the examiner can grade the amount of subluxation by the percentage of uncovering of the proximal phalanx base. This must be distinguished carefully from dorsiflexion in the plane of normal joint motion. Typically the instability produced by this maneuver also provokes the patient's pain.

The type of instability revealed by this test is thought to be the forerunner of the crossover toe and the total dislocation of the MP joint, so early treatment is important to prevent the unfolding of the natural history of this disorder (Fig. 2).

Conservative treatment consists of offering external support to prevent subluxation of the joint and healing of the presumably stretched volar plate. Adhesive tape over the dorsal base of the toe and crossed under the plantar aspect of the foot or an elastic ring toe retainer should be worn assiduously for several months. If pain and instability persist, as may happen despite the patient's conscientious efforts to be compliant, surgical stabilization is indicated.

By the time the patient elects surgical correction of the unstable second MP joint, other problems may be present that may have to be addressed at the same time such as hallux valgus, hammer toe deformity, and/or neuroma. If the hallux is in the way of where the second toe should be, it should be corrected at the same time. The hammer toe can be attended to with a resection arthroplasty at the same time if it is a fixed deformity.

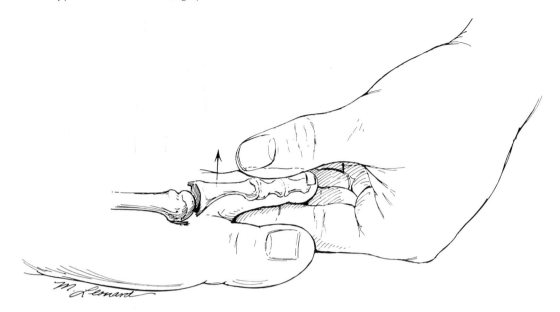

Figure 1   Dorsal subluxation test for instability of the MP joint is performed by grasping the base of the proximal phalanx and attempting to subluxate or dislocate the joint with a dorsally directed force.

Sometimes a neuroma has developed secondary to the subluxation, with the digit pulling the nerve against the sharp fibers of the deep intermetatarsal ligament. A concomitant neurectomy usually is efficacious.

The preferred approach to the unstable second MP joint is to perform a flexor-to-extensor transfer of the flexor digitorum longus (FDL) tendon to the dorsum of the base of the proximal phalanx (the Girdlestone-Taylor procedure). Under ankle block anesthesia with an ankle tourniquet, the flexor tendon is harvested through a transverse incision at the base of the plantar aspect of the toe, at the proximal volar crease. The FDL tendon lies in its sheath superficial to the flexor digitorum brevis tendon slips in this volar approach. The tendon sheath is incised vertically, and a small mosquito curved clamp is slipped under the FDL tendon to place it under tension. The tip of the toe then is grasped and manipulated into hyperextension at the distal interphalangeal (DIP) joint, and a scalpel blade tip is introduced from lateral or medial in the fat pad of the volar toe tip and aimed at the FDL insertion just distal to the DIP joint. An assistant provides traction on the tendon by way of the mosquito clamp placed under it in the proximal incision. In this way the long flexor tendon is delivered into the proximal wound.

The median raphe divides the FDL tendon into its two slips. An incision is made down the raphe, and the tendon is separated gently with traction as far down as the base of the proximal phalanx. The medial and lateral slips are clamped with a straight and a curved clamp, respectively, to distinguish them when they are transferred dorsally later.

The dorsum of the foot is approached. A zig-zag incision from 2 cm proximal to the MP joint is continued over the toe to distal to the proximal interphalangeal (PIP) joint if the hammer toe needs to be corrected; otherwise the incision is stopped at the base of the toe.

The extensor tendons are retracted, or if contracted, the brevis is divided, and the longus is cut longitudinally for a Z-plasty lengthening. The joint capsule is opened, a synovectomy performed, and the joint is checked for reduction of the base of the proximal phalanx on the metatarsal head. The collateral ligaments on either side are divided if it is necessary to obtain a reduction.

At this time the hammer toe correction can be performed by resecting the head of the proximal phalanx. The dorsal base of the proximal phalanx is exposed between the skin and the extensor hood. Using a small curved hemostat, a tunnel is burrowed *under* the neurovascular structures and *next to* the periosteum, from dorsal to plantar. The jaws of the clamp are opened, and the medial or lateral slip of the FDL tendon is grasped and pulled through to the dorsum. The clamp is left on while the other tendon is pulled up similarly.

A decision now must be made whether the reconstruction requires stabilization with a Kirschner (K-) wire. Clearly this is a judgment based on the surgeon's experience, but in general, if the joint has been unstable, if more extensive release of collateral structures or resection of bone for fixed hammer toe deformity have been performed, a K-wire may be useful for the first 2 or 3 weeks postoperatively.

A 0.62 K-wire is loaded in a small battery-powered wire driver and drilled retrograde from the articular surface of the middle phalanx of the PIP joint distally out the tip of the toe just under the toenail. It then is driven down the shaft of the proximal phalanx. Leave it long at this stage.

To set the appropriate tension on the transferred tendon slips, the foot must be held in a plantigrade position. The desired position of the toe is a few degrees of plantar flexion at the MP joint. The extensor slips are crossed over each other and sutured to the underlying extensor hood with 4-0 nonabsorbable sutures, prefera-

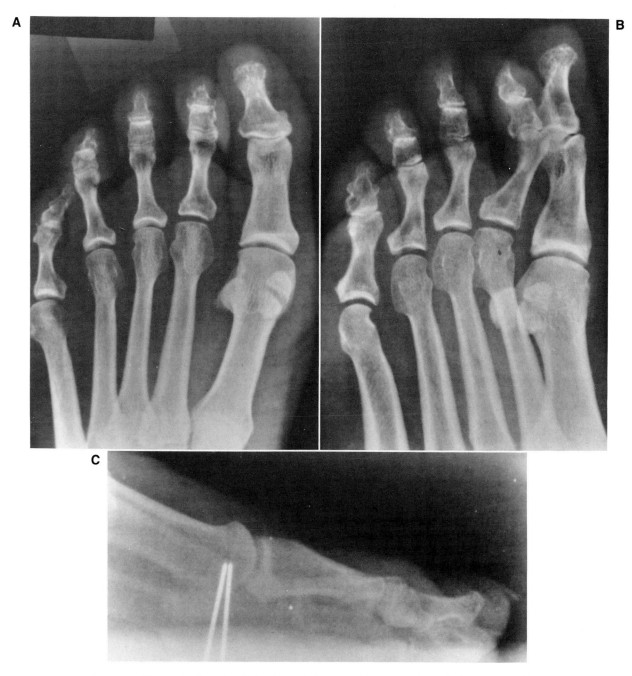

Figure 2 The evolution of a dislocation. A 64-year-old woman with pain in the second MP joint and a positive vertical stress test, which reproduced pain. *A,* Note the slight asymmetry of the second MP joint on anteroposterior (AP) view, and slight sausage-shaped digit compared to the third and fourth digit. *B,* Note the slight dorsiflexion on oblique view with hammering at the PIP joint. *C,* Lateral radiograph shows stability in stance with slight hammering at the PIP joint. Despite use of a toe retainer over 6 months, pain and deformity progressed.   *Continued.*

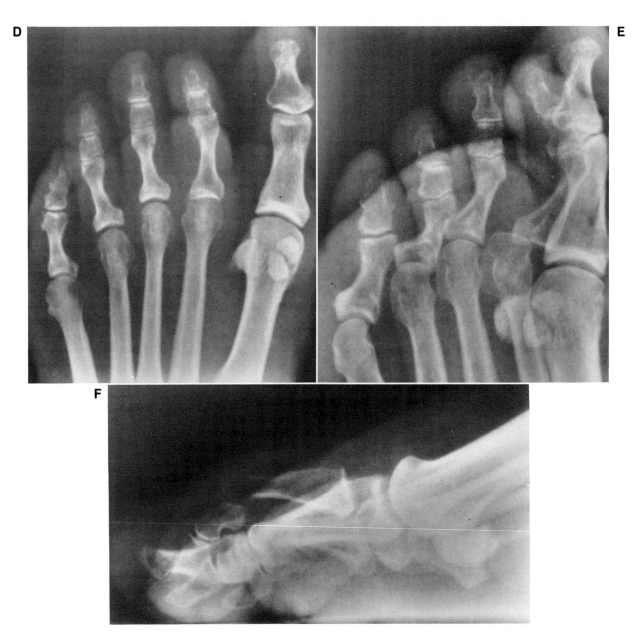

Figure 2, cont'd. *D,* AP radiograph shows overlap of the second proximal phalanx on the metatarsal head, with further soft tissue swelling of the digit. *E,* Oblique view shows dorsal subluxation of the joint. *F,* Lateral view shows dorsal displacement of the second toe, which is close to dislocating completely to a bayoneted position on the dorsum of the metatarsal head.

bly colorless so the sutures do not show through fair skin. Three such sutures are placed for each tendon slip. The position of the toe must be as desired at this time, because holding it corrected in the dressing is not going to correct a position that is not corrected at surgery.

When the toe is in the correct position, the K-wire may be driven across the MP joint. The K-wire is grasped at the tip of the toe with a needle-nosed plier, and a metal suction tip is placed over the wire and gently bent nearly 180°, then cut with a wire cutter.

After thorough irrigation, the soft tissues are closed over any exposed metatarsal head with interrupted 3-0 plain sutures. The extensor longus tendon is sutured to appropriate length if it was divided previously in a Z-plasty lengthening. The incision on the volar surface of the toe is closed with 3-0 plain chromic sutures to obviate the necessity to remove sutures from a tender, hard to reach area later. The dorsal incisions are closed as the surgeon prefers.

The patient is placed in a well-padded compressive dressing, and the tourniquet is released before surgical scrub is broken. Return of blood flow to the operated toe is observed carefully. If after 10 to 15 minutes the toe with a K-wire still is white, the K-wire should be removed.

The patient is allowed to ambulate with weight bearing as tolerated in a wood-soled postoperative shoe. However, for the first week or so, "toes above the nose" elevation is encouraged when the patient is not making a trip to the bathroom or dinner table. The sutures are removed at 2 weeks, and at that time or a week later the K-wire is removed. At this time the patient should start gentle passive dorsiflexion of the MP joint, with the eventual goal to equal the dorsiflexion of the neighboring toes. The dressing can be maintained, and the toe retainer used as well to counter any tendency for the toe to displace vertically. At 3 to 4 weeks the patient may wear a sports shoe for walking. The dressing can be discontinued at 4 weeks, but the toe retainer should be used for 6 months. Strenuous sports activities should be avoided, but an active patient can use a stationary bike with the pedal placed at the midfoot level. At 6 weeks the patient should start active plantar flexion exercises such as towel wrinkling or picking up marbles with the toes. At 3 months strenuous marathon training or racquet sports may be resumed.

The most common problem postoperatively is stiffness in dorsiflexion. For this reason the surgeon must examine the patient every 7 to 10 days in the first 6 to 8 weeks to reinforce the postoperative mobilization previously described.

CROSSOVER TOE

Crossover toe is a variant of the subluxated to dislocated MP joint. Usually the toe deviates in a medial direction first, and then begins to subluxate dorsally as well, finally resulting in a dorsomedial dislocation with the second toe resting on top of the hallux. Most often this is associated with a hallux valgus deformity, which must be corrected at the same time. By the time the second toe crosses over the hallux, there usually is a fixed hammer toe as well. The goal of surgery is to bring the second toe into the space between the hallux and the third toe, so that all toes lie in the same plane, with none pressing against the toe box of the shoe, and retain passive dorsiflexion and some active range of motion. It cannot be expected that the toe will function as it did before it crossed over, and the patient must understand that the postoperative toe will not act as a normal toe even if it looks like one. The toe may not look the same to the patient either, because there is expected toe molding after bone resection: often the toes are shorter, more sausage-shaped, and sometimes assume the shape of the space left between the hallux and the third toe.

The preferred surgical correction for the crossover toe is as described for subluxation, with some additions. Because there is usually attrition of the lateral collateral ligaments, it is desirable to reinforce the soft tissues on the lateral side with some 0 chromic sutures in the lateral capsular structures. This is, however, not always possible since the lateral juxta-articular soft tissues are poor, and because of the attritional changes, the sutures do not hold. When the dorsal dislocation has been marked, it may be necessary to include a DuVries arthroplasty of the MP joint itself, with or without a plantar condylectomy, depending on the presence of a severe callosity under the metatarsal head. Other options for treatment of the crossover toe are described in the subsequent chapter by Myerson.

The postoperative regimen is the same as that described for subluxation.

DISLOCATION OF THE SECOND METATARSOPHALANGEAL JOINT

Dislocation of the second MP joint is the end stage of the processes that start with synovitis and vertical instability. By the time the patient presents de novo with this late stage, the pain may be limited only to the dorsum of the clawed second toe where the toe meets the toe box of the shoe.

When the patient is elderly and not highly active, there may be some resistance to the concept of a total forefoot reconstruction including correction of the hallux valgus and clawed toe. Amputation of the involved digit is possible if the patient understands that the *only* result expected is the elimination of pain over the PIP joint of the second toe; metatarsalgia will not be improved, and may worsen, and similar problems may emerge in the third toe as the hallux translates laterally to fill the space made available by amputating the second toe. I reserve this procedure for the frail, elderly patient at risk for recurrent infections from skin breakdown on the dorsum of the toe.

Some patients present with dislocations of the second and third toes, with both being clawed, and the question arises as to whether the asymptomatic hallux valgus should be corrected as well. In the over-50 patient, it is possible to consider limiting surgery to the dislocations alone if the patient fully accepts the limitations including recurrence of the dislocations or incomplete reduction, continued severe valgus alignment of the toes, and continuing deformity secondary to the uncorrected hallux valgus. Men are more accepting of this than women.

Most often the preferred approach is to correct the hallux valgus, thus restoring more normal weight bearing through the medial ray and providing space in the appropriate direction for a more successful correction of the second MP joint. When shortening secondary to dorsal bayoneting of the second toe on the metatarsal neck is present, a DuVries arthroplasty is the preferred method of correction, because it allows bony resection to compensate for the significant soft tissue contracture that occurs with a long-standing dorsal dislocation. It is difficult to predict in every case which toe will require bony resection and which will not, so it is best to proceed in a stepwise fashion, assessing at each step if a stable reduction has been obtained.

The dorsum of the foot is approached. A zig-zag incision from 2 cm proximal to the MP joint is continued over the toe to distal to the PIP joint. The extensor tendons are contracted, so the brevis is divided, and the longus is cut longitudinally for a Z-plasty lengthening.

The thinned-out joint capsule is opened transversely, and the joint is checked for reduction of the base of the proximal phalanx on the metatarsal head, which is unlikely if the dislocation has been severe. To obtain this reduction, it is necessary to divide the collateral ligaments on either side.

The hammer toe correction now can be performed by resecting the head of the proximal phalanx. Because of the contracture of the clawed toe, it usually is necessary to divide the FDL tendon at this time. Make a transverse incision in the volar plate of the PIP joint. Using a small curved mosquito clamp, spread the slips of the flexor brevis tendon apart, and fish out the FDL tendon, pulling it dorsally and observing the hyperflexion of the DIP joint to confirm that the correct tendon has been selected. Cut it sharply and check for limp floppiness of the toe. If residual flexion is observed at the tip, it may be that only half the FDL tendon has been cut, and further search for the other half is needed.

At this time check the reduction of the base of the proximal phalanx on the metatarsal head. If it still is pulling proximally on the dorsum of the metatarsal head when the foot is held in a plantigrade position, a complete DuVries arthroplasty is required. The distal 3 to 4 mm of metatarsal head is removed with an osteotome. The edges are shaped with a rongeur to mimic a rounded metatarsal head. In patients with distinct plantar callosities under the metatarsal head, a plantar condylectomy is performed as well by plantar flexing the toe, and using an osteotome to remove the condyles, taking care to remove all resected bone.

Stabilize the reduction with a 0.62 double-pointed K-wire. Using a battery-powered hand driver, center the pin in the articular surface of the middle phalanx, and drive the K-wire out the end of the toe just under the toenail. Pull it out the end of the toe until only a couple of millimeters of wire show, enough to allow the pin to be placed in the center of the intramedullary canal of the proximal phalanx. Drive the pin a couple of centimeters into the proximal phalanx so that the toe is a stable construct. Hold the foot in a plantigrade position, with the base of the proximal phalanx reduced on the metatarsal head in the desired slight valgus position, and a few degrees of plantar flexion, and then drive the pin into the metatarsal. The K-wire is grasped at the tip of the toe with a needle-nosed pliers, and a metal suction tip is placed over the wire and gently bent nearly 180°, then cut with a wire cutter.

After thorough irrigation, the soft tissues are closed over any exposed metatarsal head with interrupted 3-0 plain suture. The extensor longus tendon is sutured to appropriate length. The dorsal incisions are closed as the surgeon prefers.

The patient is placed in a well-padded compressive dressing, and the tourniquet is released before surgical scrub is broken. Return of blood flow to the operated toe is observed carefully. If after 10 to 15 minutes the toe with a K-wire is still white, the K-wire should be removed.

The patient is allowed to ambulate with weight bearing as tolerated in a wood-soled postoperative shoe. However, for the first week or so, "toes above the nose" elevation is encouraged when the patient is not making a trip to the bathroom or dinner table. The sutures are removed at 2 weeks, and at that time or a week later the K-wire is removed. At this time the patient should start gentle passive dorsiflexion of the MP joint, with the eventual goal to equal the dorsiflexion of the neighboring toes. The dressing can be maintained, and the toe retainer used as well to counter any tendency for the toe to displace vertically. At 3 to 4 weeks the patient may wear a sports shoe for walking. The dressing can be discontinued at 4 weeks, but the toe retainer should be used for 6 months. Strenuous sports activities should be avoided, but an active patient can use a stationary bike with the pedal placed at the midfoot level. At 6 weeks the patient should start active plantar flexion exercises such as towel wrinkling or picking up marbles with the toes. At 3 months strenuous impacting sports may be resumed.

The most common problem postoperatively is stiffness in dorsiflexion. For this reason the surgeon must examine the patient every 7 to 10 days in the first 6 to 8 weeks to reinforce the postoperative mobilization previously described.

SUGGESTED READING

Coughlin MJ, Mann RA. Lesser toe deformities. In: Mann RA, ed. Surgery of the foot, 5th ed. St Louis: CV Mosby, 1986:148.

Freiberg AH. The so-called infraction of the second metatarsal bone. J Bone Joint Surg 1926; 8:257.

Mann RA, Mizel M. Non-articular, non-traumatic synovitis of the metatarsophalangeal joint: A new entity? Foot Ankle 1984; 4:332.

Thompson FM, Hamilton WG. Problems of the second metatarsophalangeal joint. Orthopedics 1987; 1:83–89.

CLAW TOES, CROSSOVER TOE DEFORMITY, AND INSTABILITY OF THE SECOND METATARSOPHALANGEAL JOINT

MARK MYERSON, M.D.

We rarely use our toes for gripping surfaces. It is apparent that the main function of the toes is to enlarge the weight-bearing surface of the forefoot, particularly during toe-off when the body weight is largely borne by the metatarsal heads. The toes are in contact with the ground for approximately three-quarters of the stance phase of gait and exert peak pressures similar to those of the metatarsal heads. The toes function maximally only when they are flat on the ground, and a predictable reduction in the function of the toes occurs if any toe deformities are present.

ANATOMY AND PATHOPHYSIOLOGY OF DEFORMITIES OF THE LESSER TOES

Integral to the understanding of any of these deformities are the pathologic disturbances that occur at the level of the metatarsophalangeal (MP) joint in claw

and hammer toes (Fig. 1). The extensor digitorum longus tendon extends the toe through a fibroaponeurotic sling, since the tendon does not insert into the proximal phalanx. However, phalangeal extension can occur only when the proximal phalanx is in a flexed or neutral position. Therefore, when a hyperextension deformity of the MP joint occurs, the extensor digitorum longus tendon no longer is able to extend the proximal phalanx. The extensor digitorum brevis tendon inserts into the dorsal base of the middle phalanx and extends the digits, particularly the proximal interphalangeal (PIP) joint.

In contrast to these extensors, the intrinsic and extrinsic flexors of the MP joint are far more active. The toes function maximally when the intrinsic muscles contract synergistically with the long flexors, and not surprisingly, an imbalance in the function of the intrinsic and extrinsic tendons leads to deformities at both the MP and PIP joints. The flexor digitorum longus and flexor digitorum brevis tendons are flexors of the distal interphalangeal (DIP) and PIP joints, but are weak flexors of the MP joint. The significant plantar flexors of the MP joint are the interossei and the lumbrical tendons. The interossei pass plantar to the axis of the metatarsal head, insert onto the plantar base of the proximal phalanx and strongly flex the MP joint. Both the interossei and lumbrical tendons have a more terminal extension that passes dorsal to the axis of both the PIP and DIP joints, and therefore have a weak extensor function.

In addition to the dynamic effect of these intrinsics, the plantar aponeurosis and plantar capsule stabilize the

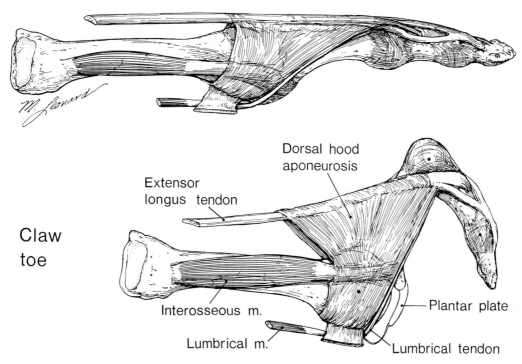

Figure 1 Normal and pathologic anatomy of the MP joint. Note the dorsal subluxation of the interosseous tendon, the tethering of the lumbrical tendon, and the dorsal bowstringing of the extensor hood.

entire MP joint. The plantar aponeurosis is attached by way of the plantar plate to the base of the proximal phalanx. This plate consists of a thick fibrocartilaginous portion that is attached to the base of the proximal phalanx and a thin, flimsy synovial attachment to the metatarsal neck. This not only stabilizes the toe, but also allows free passive motion of the MP joint during the stance and toe-off phase of gait. In addition to these musculoligamentous structures, the collateral ligaments of the MP joint are important in its stabilization.

As deformity and subluxation increase, adaptive shortening occurs in the skin and the juxta-articular soft tissue structures (Fig. 2). Dorsal to the MP joint, the skin, extensor tendons, capsule, and collateral ligaments all shorten. Since contracture occurs in the skin as well as the subcutaneous structures, transverse incisions should not be used because these gape after repositioning of the phalanx. The extensor longus tendon, dorsal capsule, and collateral ligaments account for the majority of the soft tissue deformity (Fig. 3). On the plantar aspect of the joint, the flimsy synovial attachment of the plantar plate to the metatarsal neck either lengthens or ruptures, allowing the plate to shift, and finally the toe dislocates dorsally. The axis of the intrinsic flexors of the

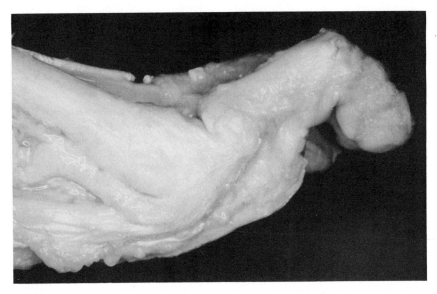

Figure 2 In this cadaver specimen with a claw toe, all the soft tissue attachments dorsally have been removed, yet an extension contracture at the MP joint persists.

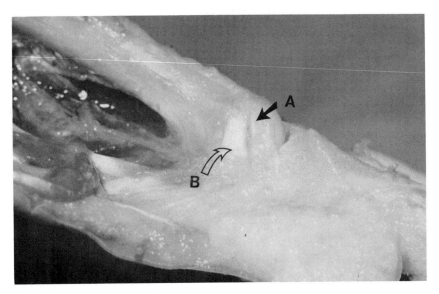

Figure 3 Two collateral ligaments. *A,* True collateral ligament; *B,* Extending to the volar plate.

MP joint changes and subluxates dorsal to the transverse axis of the metatarsal head, becoming less efficient flexors of the MP joint. The lumbrical tendons do not subluxate dorsally, since they are tethered by the deep transverse metatarsal ligament. However, they too become inefficient flexors because of the acute angulation occuring as they pass under the transverse metatarsal ligament. In addition to these pathologic disturbances, the metatarsal fat pad subluxates distal to the metatarsal head. This structure has an intimate attachment to the volar plate through vertical fibrous septae connecting the volar plate with the skin.

Under normal circumstances the toes dorsiflex passively during the final toe-off phase of gait, and the metatarsal fat pad moves with the volar plate to cover and protect the metatarsal heads. Under pathologic conditions, however, the toe is permanently extended at the MP joint, and the volar plate similarly is pulled up with the proximal phalanx. The fat pad then lies anterior to the metatarsal heads, anchored by the vertical fibrous septae. These fibers are located superficial to the metatarsal heads and arise from the sides of the plantar plate, as well as from the flexor tendon sheaths and from the sagittal septae. In between these vertical fibers, small amounts of fat are trapped forming a cushion below each metatarsal head. When the MP joint is subluxated permanently, soft tissue contractures occur both dorsally and on its plantar surfaces.

Subluxation and dislocation of the MP joint typically occurs in the sagittal plane. However, the second toe also may deviate in the horizontal plane, dorsomedially over the hallux. The pathologic process is a result of attritional rupture on the lateral aspect of the MP joint including the lateral collateral ligament and lateral capsule, as well as attenuation or rupture of the first dorsal interosseus tendon. Attenuation with or without perforation also may occur in the fibrocartilaginous plate (Fig. 4). These are accompanied by contracture on the medial aspect of the MP joint including the collateral ligament, capsule, and interossei and lumbrical tendons. Stages of this crossover toe deformity are well described, commencing with synovitis, followed by early subluxation, and finally dorsomedial dislocation. Although extension of the MP joint is present, this is but one aspect of the deformity, all which must be addressed surgically and are described subsequently.

SURGICAL TREATMENT

Treatment of deformity at the MP joint level should take into account all these contractures, and is approached sequentially, regardless of the magnitude of the deformity. Surgical planning for deformity of the second toe should take into consideration the following factors:

1. Presence of hallux valgus
2. Magnitude of the deformity
3. Whether this deformity is flexible or rigid
4. Presence of a crossover toe deformity
5. Instability of the second MP joint

Claw Toes Associated with Hallux Valgus

Hallux valgus often is associated with disorders of the second MP joint, and it is unrealistic to attempt satisfactory realignment of the second toe without correction of the hallux. The only exception to this rule is in elderly individuals in whom the bunion itself frequently is asymptomatic, and the second toe deformity is severe. It is difficult to reposition the second toe correctly without realigning the hallux. Performing a more major realignment in the elderly increases the morbidity of the procedure considerably. Severe claw toe deformity associated with hallux valgus in the elderly may be best treated with amputation of the second toe. As an alternative to amputation (of which many patients abhor the mere thought) the hallux can be moved into a neutral position by a wedge osteotomy of the proximal phalanx (Akin's procedure) without performing a bunionectomy. This is followed by soft tissue realignment at

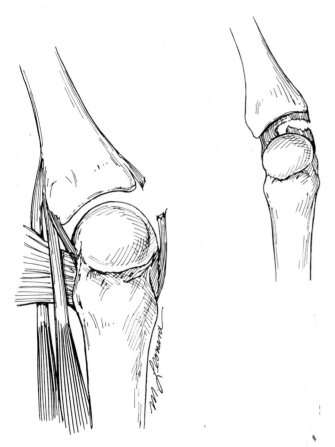

Figure 4 Pathologic anatomy of the crossover toe deformity includes rupture of the lateral collateral ligament and lateral capsule with or without perforation of the volar plate complex. On the medial aspect of the joint, the capsule, collateral ligament, and interossei and lumbrical tendons undergo adaptive contracture.

the MP joint and a PIP joint arthroplasty of the second toe. With careful patient selection, this latter procedure can be performed successfully despite hallux valgus. I find that the patient's expectations and preoperative symptoms greatly influence the success of the procedure. A severe claw toe deformity in the elderly causes pain over the dorsum of the PIP joint only, and although the toe is not satisfactorily aligned after a PIP joint arthroplasty, the symptoms abate.

Mild-to-Moderate Deformity

For mild deformity, when the complaints are predominantly over the dorsum of the PIP joint, this may be approached without dissection or release at the level of the MP joint. When performing the soft tissue release at the MP joint, it should be done in a sequential stepwise manner:

1. Extensor digitorum longus lengthening
2. Extensor digitorum brevis tenotomy or lengthening
3. Transverse dorsal capsulotomy
4. Collateral ligament release

For mild deformity, tendon lengthening and capsulotomy are sufficient to realign the toe at the MP joint. For more severe deformity at the MP joint, a more extensive release should be performed. For moderate deformity, it generally is preferable to commence the dissection at the MP joint. Once the PIP joint is addressed, whether with arthroplasty or arthrodesis, the extensor complex relaxes, and the soft tissue lengthening at the MP joint is performed less easily.

Proximal Interphalangeal Joint Resection Arthroplasty

The PIP joint arthroplasty can be performed through either a dorsal transverse or longitudinal incision. The advantage of a transverse incision is that the flexion contracture of the PIP joint can be nicely corrected. This repair, however, causes more widening at the PIP joint, and this bulbous deformity may not resolve always. I prefer to use a longitudinal incision wherever possible, following which the extensor complex is incised transversely, exposing the PIP joint. The collateral ligaments are divided sharply, and a small sharp curved gouge is used to strip the undersurface of the volar plate and the edge of either side of the collateral ligament complex. This gouge is extremely useful, since its edge hugs the bone, and no injury to the neurovascular bundle occurs. The soft tissues are pushed back and protected while the bone is cut transversely using a small bone cutter. Divide the bone transversely with a true parallel cut to prevent angular deformity of the toe postoperatively. Perhaps as important is the amount of bone resected. Ideally only the distal one-quarter of the proximal phalanx should be resected; in rare cases it is necessary to resect the distal one-third. If more bone is removed, the toe tends to be short, floppy, and unstable.

Following bone resection, the toe is dorsiflexed to check for a persistent flexion contracture. If this occurs, either more bone must be removed or the volar plate and flexor brevis tendon released off the middle phalanx. I remove as little bone as possible, and after removal of the distal one-quarter of the proximal phalanx, I prefer to free the soft tissue contracture. The extensor complex then is repaired with absorbable 4-0 sutures, removing enough of the extensor tissue to bring and hold the toe in a neutral position. I generally do not use a Kirschner (K-) wire to hold the toe unless simultaneous extensor release has been performed at the MP joint or revision surgery is performed at the PIP joint.

Arthrodesis of the Proximal Interphalangeal Joint

Arthrodesis of the PIP joint rarely is needed. However, this procedure is useful in recurrent deformity, and in cases of neuromuscular imbalance of the forefoot in which standard arthroplasty procedures are likely to result in recurrence. Generally the intrinsics, such as the lumbrical and the interossei, are not functioning well in these feet, and the arthrodesis relies on flexion of the toe through action of the long flexor tendon, a weak flexor to begin with. Patients often do not like the toe to be stiff, and for this reason, it is important to position the toe in slight flexion at the interphalangeal joint. This is not easy to achieve because of the configuration of the joint and the technique used for arthrodesis. One method that works well is to create a cup-and-cone fit at the joint by fashioning the shape of the proximal phalanx, and then burring out the center of the base of the middle phalanx. It is difficult to fix these joints in slight flexion, and it has been my experience with such cases that the rate of nonunion is high.

Severe Deformity

For moderate-to-severe deformity, particularly if rigid, a fixed flexion deformity at the PIP joint is present, requiring correction in addition to the extension deformity at the MP joint. This is accomplished with a combination of bone resection and soft tissue release. For severe deformity, repositioning of the base of the proximal phalanx at the MP joint usually is not possible without bone resection. Relocation of the proximal phalanx and reduction of the hyperextension or dislocation at the MP joint may be possible, but it places significant tension on the neurovascular structures. The deformity recurs almost immediately once the tension on the toe is released or the K-wire removed.

To avoid ischemia of the toe, bone shortening should be performed, relaxing the contracted neurovascular bundle. This bone resection may be performed at the level of the PIP joint, the proximal phalanx, the metatarsal head, or by shortening the second metatarsal. The easiest level at which to resection bone clearly is from the PIP joint, particularly when the deformity at the MP joint is moderate and is associated with fixed flexion deformity at the PIP joint. In this instance a PIP joint

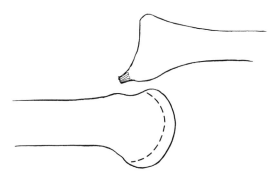

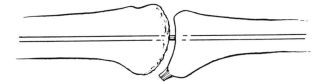

Figure 6 Following metatarsal head arthroplasty, the joint should be stabilized with a transfixation K-wire.

Figure 5 If the proximal phalanx is dislocated, significant soft tissue contracture is present. To avoid stretching the neurovascular structures, bone is shaved off the metatarsal head, preserving its contour.

resection arthroplasty decompresses the stretched neurovascular structures in addition to realigning the joint.

Alternatively, bone shortening may be accomplished either by partial shaving of the metatarsal head or by resection of the base of the proximal phalanx. The latter is not desirable, since the MP joint remains unstable, and the proximal phalanx may continue to subluxate dorsally. Syndactilization of the base of the second to the adjacent third toe has been proposed to prevent this recurrent subluxation, but it has been my experience that this does not stabilize the articulation satisfactorily, and both the second and the third toes may subluxate dorsally together. If bone decompression or shortening must be performed at the MP joint, it is preferably accomplished by a partial shaving or resection of the metatarsal head (Figs. 5 and 6). In doing so, the contour of the metatarsal head may be preserved, and the cup-and-cone stability of the joint remains. Approximately 3 to 4 mm of the articular surface and head are resected to leave the head slightly rounded.

Although this arthroplasty procedure reduces a subluxated or dislocated joint, it never is a normal joint and often is stiff. Further subluxation and recurrent deformity of the joint also may occur. A decision must be made, however, to reduce the joint somehow and preserve functional motion. In cases in which dislocation of the MP joint is not long-standing, the joint can be reduced by a shortening metatarsal osteotomy. The advantage of this osteotomy is the preservation of a portion of the collateral ligament complex, which is important in maintaining subsequent joint stability. It is difficult to ascertain exactly what is too chronic, i.e., before a shortening is insufficient to reduce the joint and maintain the position without further dislocation. I have reduced and maintained reduction of a joint that was dislocated for up to 1 year with a shortening osteotomy. Although the shortening osteotomy often reduces the proximal phalanx, a volar plate arthroplasty may be needed to pull the subluxated volar plate out of the joint. This is an important concept, and a review of the anatomy should be self-explanatory. Unless the volar

plate is reduced, the vertical fibers extending from the plate into the skin remain oriented forward, and the metatarsal fat pad remains displaced anteriorly. The volar plate can be reduced by inserting a small curved periosteal elevator under the metatarsal head, stripping it off the metatarsal neck. This theoretically detaches one of the primary restraints to dorsal dislocation (the other is the collateral ligament system); however, by repositioning the volar plate in this manner it potentially scars down to the metatarsal neck, thereby maintaining joint reduction.

Instability of the Metatarsophalangeal Joint

Once the MP joint has been reduced satisfactorily, the joint always should be assessed for stability. This is done easily by grasping the base of the proximal phalanx between the thumb and the forefinger and then attempting to subluxate or dislocate the MP joint dorsally (Fig. 7). Not infrequently, relocation of the proximal phalanx and reduction of the joint have been achieved only to find that the joint subluxates or easily dislocates with mild manipulation. Under these circumstances, it is unlikely that the joint will remain stable. Although a transfixation K-wire across the MP joint may hold the toe postoperatively, it should never be relied on to reduce it permanently. I think it is best to achieve the position of function at rest and not to rely on a K-wire to do the job, since redislocation of the joint always occurs once the wire has been removed.

In the presence of instability at the MP joint, a limited number of options are available to stabilize the base of the proximal phalanx. In many cases this can be achieved with a flexor-to-extensor tendon transfer (Fig. 8) and is described fully in the chapter *Disorders of the Second Metatarsophalangeal Joint*. An alternative method of performing the flexor-to-extensor tendon transfer is to detach the tendon distally as described, but to pull the entire tendon through the PIP joint without splitting it. This is performed in conjunction with a PIP joint resection arthroplasty. The tendon is then pulled up through the joint dorsally, sutured to the extensor complex, and secured with a transfixation K-wire. The only advantage of this flexor transfer is that it is associated with less congestion of the toe, and therefore less likelihood of injury to the neurovascular bundle. However, the more distally along the proximal phalanx that the transfer is performed, the less likely it is to

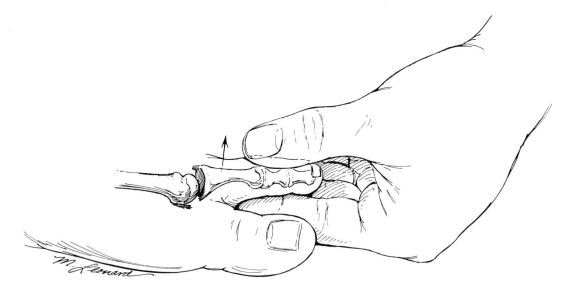

Figure 7 Dorsal subluxation test for instability of the MP joint is performed by grasping the base of the proximal phalanx and attempting to subluxate or dislocate the joint with a dorsally directed force.

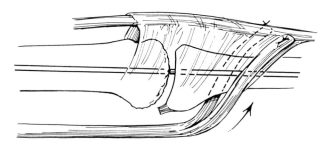

Figure 8 If the joint is markedly unstable with a positive dorsal stress test, a flexor-to-extensor tendon transfer should be performed following the metatarsal head arthroplasty and secured with a K-wire postoperatively.

reduce the base of the proximal phalanx effectively and to control an unstable MP joint. I do, however, perform the transfer in this manner if a PIP joint resection arthroplasty is done.

An alternative method for stabilizing the base of the proximal phalanx is an extensor tendon transfer using a free tendon graft to replace a completely deficient volar plate system. I have used a 2 inch portion of the peroneus tertius tendon for this purpose. The tendon is passed through a drill hole from dorsal to plantar on the base of the proximal phalanx and plantar to dorsal on the distal aspect of the metatarsal head and neck. The drill hole is made obliquely in the base of the proximal phalanx using a 2.5 mm drill bit. The drill point should exit at the nonarticular surface of the base of the proximal phalanx. The second drill hole is made obliquely from the dorsal aspect of the metatarsal neck to exit more distally on the plantar surface of the metatarsal head just posterior to the articular surface. The tendon then is passed from distal dorsal through the proximal phalanx and from

plantar to dorsal through the metatarsal neck using a large half-tapered Mayo needle. Securing the tendon at both ends obviously presents a potential problem since there is seldom strong and firm tissue other than the extensor complex dorsally. I have used sutures, but an alternative method that works extremely well is to insert a Mitek suture into the predrilled holes (preferably using the correct-sized drill for the hook device), and then anchoring the tendon at both ends to the Mitek device. The MP joint is transfixed with a 0.062 K-wire for 4 weeks postoperatively. This transfer provides a static tenodesis effect, reconstituting the deficient volar plate.

These arthroplasty procedures at the level of the MP joint are not entirely satisfactory, since the joint always is slightly stiff. Although external splinting with taping of the toe works well, the toe probably is best secured with a K-wire introduced anterograde through the toe and then retrograde across the MP joint. Joint stiffness may be minimized to some extent postoperatively by removing the K-wire earlier, but this in turn may be associated with recurrent subluxation or dislocation of the joint. The K-wire should be used only to maintain congruity following adequate soft tissue release. At times the wires have been left in place for 4 to 6 weeks, but this may be associated with joint stiffness. Alternatively, early removal at 2 to 3 weeks may be associated with recurrent laxity. Perhaps each joint should be assessed on its merits, and where scarification and fibrosis of the joint are required to hold an unstable MP joint, the wire probably should be left in for a longer period. Instability of the MP joint perhaps is best treated early before dislocation occurs.

Crossover Toe Deformity

The crossover toe deformity should be approached sequentially in a similar manner for mild-to-moderate

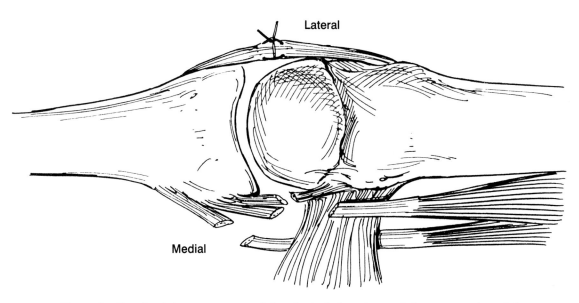

Figure 9 Repair of the crossover toe deformity includes release of the contracted medial structures and plication of the torn lateral collateral ligament.

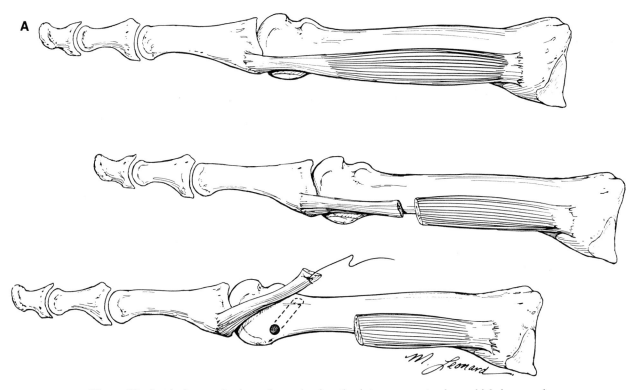

Figure 10 Intrinsic transfer is performed using the interosseous tendon, which is passed through a drill hole from lateral to medial, recreating a static lateral collateral ligament. *A,* Lateral view. *Continued.*

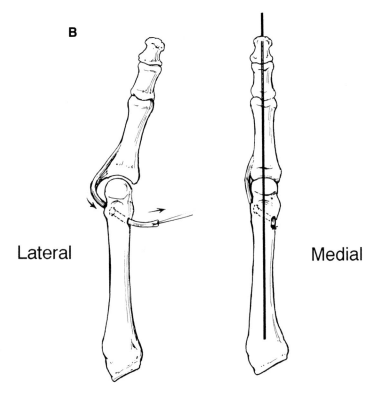

B

Lateral

Medial

Figure 10, cont'd. *B,* Anteroposterior view.

hyperextension deformity at the MP joint. Following an extensor tendon lengthening and transverse dorsal capsulotomy, the medial aspect of the MP joint is identified. The soft tissues, including the neurovascular bundle, are retracted medially and the collateral ligament and medial capsule incised. This is sufficient for a mild deformity, but for a severe deformity with subluxation and dislocation both the lumbrical and interossei tendons should be transected. On the lateral aspect at the joint, the collateral ligament usually is ruptured, and where possible, the lateral capsular structures should be repaired with a nonabsorbable suture (Fig. 9). This is difficult to achieve, since little autogenous soft tissue of substance is present to facilitate suturing. The collateral ligament often tears or avulses off the edge of the base of the proximal phalanx, and it is difficult to get a suture into the edge of the phalanx without making a small hole, which again is difficult.

If present, the first dorsal interosseous tendon may be used for a static tenodesis to replace the torn lateral collateral ligament. The tendon is harvested carefully and dissected off the muscle at the musculotendinous junction. The tendon is sutured, and an oblique drill hole is made through the metatarsal neck from dorsal-medial and proximal to plantar-lateral and distal. The suture

then is passed with the attached tendon from lateral to medial, and by pulling on the interosseous tendon, which is attached to the lateral base of the proximal phalanx, a static tenodesis is achieved (Fig. 10). Depending on the length of the tendon protruding through the bone tunnel, the tendon can be sutured to locally available tissue or attached using a Mitek suture device. If the Mitek hook and suture is used, the correctly sized drill bit should be used to anchor the hook. This is an excellent transfer provided the interosseous tendon is present and can be harvested intact. Unfortunately the tendon occasionally undergoes attritional rupture in severe grades of crossover toe deformity, and alternative methods must be implemented to stabilize the joint.

SUGGESTED READING

Coughlin MJ. Crossover second toe deformity. Foot Ankle 1987; 8:29–39.
Hughes J, Clark P, Klenerman L. The importance of the toes in walking. J Bone Joint Surg 1990; 72B:245–251.
Myerson MS, Shereff M. The pathologic anatomy of claw and hammer toes. J Bone Joint Surg 1989; 71A:45–49.
Sarrafian SK, Topouzian LK. Anatomy and physiology of the extensor apparatus of the toes. J Bone Joint Surg 1969; 51A:669–679.

BUNIONETTE DEFORMITY

MICHAEL J. COUGHLIN, M.D.

A bunionette deformity, or tailor's bunion, is characterized by a painful enlargement of the lateral condyle of the fifth metatarsal head. Friction between constricting footwear and the underlying bony abnormality leads to the development of a keratotic lesion overlying the lateral or plantar-lateral aspect of the head of the fifth metatarsal.

The anatomy of the bunionette varies significantly, and this determines the choice of the specific surgical procedure used. A prominent lateral condyle of the fifth metatarsal head may lead to symptomatic bunionette deformity (type 1 deformity). Likewise, painful symptoms over the fifth metatarsal lateral condyle may develop from divergence of the fourth and fifth metatarsals (type 3 deformity). Lateral bowing of the diaphyseal shaft of the fifth metatarsal also can lead to symptoms (type 2 deformity) (Fig. 1).

The most frequent type of deformity (type 3) is an increased 4-5 intermetatarsal angle, which occurs in approximately 50 percent of cases, whereas type 1 and type 2 deformities are less common.

Radiographic measurements that quantitate a bunionette deformity are the 4-5 intermetatarsal angle, which calculates the angle of divergence of the fourth and fifth metatarsals, and the metatarsophalangeal-5 (MP-5) angle, which calculates the magnitude of medial deviation of the fifth toe in relationship to the axis of the fifth metatarsal shaft (Fig. 2).

CLINICAL ASSESSMENT

The most frequent subjective complaint of a patient with a symptomatic bunionette deformity is pain and irritation resulting from friction between constricting footwear and the underlying bony abnormality. On physical examination, an inflamed bursa, a lateral keratosis, a plantar keratosis, or combined plantar-lateral keratosis may be present. Pain and chronic irritation overlying the fifth metatarsal head may be alleviated by well-fitted roomy shoes. Shaving of thickened calluses and padding of the prominent fifth metatarsal head also may reduce symptoms. A prefabricated or custom arch support may help to diminish pronation and reduce symptoms. Surgical intervention may be considered when conservative methods are unsuccessful.

SURGICAL TREATMENT

Numerous operative procedures have been used to correct a painful bunionette deformity surgically including (1) lateral condylectomy, (2) fifth metatarsal head resection and fifth ray resection, (3) distal fifth metatarsal osteotomy, (4) diaphyseal fifth metatarsal osteotomy, and (5) proximal fifth metatarsal osteotomy. An important principle in any conceived surgical procedure is to correct all the underlying pathology to prevent recurrence.

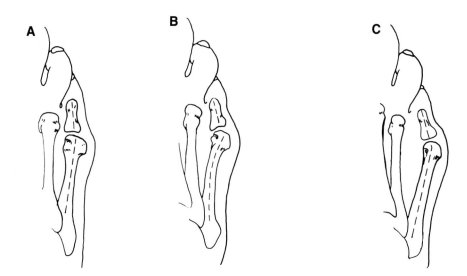

Figure 1 *A*, Type 1 bunionette deformity characterized by an enlarged fifth metatarsal head. *B*, Type 2 bunionette deformity characterized by lateral bowing of the fifth metatarsal. *C*, Type 3 bunionette deformity is characterized by an abnormally wide 4-5 intermetatarsal angle. (From Mann RA, Coughlin MJ. Video textbook of foot and ankle surgery. St Louis: Medical Video Productions, 1991; with permission.)

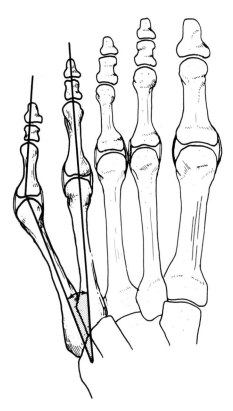

Figure 2 The MP-5 angle and the 4-5 intermetatarsal angle. The MP-5 angle is the angle subtended by the axis of the proximal phalanx and the fifth metatarsal. The 4-5 intermetatarsal angle is the angle subtended by the intersecting axis of the fourth and fifth metatarsals. (From Mann RA, Coughlin MJ. Video textbook of foot and ankle surgery. St Louis: Medical Video Productions, 1991; with permission.)

A lateral condylectomy is a simple procedure that can be used to correct a bunionette deformity but has significant limitations. It achieves almost no correction in either the 4-5 intermetatarsal angle or the MP-5 angle and may be associated with recurrent deformity. This procedure may be used for a symptomatic, enlarged lateral condyle. Correction achieved is, however, limited, and this procedure frequently is reserved for an elderly patient in whom a simple operation is the most expeditious.

A fifth metatarsal head resection and fifth ray resection rarely is indicated as a primary procedure. This procedure is performed far too frequently in the presence of hindfoot varus or cavovarus deformity, and is illogical since the pressure transfers to the fourth metatarsal head. Retraction or shortening of the fifth toe, subluxation of the fifth toe, and development of transfer lesions beneath adjacent metatarsal heads are recognized complications and occur frequently with this procedure. The 4-5 intermetatarsal angle actually may increase in magnitude after a fifth metatarsal head resection. This procedure typically is reserved for

intractable ulceration, severe deformity, infection, and for cases of rheumatoid arthritis in which multiple metatarsal head resections are performed.

A fifth metatarsal osteotomy may be used to correct alignment of the fifth metatarsal. A distal fifth metatarsal osteotomy achieves significantly more correction than a lateral condylar resection. A midshaft diaphyseal osteotomy achieves greater correction than a distal metatarsal osteotomy. Although an osteotomy in the proximal 2 cm of the metatarsal may impair the blood supply and lead to delayed union or nonunion, this has not been supported in the literature to date. With any metatarsal osteotomy, instability at the osteotomy site may lead to loss of alignment, development of transfer lesions, and recurrence of deformity. Internal fixation should be considered wherever possible.

Fifth Metatarsal Chevron Osteotomy

The chevron-type distal metatarsal osteotomy is inherently stable in comparison to oblique or transverse osteotomies. Since the capital fragment is translated in a lateral-medial plane, it is effective only in correcting a lateral keratosis and is contraindicated in the presence of a plantar keratosis.

Technique

A 3 to 4 cm longitudinal incision is centered over the lateral eminence extending from the midportion of the proximal phalanx to 1 cm above the lateral eminence. The dorsal and plantar neurovascular bundles are protected. The fifth MP joint capsule is incised along the proximal and dorsal border, creating an inverted "L" capsular flap (Fig. 3). This flap is detached from the abductor digiti quinti muscle proximally and the periosteum dorsally. The flap is reflected downward, exposing the lateral eminence, which is resected with a power saw. A 0.045 Kirschner (K-) wire is drilled in medial-lateral direction through the center of the metatarsal head to mark the apex of the fifth metatarsal osteotomy. A sagittal saw is used to create the chevron osteotomy (Fig. 4A). A saw blade with teeth that are not offset minimizes shortening at the osteotomy site. The osteotomy cut is made in a lateral-medial direction at an angle of approximately 60°. Excessive soft tissue stripping must be avoided because the remaining vascular supply to the fifth metatarsal head is from the medial aspect of the capital fragment. The metatarsal diaphysis is grasped with a towel clip, and the capital fragment is displaced medially a distance of approximately one-third to one-half the width of the metaphysis (Fig. 4B). The osteotomy then is stabilized with a 0.045 K-wire. The MP joint capsule is approximated with interrupted absorbable sutures (Fig. 5). The capsular flap frequently is secured to the metatarsal metaphysis by metaphyseal drill holes. The capsule also is approximated to the dorsal periosteum of the fifth metatarsal and to the abductor digiti quinti. The skin is approximated with interrupted sutures.

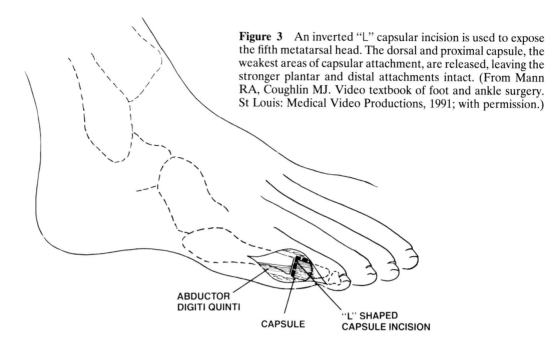

Figure 3 An inverted "L" capsular incision is used to expose the fifth metatarsal head. The dorsal and proximal capsule, the weakest areas of capsular attachment, are released, leaving the stronger plantar and distal attachments intact. (From Mann RA, Coughlin MJ. Video textbook of foot and ankle surgery. St Louis: Medical Video Productions, 1991; with permission.)

ABDUCTOR
DIGITI QUINTI

CAPSULE

"L" SHAPED
CAPSULE INCISION

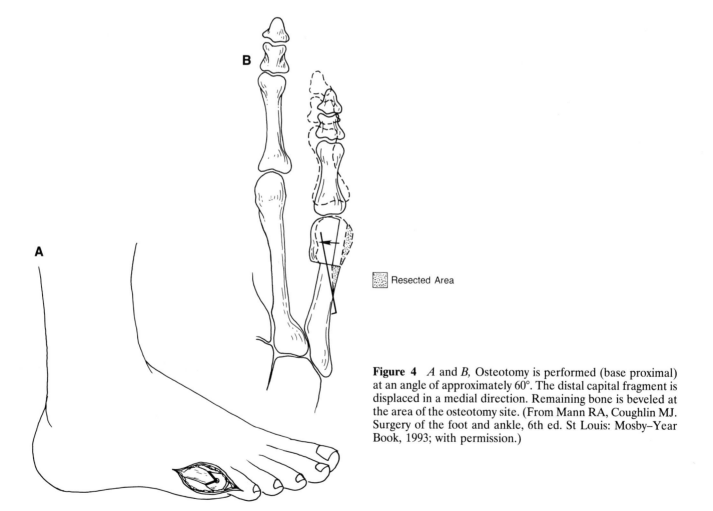

Resected Area

Figure 4 *A* and *B,* Osteotomy is performed (base proximal) at an angle of approximately 60°. The distal capital fragment is displaced in a medial direction. Remaining bone is beveled at the area of the osteotomy site. (From Mann RA, Coughlin MJ. Surgery of the foot and ankle, 6th ed. St Louis: Mosby–Year Book, 1993; with permission.)

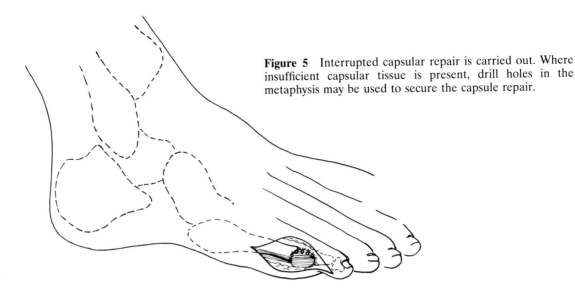

Figure 5 Interrupted capsular repair is carried out. Where insufficient capsular tissue is present, drill holes in the metaphysis may be used to secure the capsule repair.

Postoperative Care

The foot is placed in a gauze and tape dressing. The dressing is changed weekly for 6 weeks following surgery. Although a gauze and tape dressing may suffice, casting is recommended for unreliable patients. The sutures and K-wire are removed 2 to 3 weeks after surgery.

Results

Although a limited amount of correction in the 4-5 intermetatarsal angle is possible with a distal chevron osteotomy, this procedure frequently is successful from a subjective standpoint. The 4-5 intermetatarsal angle often can be diminished by 2° to 3°, and the MP-5 angle can be corrected from 7° to 10°. I would recommend internal fixation, which can be removed 3 weeks after surgery. Excessive stripping of the soft tissue on the dorsal and plantar aspect of the fifth metatarsal may be ill-advised because it may predispose it to the development of nonunion or avascular necrosis.

Diaphyseal Oblique Osteotomy

In the presence of a type 1 bunionette deformity or a mild-to-moderate type 2 or type 3 deformity, a chevron osteotomy appears to achieve adequate correction of the deformity. It is preferable to a lateral condylar resection. With a plantar keratosis, a chevron osteotomy is contraindicated. For more severe type 2 and type 3 deformities, an oblique diaphyseal osteotomy of the fifth metatarsal may be considered.

Technique

A longitudinal incision is centered over the midportion of the fifth metatarsal, extending from the proximal phalanx to the base of the fifth metatarsal. The neurovascular bundles are protected. The abductor digiti quinti is reflected plantarward, exposing the fifth metatarsal diaphysis. Care is taken to not strip the periosteum on the medial aspect of the fifth metatarsal to maintain vascular attachments. The MP joint capsule is exposed and released on the dorsal and proximal aspect with a L-type capsular incision (see Fig. 3). The lateral condyle is resected with a power saw. The fifth toe is distracted, and the medial fifth MP joint capsule is released, allowing realignment of the MP joint. In the presence of a pure lateral keratosis, a horizontal osteotomy is performed (Fig. 6A) (the saw blade is directed in a dorsal-proximal to plantar-distal direction, the saw cut is made in a medial-lateral direction). Before completion of the osteotomy, a 3.5 mm gliding drill hole is placed in the distal fragment. A 2.5 mm drill hole is created in the proximal fragment and is tapped. The drill holes are placed before completing the osteotomy, because the osteotomy often is unstable and difficult to fix afterward. The osteotomy then is completed, and the distal fragment is rotated to a point parallel with the fourth metatarsal (Fig. 6B). A small-fragment compression screw (2.7 or 3.5 mm) is used to stabilize the osteotomy site. A K-wire also may be used to stabilize the osteotomy site in addition to the screw fixation. (An alternative to screw fixation is multiple K-wire fixation.) Prominent bone protruding at the osteotomy site is removed with a sagittal saw but not if this compromises the stability of fixation.

With the fifth toe held in neutral alignment, the capsule is reefed to the abductor digiti quinti and dorsal periosteum. The capsule also may be secured to drill holes in the fifth metatarsal metaphysis. The skin is closed with interrupted sutures.

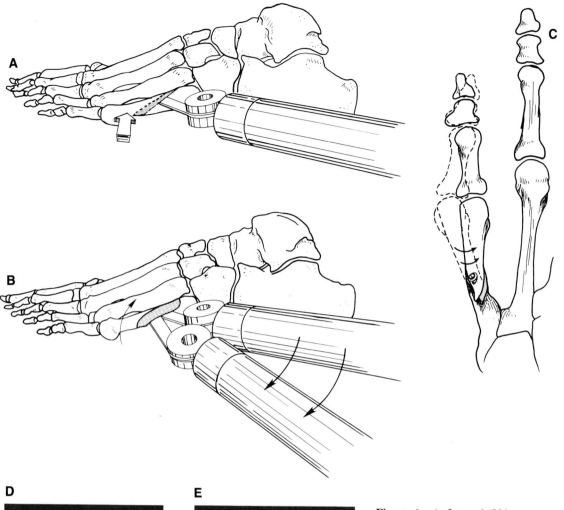

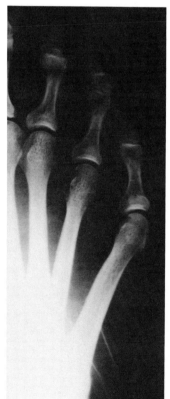

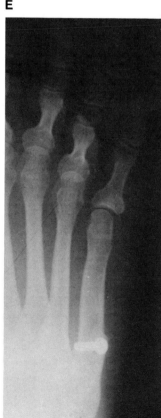

Figure 6 *A,* Lateral fifth metatarsal condyle is removed with a sagittal saw. Orientation of the diaphyseal oblique osteotomy is in a lateral-medial plane. *B,* Osteotomy site is rotated and fixed with a small-fragment screw. K-wire fixation may be added to give rotational stability. *C,* Where an intractable plantar keratotic lesion is present, the saw blade is directed in a cephalad direction. (The hand is dropped as the saw cut is created, so when the osteotomy site is rotated the fifth metatarsal head is elevated.) *D,* Preoperative radiograph demonstrating bunionette deformity with widened 4-5 intermetatarsal angle. *E,* Following diaphyseal oblique osteotomy with distal soft tissue repair, a correction of the deformity is achieved. (From Mann RA, Coughlin MJ. Video textbook of foot and ankle surgery. St. Louis: Medical Video Productions, 1991; with permission.)

Postoperative Care

Although a cast may be used in an unreliable patient, gauze and tape dressings are applied at surgery and changed on a weekly basis when possible. This allows proper alignment of the fifth toe, as well as continued compression in the midfoot.

Sutures are removed 3 weeks after surgery. Internal fixation of the osteotomy site is removed 6 weeks after surgery or after radiographic proof of healing (Fig. 6D and E).

In the presence of a combined plantar-lateral keratosis, the orientation of the oblique osteotomy is altered (Fig. 6C). Although the dorsal-proximal to plantar-distal osteotomy is made, the orientation of the cut is changed from a direct lateral-medial to a more cephalad osteotomy cut. By dropping his hand holding the saw, the surgeon cuts in an upward direction. Then when the osteotomy site is rotated, the distal fifth metatarsal is elevated. This helps to relieve pressure on the plantar aspect of the fifth metatarsal head, as well as to correct the bunionette deformity. Internal fixation is carried out as previously described, and postoperative care also is similar.

DISCUSSION

An enlarged fifth metatarsal head or lateral condyle (with or without excessive pronation of the foot) may be treated with a lateral condylar resection and fifth MP joint realignment; however, a chevron osteotomy is preferred because it achieves greater correction. Realignment of the MP joint and meticulous capsular closure are important to prevent later subluxation or dislocation of the MP joint. A distal chevron osteotomy is inherently stable; however, K-wire fixation tends to increase stability until the osteotomy site has healed. In the presence of a plantar or a plantar-lateral keratosis, or a moderate-or-severe type 2 or type 3 deformity, a diaphyseal oblique osteotomy is the preferred procedure. The diaphyseal osteotomy is combined with a distal soft tissue realignment of the MP joint because it corrects the MP-5 angle as well.

SUGGESTED READING

Coughlin MJ. Etiology and treatment of the bunionette deformity. AAOS Inst Course Lectures 1990; 39:37–48.

Coughlin MJ. Treatment of bunionette deformity with longitudinal diaphyseal osteotomy with distal soft tissue repair. Foot Ankle 1991; 11:195–203.

Fallat LM, Buckholz J. An analysis of the Tailor's bunion by radiographic and anatomical display. J Am Podiatr Assoc 1980; 70:597–603.

Shereff MJ, Yang QM, Kummer FJ, et al. Vascular anatomy of the fifth metatarsal. Foot Ankle 1991; 11:350–353.

Throckmorton JK, Bradlee N. Transverse V. sliding osteotomy: A new surgical procedure for the correction of Tailor's bunion deformity. J Foot Surg 1978; 18:117–121.

RHEUMATOID FOREFOOT

MARK E. SCHAKEL II, M.D.

In 16 percent of patients with rheumatoid arthritis, the foot is the initial site of involvement, and the foot eventually is involved in upward of 90 percent of patients. A certain percentage of these patients develop significant involvement and progressive deformity. The metatarsophalangeal (MP) joints are affected preferentially, with less involvement of the proximal interphalangeal (PIP) joints. Synovitis causes attenuation of the capsular structures, particularly in a juxta-articular location. Combined with the forces applied to the joints by standing and walking, this erosive synovitis results in subluxation and frank dislocation of the lesser MP joints. The PIP joints are involved secondarily. Hallux valgus deformity develops as a result of the same soft tissue pathology and the combined forces of shoe wear and walking. The clawing of the toes causes distal migration of the plantar fat pad, increased plantar prominence of the metatarsal heads, painful plantar callosities, and bursa formation. The flexion deformities of the PIP joints result in dorsal irritation in shoes. The hallux valgus, with accompanying metatarsus primus varus, leads to pain over the prominent medial eminence.

THERAPY

Treatment of rheumatoid forefoot deformities is directed toward pain relief but is determined by the stage of the disease and the magnitude of the deformity. Nonoperative treatment involves optimization of the medical management of the disease process and shoe wear modifications to accommodate the deformities. For severe deformities this entails a custom-molded Plastizote insert and an extra-depth shoe.

Surgical treatment of mild isolated soft tissue (particularly nodule formation) or bony problems should be limited. The progressive nature of the disease increases the risk of recurrence, particularly since the isolated symptomatic rheumatoid nodules are a response to underlying pressure, i.e., deformity and nodule formation in the forefoot are best treated by first correcting the underlying deformity.

When significant forefoot joint involvement and deformity have developed, soft tissue and limited bony procedures such as ostectomy no longer are indicated because of the high rate of recurrence of deformity. Numerous techniques for rheumatoid forefoot reconstruction have been reported. Hoffman described resection of all the metatarsal heads, and Clayton added resection of the proximal phalangeal bases. This treatment of the hallux has been modified to a Keller-type arthroplasty, maintaining the metatarsal head and resecting the base of the proximal phalanx. Silastic implants have been used in the hallux and even the lesser MP joints. Good results have been reported with all these procedures; however, in a number of reports a significant rate of recurrence of deformity with redislocation and resultant callosity formation under the lesser metatarsals and up to a 50 percent hallux valgus recurrence have been noted. There is no doubt that some patients may benefit from these alternative procedures, particularly on the hallux.

However, the combination of resection of the lesser metatarsal heads with arthrodesis of the first MP joint appears to minimize the risk of recurrent deformity, allows the almost uniform return to regular shoe wear, significantly diminishes pain, and improves the patient's ability to stand and walk. Arthrodesis results in an earlier lift-off of the foot, thereby decreasing the dorsiflexion and lateral deviation forces on the lesser toes. This plays a major role in the prevention of recurrent deformities.

The hallux MP joint is fused in 15° to 20° of valgus, 20° to 30° of dorsiflexion with respect to the line of the first metatarsal, or 0° to 10° of dorsiflexion with respect to the floor. Pronation or supination is corrected. It is essential to the supinate the hallux into a neutral position since pronation is tolerated poorly.

The lesser MP joint deformities are corrected by resection of the metatarsal heads. Retention of the phalangeal bases results in a more cosmetic appearance, since the length of the toes is preserved. The interphalangeal joint deformities can be corrected by manual manipulation without further bony resection. Kirschner (K-) wires occasionally are used to maintain alignment with the metatarsal in the postoperative period.

Although controversial, even if the first MP joint is essentially uninvolved, an arthrodesis probably should be performed. A high incidence of hallux valgus development occurs if the joint is left intact. This is probably from the loss of lateral support, resulting from lesser metatarsal head resection. Similarly, sparing of uninvolved lesser MP joints is not advisable, because it almost uniformly results in a callosity and metatarsalgia under the retained metatarsal head. This is an important decision in early disease when a few MP joints are dislocated, and the hallux is involved minimally.

SURGICAL TECHNIQUE

The surgery can be performed under either ankle block or general anesthesia. A pneumatic tourniquet may be used, but usually is not necessary. When an ankle block is employed, an ankle tourniquet is used in the supramalleolar region. I use a sterile tourniquet, but this is not essential. Bilateral procedures should be spaced at least 2 weeks apart, since patients should be ambulating comfortably before surgery is performed on the opposite foot. Aspirin should be discontinued 2 weeks before surgery, other nonsteroidals 5 to 7 days preoperatively. Methotrexate and other medications are not withheld routinely. Oral corticosteroid medications should have a burst and taper to routine levels.

Three longitudinal dorsal incisions are employed, one centered over the first MP joint and one in the second and fourth interspaces, respectively. Before any incisions are made, manual manipulation of the interphalangeal joints into extension is performed. This is best accomplished now when all bony structures still are intact. Gentle passive extension on the digits is performed, tearing at the plantar PIP capsuloligamentous contracture.

The hallux MP joint incision is made first; it extends from the midmetatarsal to the interphalangeal joint. The extensor hallucis longus tendon is retracted, a dorsal capsulectomy is performed, and the capsule is dissected from the metatarsal head and the base of the proximal phalanx. On the medial aspect this dissection is extended even further proximally and distally to allow for later resection of the medial eminence and transarticular screw placement. A sagittal saw is used to resect the articular surfaces. Minimal bone is removed initially. The first cut is made on the first metatarsal, resecting the joint surface in 15° to 20° of valgus and 20° to 30° of dorsiflexion with respect to the line of the metatarsal shaft, or 0° to 10° of dorsiflexion with respect to the line of the floor. The hallux then is held in the desired alignment, and the articular cartilage and subchondral bone of the proximal phalangeal base are resected perpendicular to the axis of the proximal phalanx. Care should be taken to avoid excessive bone resection because this may compromise fixation of the arthrodesis. A provisional reduction is performed to confirm the alignment and the presence of adequate coaptation of the surfaces. If further resection is necessary, this should be performed on the metatarsal side. An alternative technique of arthrodesis site resection uses commercially available reamers to fashion a cup and cone. This technique allows simpler alignment in the desired position. One must resect the cartilage and subchondral bone with a saw before reaming. This technique results in more shortening of the hallux, but this generally is not a problem when one is combining the arthrodesis with resection of the lesser metatarsal heads.

The second incision is made in the second interspace. Dissection is performed down to the second and third MP joints in turn. The extensor tendon is transected and a dorsal capsulectomy is performed transversely in the MP joint. Longitudinal traction is placed on the toe, and the capsule and collateral ligaments are dissected from the metatarsal head and neck. Even with significant dislocation at this joint, with persistence this exposure can be accomplished and the proximal phalangeal base can be left intact. A third skin incision is made in the fourth interspace, and the process is repeated on the fourth and fifth MP joints.

The lesser metatarsal heads are next resected at the neck with a sagittal saw, beginning with the second and progressing laterally, attempting to make a smooth arc from medial to lateral. Slight inclination of the saw in a dorsoplantar direction ensures that a bone spike is not present on the plantar surface of the metatarsal neck. By grasping the metatarsal heads with an adequate-size rongeur and using a rolling action, one usually can peel the bone from the volar soft tissues. The wound is inspected for rheumatoid cysts, which are incised and debrided. No attempt is made to excise them completely.

After resection of the lesser metatarsal heads, attention is directed back to the first MP arthrodesis, which is reduced again. If the hallux is more than 0.5 cm longer than the second toe, further bone is resected from the metatarsal. The arthrodesis is fixed provisionally with two 0.045 inch K-wires placed from the medial aspect of the metatarsal. These K-wires are placed relatively dorsally so as not to interfere with later screw placement. The alignment of the arthrodesis then is checked with respect to valgus, dorsiflexion, and rotation.

Once adequate alignment of the arthrodesis has been attained provisionally, rigid internal fixation is performed. This is accomplished with an oblique transarticular screw placed from the medial aspect of the base of the proximal phalanx and a ¼ tubular AO minifragment plate placed dorsally. The type of screw used depends on bone quality. If the bone is reasonably hard, 2.7 mm cortical screws with their less prominent screw heads can be used. If bone quality is poor, 3.5 mm cortical or 4.0 mm fully threaded cancellous screws can be used. Often a combination is used, with the 2.7 mm screws in the stronger cortical bone of the metatarsal and the 4.0 mm screws in the metaphyseal region and proximal phalanx. The plate is not always necessary, but using it in combination with the screw is my preferred approach to the rheumatoid MP fusion. It enhances stability in osteopenic bone and allows for immediate ambulation. On its own, the plate is inadequate fixation, since it is placed on the compression and not the tension side of the MP joint. The screw is inserted first to act as a tension band against the dorsally applied plate.

The first screw placed is the oblique screw across the arthrodesis in a lag fashion from the medial aspect of the proximal phalanx. A washer often is used. The provisional K-wires can be removed at this time. A six or seven hole ¼ tubular plate then is contoured to the dorsum of the arthrodesis and fixed with AO 2.7 mm, 3.5 mm, or 4.0 mm screws. The phalangeal screws typically are placed first. Upon completion of fixation a generous resection of the medial eminence of the first metatarsal is performed.

The lesser toes are fixed using long double-ended 0.045 inch K-wires. These are retrograded out the toes with the interphalangeal joints held straight. The K-wires then are inserted antegrade up the medullary canals of the metatarsals until firm fixation in the base is noted. The pins then are bent and cut to protrude out the tips of the toes (Fig. 1).

The tourniquet is deflated, hemostasis is obtained, and the incisions are closed. A bulky gauze dressing is placed. Not infrequently, after deflation of the tourniquet, return of circulation to the lesser toes is slow. If evidence of ischemia to a given toe persists, the dressing should be loosened; if ischemia persists, that K-wire should be removed. This almost always allows return of

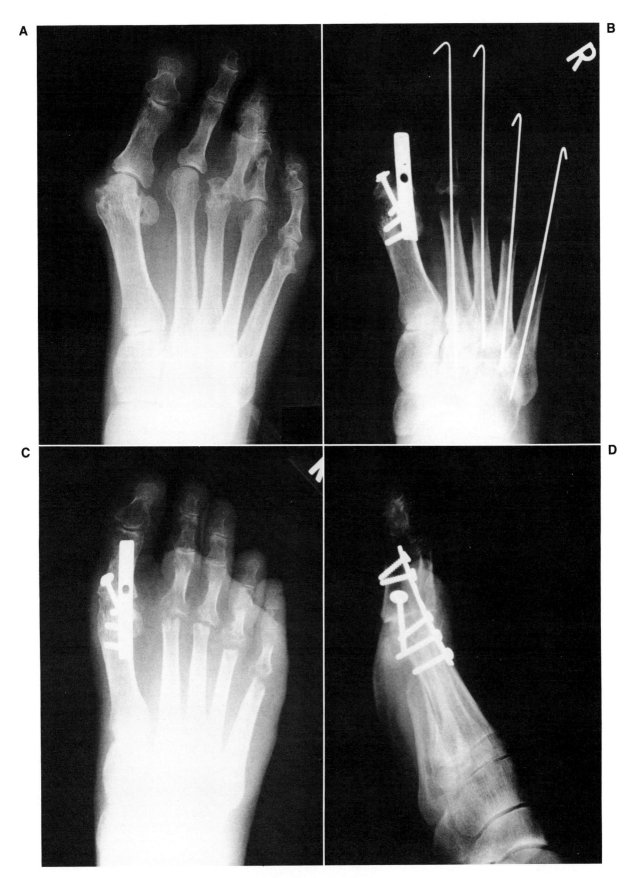

Figure 1 *A*, Rheumatoid forefoot deformities. *B*, Immediate postoperative view with plate and screw fixation of the first MP joint arthrodesis and K-wire fixation of the lesser toes resection arthroplasties. *C* and *D*, Alignment 3 months postoperative.

circulation. Toe alignment then is maintained by the dressing.

POSTOPERATIVE CARE

The bulky gauze dressing placed during surgery is changed on the first postoperative day to a gauze and tape dressing to the midfoot to help control swelling. Dressings are maintained for 2 to 4 weeks. Sutures are removed at 10 to 14 days based on healing. Weight bearing in a postoperative wooden shoe is permitted immediately. The shoe is worn for all standing and walking until solid union of the arthrodesis is demonstrated. The lesser toe K-wires are removed at 6 weeks. If a pin tract infection develops or a pin begins backing out before that time, that pin can be removed. The infection usually can be managed by local wound care and oral antibiotics.

Arthrodesis of the first MP joint usually is completed 8 to 12 weeks postoperatively. When this is confirmed radiographically, the patient may go into a regular shoe as swelling and comfort permit.

SPECIAL CIRCUMSTANCES

In patients who have had a previous Keller or Silastic interposition arthroplasty of the first MP joint,

screw and plate fixation for the arthrodesis may not be feasible. If this is the case, fixation using either two heavy threaded Steinmann pins ($\%_2$ and $\frac{1}{8}$ inch) retrograded out the tip of the toe and then antegraded across the arthrodesis or smaller threaded 0.062 inch K-wires placed in a crossed fashion, can be used (Fig. 2). Bone graft from the lesser metatarsal heads may be used to fill the defect from the Silastic implant.

Occasionally patients have significant rheumatoid nodules under the first metatarsal head and sesamoids. These should be excised by way of a separate medial incision made just dorsal to the plantar skin. If the sesamoid or sesamoids are prominent, they should be excised through the same surgical approach. One should ensure that the sesamoids retract proximal to the metatarsal head, since they invariably cause pain if they stick down under the metatarsal head.

COMPLICATIONS

About 20 percent of patients have some symptoms about the first ray, either symptomatic callosities under the sesamoids or symptoms about the interphalangeal joint. Painful callosities under the sesamoids often can be relieved by felt pads or inserts that distribute the pressure away from them. If this is unsuccessful, one or both sesamoids can be excised.

Rheumatoid cysts can develop at the interpha-

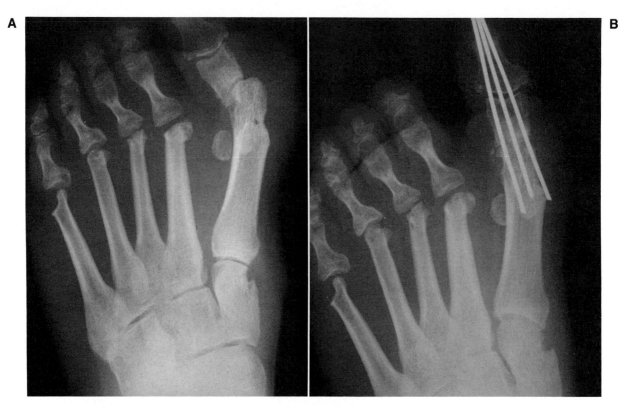

Figure 2 *A,* Recurrent forefoot deformity is not easy to stabilize. *B,* Technique of fixation using threaded 0.062 inch K-wires.

langeal joint of the hallux. If they are symptomatic, simple excision often is successful. In cases in which they are recurrent or significant symptomatic arthritis develops, the interphalangeal joint can be fused without significant loss of function.

Nonunion of the first MP joint arthrodesis occurs about 5 to 10 percent of the time. Frequently a stable fibrous ankylosis is observed, which is asymptomatic. The rare symptomatic pseudoarthrosis requires a second attempt at fusion with iliac crest bone graft and rigid internal fixation.

It is not unusual to have some heterotopic ossification at the ends of resected lesser metatarsals. Generally this causes no problems, but occasionally is significant enough to result in a symptomatic callus. Resection of the symptomatic bone is uniformly successful in alleviating the problem. Persistent or recurrent hammer toes are rare. If they do occur, however, a resection arthroplasty-type hammer toe correction usually is successful. Arthrodesis is successful less often and should be avoided.

SUGGESTED READING

Hoffman P. An operation for severe grades of contracted or clawed toes. Am J Orthop Surg 1912; 9:441–449.

Mann RA, ed. Surgery of the foot. St Louis: CV Mosby, 1986:171.

Mann RA, Thompson FM. Arthrodesis of the first metatarsophalangeal joint for hallux valgus in rheumatoid arthritis. J Bone Joint Surg 1984; 66A:687–692.

McGarvey SR, Johnson KA. Keller arthroplasty in combination with resection arthroplasty of the lesser metatarsophalangeal joints in rheumatoid arthritis. Foot Ankle 1988; 9:75–80.

TRANSPOSITIONAL BIPLANAR CERVICAL OSTEOTOMY FOR METATARSUS PRIMUS VARUS

MELVIN H. JAHSS, M.D.

PATHOLOGIC ANATOMY AND BIOMECHANICS

The prime cause of hallux valgus (HV) and bunions is metatarsus primus varus (MPV), along with other factors such as pes planus and hypermobile joints. Conversely, MPV is aggravated by the HV because as the distal portion of the first metatarsal displaces medially, it leaves behind the sesamoids and the conjoined tendons. At the same time, the extensor hallucis longus (EHL) and flexor hallucis longus (FHL) become tightly bowstrung laterally, which further accentuates the MPV. The HV deformity becomes fixed, augmented by contracture of the lateral capsule and adductor tendons. The hallux also rotates medially, causing the abductor hallucis to function as a flexor.

The hallux ultimately pushes under the second toe, which begins to deform by subluxation at the metatarsophalangeal (MP) joint. This in turn forces down the second metatarsal head. In addition, the hallucal deformity and the MPV both decrease the weight bearing under the first ray, causing further excess weight bearing under the middle metatarsal heads.

The entire pathologic anatomy must be considered to correct the deformity surgically. In addition, two other factors, often not considered, must be evaluated. The first is that excessive joint hypermobility combined with hallucal pressure from inappropriate shoes may cause recurrence of the deformity at the MP joint, as well as abnormal angulation at the first metatarsal medial cuneiform joint (Fig. 1). Such joint laxity is recognized readily preoperatively by hypermobile finger joints, hypermobile pes planus, and excess laxity of the second and third metatarsals.

The second factor is that any corrective osteotomy must be biplanar. A mere 2 mm of shortening of the first metatarsal following osteotomy may result in painful transfer of weight bearing under the second and third metatarsal heads. Any shortening—whether from the thickness of the saw blade, upward tilt of the osteotomy,

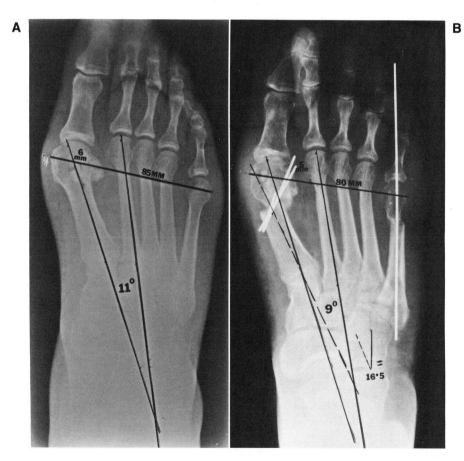

Figure 1 Hypermobility at first metatarsal medial cuneiform joint. *A,* Metatarsus primus varus of 11°. *B,* A 4 mm lateral displacement cervical osteotomy was done, but increasing angulation at the first metatarsal medial cuneiform joint of 5.5° obviated the correction.

or an ill-conceived osteotomy—contributes to the shortening. Measuring the amount of needed correction by radiographs is not accurate. However, objective guidelines have been established from mathematic formulas for corrections in both the transverse and sagittal planes for each type of metatarsal osteotomy.

SHORTENING

Shortening of the first metatarsal causes elevation of the metatarsal head from the ground with decrease in its weight-bearing function. This results in weight-bearing transfer to the middle metatarsal heads. Shortening as little as 1 to 2 mm may result in painful transfer.

Shortening is inherent in any osteotomy as a result of the thickness of the power saw blade (1 to 2 mm), the bone necrosis at the osteotomized surfaces (2 mm), and the process of union of the osteotomy. Delayed union and nonunion may result in up to 10 mm of shortening. In general, unacceptable shortening is inherent in the Mitchell stepcut procedure, oblique sliding osteotomies,

e.g., Wilson's (Fig. 2), and lateral closing wedges. Other causes of decreased weight bearing under the first metatarsal head include unrecognized dorsal slipping or tilting of the distal fragment (metatarsal head) (Fig. 3). Similarly, unrecognized medial tilting of the metatarsal head results in less weight bearing and poor correction of the MPV.

Shortening may be corrected partially by plantar displacement or angulation of the distal fragment. Lengthening procedures are not advisable because tension on contracted soft tissues may increase the deformities.

Since correction of HV and MPV involves both the transverse and sagittal planes, as well as rotation, any first metatarsal osteotomy must be biplanar in its effect in addition to minimizing shortening. With respect to cervical osteotomies, only the chevron and the biplanar lateral transpositional osteotomy result in minimal shortening. However, the chevron is uniplanar so that the distal fragment cannot be displaced plantarward or rotated and has the potential danger of aseptic necrosis since the cuts enter the head (Fig. 4). The chevron is

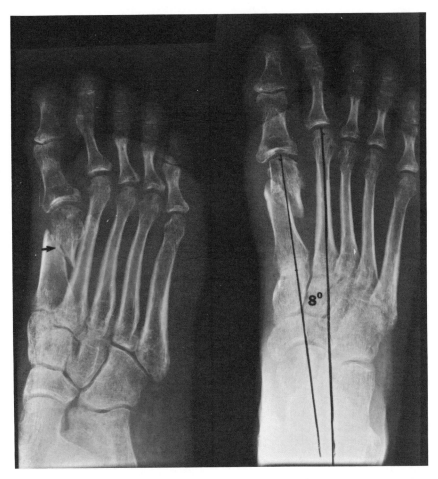

Figure 2 Typical Wilson oblique cervical osteotomy with unacceptable shortening. The more oblique the cut, the less correction and the greater shortening per millimeter of lateral shift.

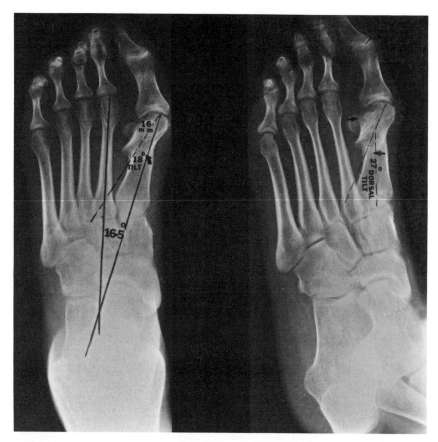

Figure 3 Unrecognized intraoperative medial and dorsal tilt of the first metatarsal head. An increase over the original degree of MPV and loss of first metatarsal weight bearing was observed with transfer metatarsalgia. It was corrected by a reosteotomy through the neck with plantar displacement of the distal fragment.

more stable than the simple transpositional osteotomy, but the head may slip back medially. Although the chevron osteotomy is stable, internal fixation avoids slippage or shifting of the osteotomy. Finally, if the chevron cut is taken too distally, the head fragment will be highly unstable or the head may split.

BIOMECHANICS OF THE SAGITTAL PLANE

The angle of declination of the first metatarsal is the angle in which it subtends the ground as seen in the sagittal plane. It averages 25° and is greater with high arches. Trigonometric calculations indicate that with this 25° angle, for each 1 mm of shortening of the metatarsal secondary to any procedure (or its complications), there is an elevation of the metatarsal head of 0.42 mm from the ground. Any significant shortening results in weight-bearing transference under the rigid second and third metatarsals with resultant anterior metatarsalgia. Inadvertent dorsal tilting is even more significant with respect to its sagittal effect. A 10° dorsal tilt of a cervical

osteotomy elevates the head 1.64 mm, and a 20° tilt elevates it 3.35 mm (see Fig. 3). Even more serious is that 10° and 20° tilts from basilar osteotomies elevate the head 4.91 and 10.1 mm, respectively.

Above all, it must be stressed that lateral transfer of weight bearing with painful anterior metatarsalgia is much more disabling than an uncorrected HV and MPV.

BIPLANAR CERVICAL OSTEOTOMY

Indications

The average width of the first metatarsal neck is 13 mm. My experience indicates that lateral transposition of the distal fragment a maximum of one-third the diameter of the neck prevents such complications as nonunion and aseptic necrosis of the first metatarsal head. This transposition therefore would be approximately 4.5 mm. Since each millimeter shift results in 1° correction of the MPV, the maximal MPV correction with this operation is 4.5°. Since 9° is normal, any MPV

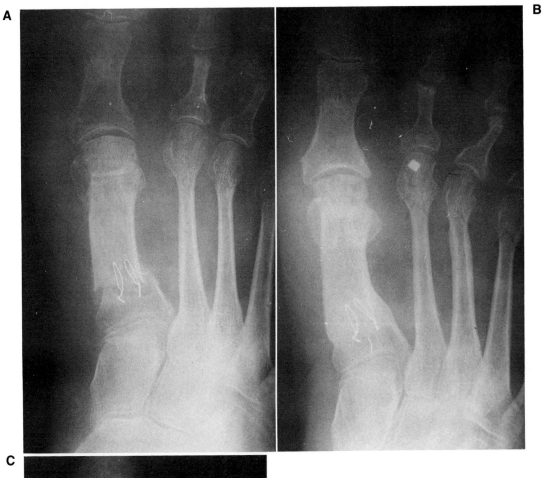

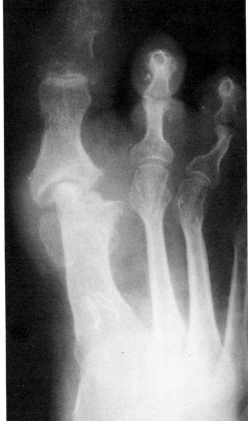

Figure 4 Aseptic necrosis of the first metatarsal head following a high cervical osteotomy combined with a basilar closing wedge. *A,* Double osteotomy. *B,* Six months later. Spotty osteoporosis in the metatarsal head. *C,* Eighteen months later. Massive aseptic necrosis with absorption of the lateral two-thirds of the head.

over 13° cannot be corrected fully by a cervical transpositional osteotomy. I prefer to use the cervical osteotomy for MPV between 10° and 12°.

The contraindications and limitations of the biplanar cervical osteotomy are clear cut as noted in Table 1.

Advantages

Excluding the foregoing contraindications, the biplanar osteotomy is the simplest of the cervical osteotomies with minimal complications. It avoids shortening, provides a biplanar correction, prevents aseptic necrosis, and minimizes delayed union and nonunion.

Table 1 Contraindications to Biplanar Cervical Osteotomy

Contraindications	Surgical Choice
MPV over 12°	Basilar crescentic
Hypermobile foot	Lapidus' procedure
OA first MP	Arthrodesis
Rheumatoid arthritis	Exostectomy/Hoffman's arthrodesis
Tight (fixed) adductor	Basilar crescentic and lateral release
Professional athlete or dancer	No surgery

MPV, metatarsus primus varus; OA, osteoarthritis; MP, metatarsophalangeal.

Surgical Technique

No tourniquet is used. Ankle block is acceptable, but the patient may require additional sedation and must be prepared for general anesthesia should the block be less than optimal.

A longitudinal medial skin incision is made and then a Y-shaped capsular flap with its base attached distally. The bunion is excised in line with the metatarsal neck and not in the plantar sagittal groove, which removes excess articular surface. The periosteum about the neck is stripped partially, leaving the lateral portion intact. The osteotomy is done with a power saw at right angles through the neck (Fig. 5A). The distal fragment is shifted laterally, depending on the amount of MPV. Since the average neck width is 13 mm, a maximal lateral shift of one-third the diameter is about 4.5 mm. Since one would like final correction of 8° MPV or less, an MPV of up to 12° is fully correctable by a cervical osteotomy. As an operative guideline, the thickness of the cortex of the neck is 2 to 3 mm. Doubling this shift usually gives satisfactory correction, which should be verified by direct measurement after Kirschner (K-) wire fixation. At the same time that the head is shifted laterally, it is displaced

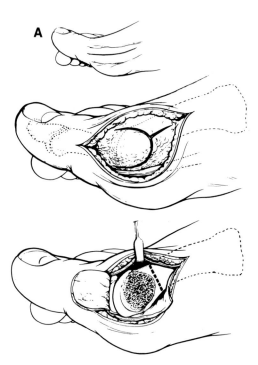
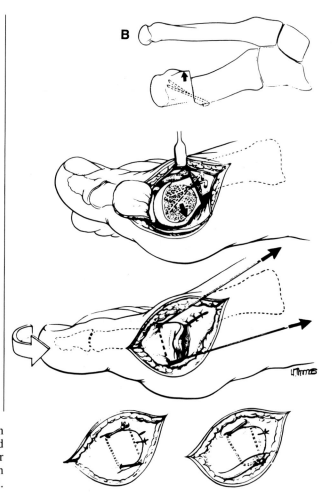

Figure 5 Biplanar transverse cervical osteotomy. *A,* From top to bottom: incision, capsular flap, bunionectomy, and osteotomy site. *B,* From top to bottom: lateral shift, plantar displacement and fixation, and capsular advancement. (From Jahss MH, ed. Disorders of the foot and ankle, 2nd ed. Philadelphia: WB Saunders, 1991:1005; with permission.)

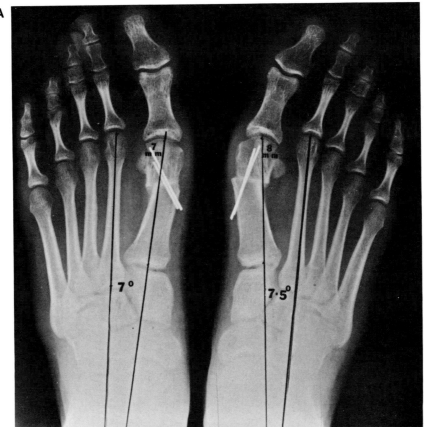

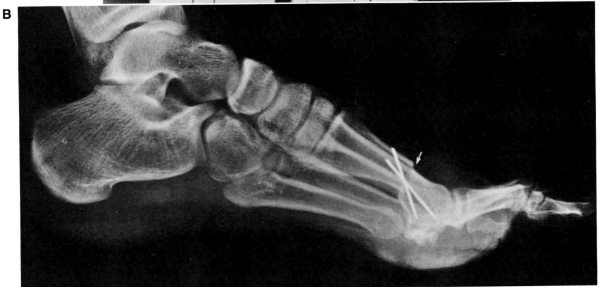

Figure 6 Roentgenographic appearance of a biplanar cervical osteotomy. The anteroposterior (AP) must be taken with the feet flush on the plate, because slight foot rotation results in misleading radiographic distortion. *A,* AP view illustrating lateral displacement and K-wire fixation. *B,* Lateral view illustrating plantar displacement *(arrow).*

plantarward 2 to 4 mm, depending on the amount of weight-bearing insufficiency of the first ray (Figs. 5B and 6). This is determined preoperatively by the degree of soft "baby skin" palpable under the head of the first metatarsal and the presence or absence of callus (excess weight bearing) under the second metatarsal head. Also the head is rotated externally to compensate for any medial rotation. The fragments are held by two 0.045 K-wires inserted proximal to distal. The first MP joint is moved to determine if either wire has crossed the joint. If the fragments are not satisfactorily shifted or aligned, the wires are removed and the process repeated. The pins are bent and cut short under the skin to prevent migration, loosening, and infection. The protruding medial edge of the proximal fragment at the osteotomy site is beveled with a power saw. The K-wires are removed under local anesthesia in 6 weeks. I prefer non–weight bearing during this period since a mere 1 to 2 mm of upward displacement of the distal fragment with weight bearing causes 50 percent loss of correction of a 2 to 4 mm plantar shift.

After the K-wire insertion the capsular flap is advanced and tightly sutured to the proximal periosteum (see Fig. 5B) or to the abductor hallucis tendon, which is located in a fibrous canal plantar medially. The tendon sheath is opened and the tendon displaced more medially and sutured with two vertical mattress sutures (0-0 chromic) to the capsular flap, tight enough to obtain 10° to 15° of hallux varus (Fig. 7). The skin is closed with interrupted 5-0 chromic sutures. With respect to adductor release, the lateral shift of the distal fragment usually relaxes the lateral conjoined tendon to permit correction of the HV along with the capsular plication. Earlier reports of increased incidence of aseptic necrosis of the first metatarsal head with cervical osteotomies associated with adductor release now have been disproven conclusively. Despite this, I prefer to do a basilar concentric osteotomy in lieu of a cervical osteotomy when the adductor is unduly tight and fixed on preoperative evaluation. This applies to any degree of MPV.

The hallux is bandaged weekly to hold the corrected position for approximately 3 to 4 weeks.

Complications and Salvages

Early in the postoperative period, if the wires are found to be inadequately displaced, the wound is opened, the osteotomy adjusted if necessary, and the wires replaced.

A poorly corrected united cervical osteotomy (see Fig. 3) is reostomized with the appropriate lateral displacement. Because associated shortening usually is observed with both the original and the salvage procedures, plantar shift may have to be accentuated to about 4 to 5 mm. Fixation and aftercare are similar.

In cases of delayed union (Fig. 8), weight bearing still is permitted after 6 weeks. It may take up to 1 year for roentgenographic union to occur. In cases of nonunion, conservative freshening up of the pseud-

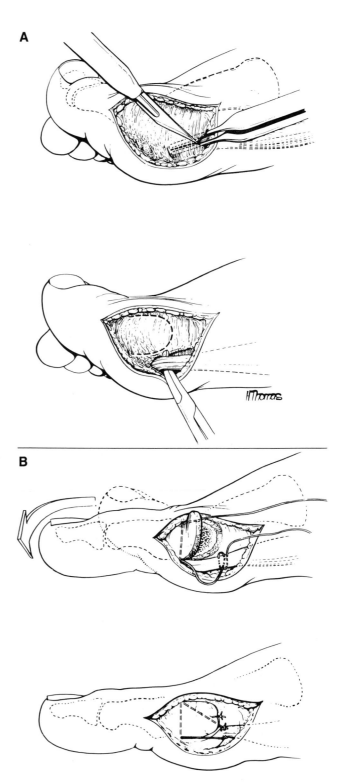

Figure 7 Capsular advancement and plication to the abductor hallucis tendon. *A,* Uncovering the abductor hallucis tendon from its sheath and "hooking" it into view with a small curved clamp. *B,* Releasing the abductor from its sheath without transecting it and plicating it to the advanced capsular flap. The tendon is now located more medially. (From Jahss MH, ed. Disorders of the foot and ankle, 2nd ed. Philadelphia: WB Saunders, 1991:993; with permission.)

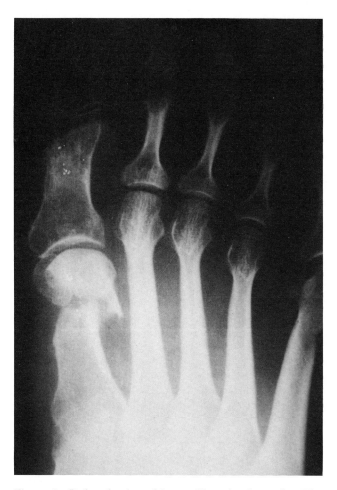

Figure 8 Delayed union of 1 year. Note the shortening. The bone ends are starting to sclerose and smooth off, but spontaneous union still may occur.

arthrosis without causing undue shortening in addition to bone grafting and wire fixation are done along with sufficient plantar displacement to accommodate for any shortening that may be significant. Before the surgery, make sure the pain is coming from the pseudoarthrosis and not from the MP joint.

SUGGESTED READING

Carr CR, Boyd BM. Correctional osteotomy for metatarsus primus varus and hallux valgus. J Bone Joint Surg 1968; 50A:1353–1367.

Hawkins FB, Mitchell CL, Hedrick DW. Correction of hallux valgus by metatarsal osteotomy. J Bone Joint Surg 1945; 27:387–394.

Inman VT. Hallux valgus: A review of etiologic factors. Orthop Clin North Am 1974; 5:59–66.

Jahss MH. LeLièvre bunion operation. In: Instructional course lectures, American Academy of Orthopaedic Surgeons, Vol 21. St Louis: CV Mosby, 1972:285.

Jahss MH. Disorders of the hallux and the first ray. In: Jahss MH, ed. Disorders of the foot and ankle: Medical and surgical management. 2nd ed. Philadelphia: WB Saunders, 1991:943.

Jahss MH, Troy AI, Kummer F. Roentgenographic and mathematical analysis of first metatarsal osteotomies for metatarsus primus varus: A comparative study. Foot Ankle 1985; 5:280–321.

Kinnard P, Gordon D. A comparison between Chevron and Mitchell osteotomies for hallux valgus. Foot Ankle 1984; 4:241–243.

Kummer FJ. Mathematical analysis of first metatarsal osteotomies. Foot Ankle 1989; 9:281–289.

Lapidus PW. The author's bunion operation from 1931 to 1959. Clin Orthop 1960; 16:119–135.

Lindgren U, Turan I. A new operation for hallux valgus. Clin Orthop 1983; 175:179–183.

Meier PJ, Kenzora JE. The risks and benefits of distal first metatarsal osteotomies. Foot Ankle 1985; 6:7–17.

Merkel KD, Katoh Y, Johnson EW, Chao EYS. Mitchell osteotomy for hallux valgus: Long-term follow-up and gait analysis. Foot Ankle 1983; 3:189–196.

CHEVRON OSTEOTOMY FOR HALLUX VALGUS

MICHAEL J. SHEREFF, M.D.

The hallux valgus deformity consists of lateral deviation of the great toe, medial deviation of the first metatarsal, attenuation of the medial capsule, and contracture of the lateral capsule and soft tissue structures. The valgus deflection of the hallux combined with metatarsus primus varus causes the medial aspect of the metatarsal head to become prominent. Patients note pain, because this prominent medial eminence impinges against the toe box of the shoe. As one might expect, patients describe difficulty fitting shoe wear. Physical examination reveals the deformity as described. Erythema may be identified at the skin overlying the prominent medial eminence.

The chevron procedure is a distal osteotomy of the first metatarsal used for correction of the hallux valgus deformity. This procedure consists of a transverse V-shaped osteotomy made at the distal aspect of the bone. This operation includes resection of the prominent medial eminence, which reduces forefoot width. Lateral translocation of the distal fragment following osteotomy corrects metatarsus primus varus, and medial capsulorrhaphy corrects lateral deviation of the hallux.

The chevron osteotomy has numerous advantages as compared with other distal osteotomies. The V-shaped osteotomy provides some degree of inherent stability, thereby reducing malunion postoperatively. Although the original descriptions of this operation did not include internal fixation, the use of percutaneous single-pin fixation is thought to add stability during the healing period. The osteotomy itself provides a large contact area between the osteotomy fragments as compared with other types of distal metatarsal osteotomies. This factor provides for rapid healing. Delayed union and nonunion of this osteotomy is uncommon. The chevron osteotomy is associated with minimal bone loss, leading to minimal shortening. Other osteotomies that shorten the first ray may lead to decreased loading of the first metatarsal, with subsequent transfer metatarsalgia.

PATIENT SELECTION

Indications

The chevron osteotomy provides correction of the common acquired forefoot disorder consisting of hallux valgus, metatarsus primus varus, and a prominent medial eminence. This procedure is best suited for patients who display a mild-to-moderate deformity. This includes those individuals in whom anteroposterior (AP) standing radiographs of the foot reveal an intermetatarsal angle of 14° or less. This procedure is best suited for those who display a metatarsophalangeal (MP) angle of 35° or less. The chevron osteotomy is best suited for a patient who is less than 60 years of age.

Contraindications

Long-standing deformities associated with subluxation of the MP joint may lead to subsequent intra-articular arthrosis. Patients with arthritis of that joint are best treated with other surgical procedures such as resection arthroplasty or arthrodesis. Severe metatarsus primus varus (an intermetatarsal angle greater than 15°) is better treated with a proximal metatarsal osteotomy or metatarsocuneiform MP arthrodesis.

TIMING OF SURGERY

Surgical intervention should be reserved for those patients who fail to respond to conservative methods of treatment. Patients should be counseled regarding reasonable footwear. In general, patients should be asked to wear shoes made of soft pliable leather and directed toward shoes with a high wide toe box, which allows ample room to accommodate the forefoot deformities. Patients should be asked to lower the height of their heels, since high-heeled shoes tend to propel the foot forward into the toe box and thus lead to mechanical impingement.

PREOPERATIVE PREPARATION

Preoperative workup requires radiographic evaluation of the foot. This generally includes AP and lateral radiographs. An AP weight-bearing view is taken with the patient erect, standing on the cassette. The x-ray source is centered on the midfoot and tilted 15° toward the ankle joint. Objective radiographic parameters may be measured. The MP angle, often referred to as the hallux valgus angle, is one of the most common measurements made in the evaluation of forefoot deformities. This parameter is determined by measuring the angle formed by the intersection of the midlongitudinal axis of the first metatarsal and the proximal phalanx. The first intermetatarsal angle is formed by the intersection of the lines bisecting the shafts of the first and second metatarsals as measured on the AP weight-bearing radiographs.

Preoperative preparation also includes extensive discussions with the patient regarding the nature of the surgical procedure, as well as alternative modes of treatment. Most important the patient must be provided with realistic expectations as to the possible results of the surgical procedure. Potential problems and complications of the surgery are reviewed.

OPERATIVE PROCEDURE

A medial-longitudinal incision is made approximately 6 cm in length. The incision is positioned just dorsal to the midline and extends from the region of the midpoint of the proximal phalanx to several centimeters proximal to the prominent medial eminence (Fig. 1*A*). Subcutaneous tissue is divided along the line of the skin incision. Care is taken to prevent injury to the dorsal cutaneous nerve.

Skin and subcutaneous tissue are reflected to visualize the joint capsule. A Y-shaped capsular incision is made based distally. The apex of the V-portion lies just proximal to the prominent medial eminence (Fig. 1*B*). The V-portion is reflected distally to expose the head and neck of the metatarsal. The prominent medial eminence is resected parallel to the medial border of the foot with a microsagittal saw (Fig. 1*C*).

A transverse V-shaped osteotomy is made distally

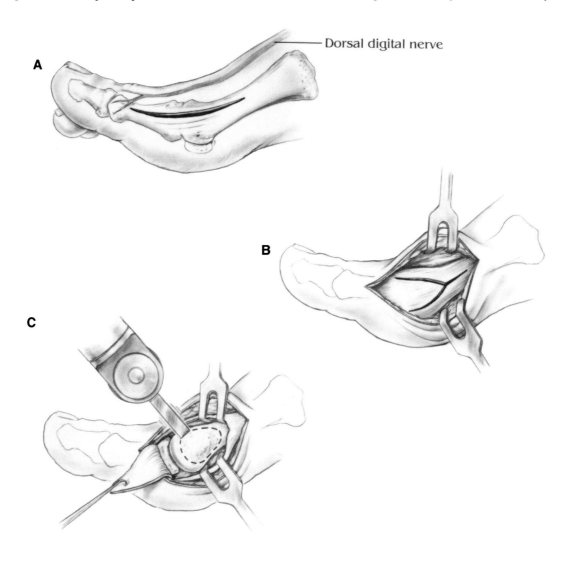

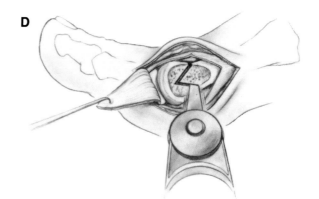

Figure 1 *A through H,* Chevron osteotomy. See text description. (From Shereff MJ. Atlas of Foot and Ankle Surgery. Philadelphia: W.B. Saunders, in press; with permission.)

Continued.

with the microsagittal saw (Fig. 1D). It is recommended that the angle of the osteotomy is less than 60° to provide inherent stability.

The distal fragment is translocated laterally for 2 to 4 mm (Fig. 1E) and depends on the width of the metatarsal neck. The osteotomy is fixed with a percutaneous 0.045 inch Kirschner (K-) wire. The K-wire is inserted lateral to the extensor hallucis longus tendon and is oriented obliquely from dorsodistal to plantar proximal (Fig. 1F). The K-wire is cut off and bent over

the skin. The resulting medial bony projection is resected with the microsagittal saw (Fig. 1F). The cut surface is smoothed with a rasp.

While holding the hallux in slight overcorrection of varus and plantar flexion, the capsule is closed with a horizontal mattress tension suture of 2-0 Vicryl (Fig. 1G). The remainder of the capsule is closed with interrupted simple 2-0 Vicryl sutures. The skin is closed with a running subcuticular suture of 3-0 Prolene (Fig. 1H).

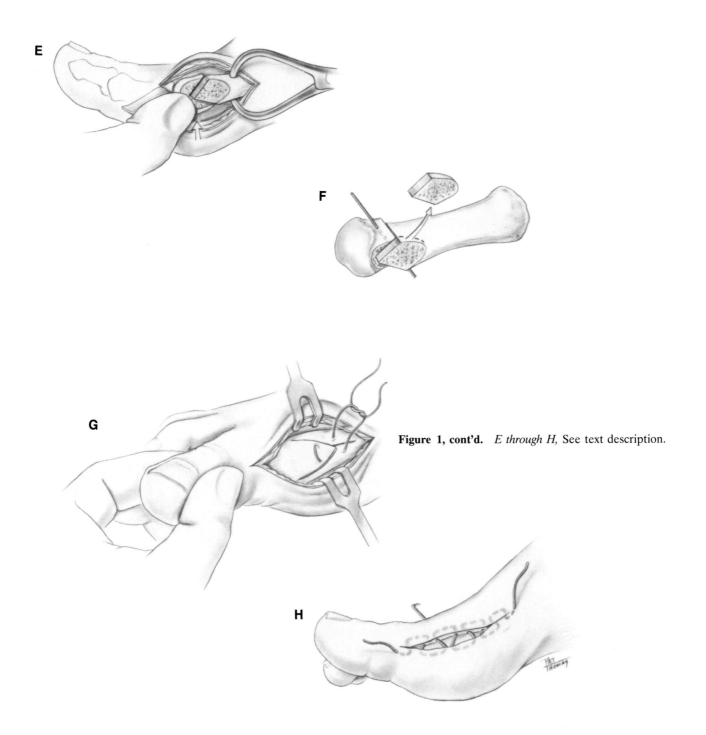

Figure 1, cont'd. *E through H,* See text description.

POSTOPERATIVE COURSE

A sterile dressing and soft compression dressing are applied for 48 hours. This dressing then is changed and replaced with a short-leg walking cast for 3 weeks, at which time the cast is taken off and the sutures and percutaneous pin are removed. A smaller dressing is applied, and the patient is allowed to ambulate in a stiff-soled postoperative shoe. At 6 weeks after surgery, the patient is allowed a slow, gradual, progressive return to weight-bearing activities and shoe wear within limits of discomfort.

TECHNICAL PITFALLS

It is recommended that soft tissue stripping be minimized to prevent avascular necrosis of the first metatarsal head. Excessive resection of the prominent medial eminence may lead to postoperative instability of the first MP joint. Prevent injury to the articular surface of the MP joint. Metatarsal osteotomy at an angle of greater than 60° is associated with osseous instability. If the apex of the osteotomy is made too far distal, the structural integrity of the metatarsal head may be jeopardized. If the osteotomy is positioned too far proximal, and is located in the diaphyseal bone, impairment of osseous union may result. The osteotomy must be made parallel in the medial-lateral plane.

COMPLICATIONS AND THEIR TREATMENT

Nonunion of the osteotomy may be associated with excessive soft tissue stripping to expose the first metatarsal head. Nonunion also may occur if the osteotomy is positioned too far proximal in an area of diaphyseal bone. Treatment of nonunion may include prolonged cast immobilization and non–weight bearing until osseous union is identified on radiographs. Persistent symptomatic nonunion may require open reduction and internal fixation using cancellous bone graft.

Avascular necrosis of the metatarsal head may be associated with excessive soft tissue stripping, particularly on the dorsal and lateral aspects of the first metatarsal head. This disorder may be associated with cystic erosion and collapse of the metatarsal head, with subsequent articular incongruity and degenerative arthritis. Nonoperative treatment includes the use of antiarthritic medication as well as shoe modifications. The use of a lightweight rubber-soled shoe with a wedge-shaped configuration may decrease the impact loading during the stance phase of gait. The addition of a ¼ inch tapered inflexible rocker sole to the outer sole of the shoe may decrease the painful grinding of the incongruous articular surface during toe-off. If conservative measures fail to provide relief, surgical intervention may require arthrodesis of the first MP joint.

Recurrence of deformity is a well-known problem associated with this procedure. Patients should be told to wear appropriate footwear even after surgery. Shoes with high heels or a narrow pointed toe box will most likely lead to recurrence of deformity with time. Even if some degree of hallux valgus occurs, most patients are asymptomatic. If symptoms do occur, and conservative modalities of treatment fail, other surgical procedures may be considered. If metatarsus primus varus is a major factor, proximal osteotomy may be required. If recurrent hallux valgus occurs without metatarsus primus varus, an Akin-type osteotomy at the base of the proximal phalanx may be indicated.

Late degenerative changes at the first MP joint leading to recurrent symptoms may require resection arthroplasty or arthrodesis of that joint, depending on the age and activity level of the patient.

SUGGESTED READING

Hattrup SJ, Johnson KA. Chevron osteotomy: Analysis of factors in patient's dissatisfaction. Foot and Ankle 1985; 5:327–332.

Johnson KA. Chevron osteotomy of the first metatarsal: Patient selection and technique. Contemporary Orthopaedics 1981; 3:707–711.

Johnson KA, Cofield RH, Morrey BF. Chevron osteotomy for hallux valgus. Clinical Orthopaedics 1979; 142:44–47.

HALLUX VALGUS CORRECTION USING THE DISTAL SOFT TISSUE PROCEDURE AND PROXIMAL CRESCENTIC OSTEOTOMY

ROGER A. MANN, M.D.

This versatile procedure can be used in patients with a wide range of hallux valgus deformity. The main indication is moderate-to-severe hallux valgus deformity with a subluxed metatarsophalangeal (MP) joint.

It is my belief that a proximal crescentic osteotomy is indicated when a fixed intermetatarsal angle is present that cannot be corrected by releasing the soft tissues about the MP joint, and a fair degree of rigidity exists between the first and second metatarsals at the time of surgery. The patient's age is not thought to be a significant consideration in using this procedure. In the juvenile patient, it is imperative that the osteotomy is performed distal to the epiphyseal plate. The procedure has been used in patients into the eighth decade with a satisfactory clinical result.

The contraindications to the procedure consist of the following:

1. A congruent MP joint
2. The presence of significant arthrosis
3. A distal metatarsal articular angle greater than 15°
4. Spasticity of any type, whether it is secondary to a head injury, stroke, or cerebral palsy

SURGICAL TECHNIQUE (FIG. 1)

Lateral Capsular Release

The initial skin incision is made in the first dorsal web space and is carried down through subcutaneous tissue and fat, staying in the midline. By blunt dissection the soft tissue of the interspace is pushed aside, and a Weitlaner retractor is inserted between the first and second metatarsal heads. The adductor tendon is identified as it inserts into the lateral aspect of the sesamoid and base of the proximal phalanx and is released from its lateral capsular attachment along the side of the metatarsal. The release of the adductor tendon then is extended distally to remove it from the base of the proximal phalanx. Once this is achieved, the tendon is removed from the lateral aspect of the fibular sesamoid back to the junction of the fleshy portion of the adductor hallucis and flexor hallucis brevis muscles. The Weitlaner retractor now is reinserted at a deeper level,

placing the transverse metatarsal ligament on stretch. The transverse metatarsal ligament then is sectioned, using the tip of the knife blade. One must be cautious here, because the nerve and vessel to the first web space are present just beneath the ligament. Finally, the lateral joint capsule is perforated and torn by bringing the great toe into approximately 25° of varus, which completes the release of the lateral joint capsular structures.

Preparation of the Medial Aspect of the Metatarsophalangeal Joint

A longitudinal incision is made in the midline along the first MP joint. The incision begins at the midportion of the proximal phalanx and is brought about 1 cm proximal to the medial eminence. The incision is deepened down to the plane of the capsule.

Along the capsular plane, a full-thickness dorsal and volar flap are created. It is imperative as the flap is created that caution is taken to identify the dorsomedial cutaneous nerve so it can be retracted and protected. In the plantar flap, the dissection stops after the abductor hallucis tendon is identified. One must be cautious in the plantar flap that the plantar-medial cutaneous nerve to the great toe is not injured inadvertently.

A wedge of capsular tissue now is removed. The first incision starts 2 to 3 mm proximal to the base of the proximal phalanx and is carried full thickness through the joint capsule, perpendicular to the long axis of the metatarsal. A second incision is made parallel to this and 3 to 8 mm more proximal to it, depending on the degree of deformity present. Approximately a 5 mm wedge of capsular tissue usually is removed. After this wedge is created, it is V'd dorsally, ending about 1 cm medial to the extensor hallucis longus tendon. On the plantar aspect, the capsule is V'd down through the abductor hallucis tendon, stopping at the sesamoid. As this wedge of capsule is removed, the knife blade must be kept inside of the joint, so that as the tip of the knife proceeds plantarly through the abductor hallucis tendon, it strikes the sesamoid bone and does not inadvertently cut the plantar-medial cutaneous nerve to the great toe.

The exposure of the medial eminence now is facilitated by making an incision along the dorsomedial aspect of the metatarsal. A flap of capsular tissue now is created and brought back proximally and plantarward, exposing the medial eminence. The medial eminence is removed in line with the medial aspect of the metatarsal, starting approximately 1 to 2 mm medial to the sagittal sulcus. It is important, when taking off the medial eminence, that an excessive amount is not removed and an adequate medial buttress is left intact. Following the removal of the medial eminence, the edges are smoothed with a rongeur.

Decision Making Pertaining to Creation of a Proximal Crescentic Osteotomy

After release of the lateral joint capsule, preparation of the medial joint capsular tissue, and excision of

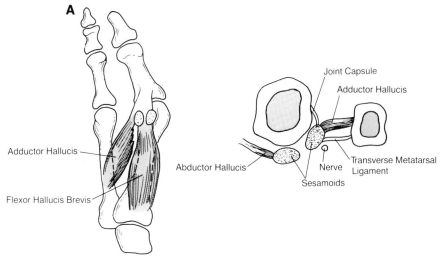

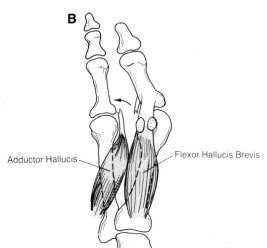

Figure 1 Distal soft tissue procedure. *A*, The adductor tendon inserts into the lateral aspect of the fibular sesamoid and into the base of the proximal phalanx. *B*, The adductor tendon has been removed from its insertion into the lateral side of the fibular sesamoid and base of the proximal phalanx. *C*, The transverse metatarsal ligament is noted to pass from the second metatarsal into the fibular sesamoid. *D*, The transverse metatarsal ligament has been transected. *E*, The three contracted structures on the lateral side of the metatarsophalangeal joint have been released. *F*, The medial capsular incision begins 2 to 3 mm proximal to the base of the proximal phalanx, and a flap of tissue measuring 3 to 8 mm is removed.

Continued.

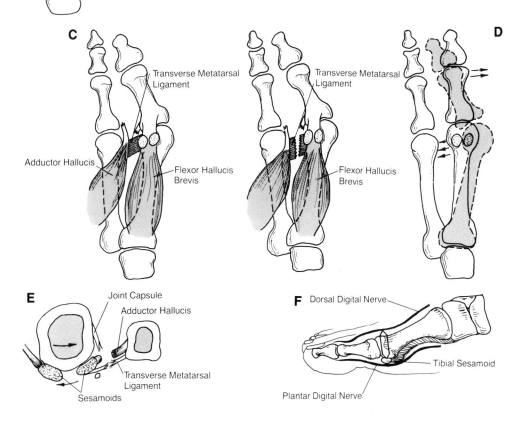

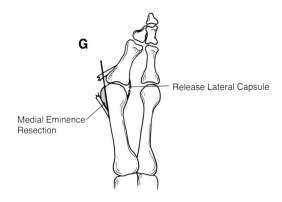

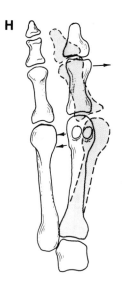

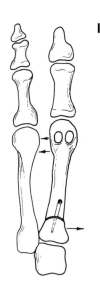

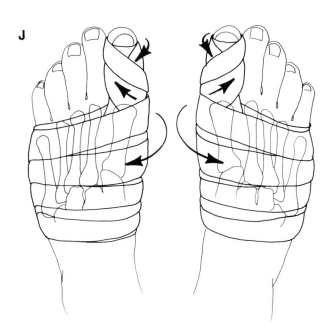

Figure 1, cont'd Distal soft tissue procedure. *G,* The medial eminence is removed in line with the medial aspect of the first metatarsal. *H,* To determine whether an osteotomy is necessary after the soft tissue release has been carried out, one pushes the first metatarsal head laterally. If there is any tendency for the metatarsal head to spring open, an osteotomy should be considered. We perform an osteotomy about 85 percent of the time. *I,* The osteotomy site is reduced by totally freeing the soft tissue about the osteotomy, then pushing the proximal fragment medially with a small Freer elevator, while pushing the metatarsal head laterally. This locks the lateral side of the osteotomy site so the internal fixation can be inserted. *J,* The postoperative dressings are critical. Note that the metatarsal heads are firmly bound with the gauze, and that the great toe is rotated so as to keep the sesamoids realigned beneath the metatarsal head. This necessitates dressing the right toe in a counterclockwise direction and the left great toe in a clockwise direction when one is standing at the foot of the bed. (Reprinted with permission from Mann RA, Coughlin MJ. Videotextbook of foot and ankle surgery. St. Louis: Medical Video Productions, 1991.)

the medial eminence, the first metatarsal head is pushed toward the second metatarsal. If there is any tendency for the first metatarsal to spring away from the second metatarsal, I believe this demonstrates a certain element of a fixed bony deformity, and as such, a proximal metatarsal osteotomy should be added to the distal soft tissue procedure. As a general rule, I carry out an osteotomy in about 85 to 90 percent of cases.

Technical Aspects of a Proximal Metatarsal Osteotomy

The incision to expose the proximal portion of the metatarsal is dorsal, starting at the level of the metatarsocuneiform joint and proceeding distally for a distance of about 3 cm. The extensor tendon is moved either medially or laterally, whichever is simplest. The metatarsocuneiform joint is identified with a knife blade,

following which the osteotomy site is selected about 1 cm distal to it, just distal to the flare at the base of the first metatarsal. A second mark is made about 1 cm distal to the osteotomy site if a screw is to be used for fixation. I prefer using a screw for fixation to avoid the problem associated with inflammation about an external pin.

If a screw is to be used for fixation, the drill hole is created in the metatarsal before creating the osteotomy. The glide hole is produced with a 3.2 mm drill bit, which is directed in the long axis of the first metatarsal and penetrates the bone only about 4 to 5 mm. It is important that one does not create a large hole that crosses the osteotomy site, because it makes it difficult to maintain adequate alignment of the osteotomy site after it has been reduced. A countersink is used to lower the profile of the screw head.

The osteotomy site is prepared using a crescentic-shaped blade, with the concavity of the cut directed toward the heel. As this cut is made, it is important that the saw exit the lateral aspect of the metatarsal. If a bone island is left along the medial side, this is cut easily with an osteotome following the creation of a crescentic osteotomy. If, however, the saw cut does not exit the lateral aspect of the metatarsal, the osteotomy site cannot be rotated—which is necessary to correct the intermetatarsal angle.

Once the osteotomy has been completed, it must be mobilized completely. This is checked by placing a Freer elevator into the drill hole and pushing against it, thereby assuring that all the periosteum and bone has been cut. If there appears to be a bony hinge, it should be released at this time.

Repair of the Hallux Valgus Deformity

Now that the lateral capsular tissue has been released, the medial joint capsule prepared, and the osteotomy created, it is time to repair the hallux valgus deformity. This is carried out by first placing sutures in the first web space, stabilizing the osteotomy site, and then plicating the medial capsular tissue.

Technical Aspects of the Repair

Three sutures are placed in the first web space between the first and second metatarsals incorporating the adductor tendon. In this manner the adductor tendon is brought off the plantar aspect of the foot and helps scar down the capsular tissue along the lateral aspect of first MP joint.

The osteotomy site now is reduced. This is carried out by placing a Freer elevator on the proximal portion of the metatarsal and displacing the fragment, and therefore the metatarsocuneiform joint, as far medially as possible. Stabilizing this basilar fragment, the distal portion of the metatarsal is brought around on it by applying pressure on the metatarsal head. In this way the osteotomy site is "rotated" around on itself along the curve. As this occurs, the first and second metatarsal heads are placed adjacent to one another. The common error that is made at this step of the procedure is that the basilar (proximal) fragment is not displaced medially, as the distal portion of the metatarsal is pushed laterally, to correct the intermetatarsal angle.

Holding the metatarsal in this corrected position, an assistant now places the sleeve guide (mushroom) into the drill hole, and the hole is redrilled using a 2.5 mm drill bit. In an older patient with soft bone, a 2 mm drill bit often is used. A 26 mm, fully threaded, 4.0 mm cancellous screw routinely is used. The drill hole is not measured routinely. The hole, however, is tapped and the screw inserted. As the screw is tightened, one must be cautious not to crack the small fragment between the drill hole and the osteotomy site.

If a problem is encountered at the time the screw is being placed, the fixation can be carried out by using multiple Kirschner wires. If the surgeon does this procedure without a trained assistant, the osteotomy site can be reduced and pins placed across the osteotomy

site, holding it in place, following which the surgeon can insert the screw.

An alternative method of fixation is to place an oblique 5/64 inch Steinmann pin across the osteotomy site. If this is done, it is important to predrill a hole with a 1/16 inch bit along the medial side of the metatarsal; using a trochar-tipped Steinmann pin prevents sliding out of the hole in the metatarsal shaft while trying to gain fixation.

The plication of the medial capsular tissue is carried out by holding the great toe in neutral position as far as extension and flexion are concerned. The pronation is corrected by rotating the great toe in such a way that the sesamoids are twisted back underneath the metatarsal head and the toe is held in about 2° to 3° of varus.

Four stitches are placed in the medial joint capsule, holding the great toe in alignment. If undercorrection has been achieved, one needs to remove the capsular sutures, excise more capsule, and repair it once again.

At the end of the procedure, the toe should be in satisfactory alignment, and if it is not, one needs to determine why.

POSTOPERATIVE MANAGEMENT

The initial dressing from the time of surgery is changed approximately 24 to 36 hours after the operation. The patient then is placed into a firm compression dressing consisting of a 2 inch Kling bandage and 1/2 inch adhesive tape. This dressing binds the metatarsal heads together, supporting the osteotomy site, and allows sufficient purchase on the great toe to keep it corrected for rotation and varus valgus.

The dressing is changed 1 week after surgery is carried out in conjunction with a radiograph taken as weight bearing as possible. This permits the surgeon to see the alignment of the MP joint and make any corrections with the dressing as necessary. The same type of dressing is applied on a weekly basis for a total of 8 weeks, until the osteotomy site is healed and the soft tissues have gained sufficient strength that the patient can ambulate safely without causing recurrence of the deformity.

Care Following Removal of the Dressings

After 8 weeks, patients are started on a vigorous course of range-of-motion exercises that they usually carry out on their own. The patient is encouraged to wear broad soft shoes or sandals. During the postoperative period, the patient is allowed to ambulate in a postoperative shoe.

SUGGESTED READING

Mann RA, Coughlin MJ. Videotextbook of foot and ankle surgery. St. Louis: Medical Video Productions, 1991.

Mann RA, Rudicel S, Graves SC. Repair of hallux valgus with distal soft tissue procedure and proximal metatarsal osteotomy. J Bone Joint 1992; 74A:124–129.

AKIN'S PHALANGEAL OSTEOTOMY FOR BUNION REPAIR

JAMES L. BESKIN, M.D.

In 1925 Akin published his technique for bunion repair. The procedure involved simple exostectomy and a medial closing-wedge osteotomy of the proximal phalanx for hallux valgus correction. The popularity of the Akin procedure has waxed and waned over the years; but with current modifications, it remains an important tool in bunion surgery.

Present use of the procedure as described by Akin is highly limited. As an isolated procedure, it is best used for angular deformities of the proximal phalanx such as hallux interphalangeus. Its use as the primary means to correct a bunion and hallux valgus deformity is restricted to those patients in whom there is no significant metatarsus varus, sesamoid subluxation, or hallux valgus deformity greater than 30°. In addition, the procedure is contraindicated in patients with significant incongruence or arthritic involvement of the metatarsophalangeal (MP) joint.

Despite these limitations, Akin's osteotomy can be a practical adjunct in other bunion operations. Specifically, when metatarsus varus and sesamoid subluxation are adequately corrected by metatarsal osteotomy, Akin's procedure offers improved correction of residual valgus, but more importantly pronation deformities of the hallux. Severe pronation is particularly difficult to correct despite correct metatarsal osteotomy and capsular closure. This may be important particularly in a patient with a laterally deviated articular surface of the distal metatarsal, in which full correction of the hallux valgus deformity by capsular repair would result in an incongruent joint (Fig. 1). Akin's osteotomy preserves the orientation of the distal metatarsal and basilar phalanx articular alignment, and improves cosmetic valgus correction through the osteotomy site. The procedure is also useful in elderly patients with symptomatic second toe deformity, but asymptomatic hallux

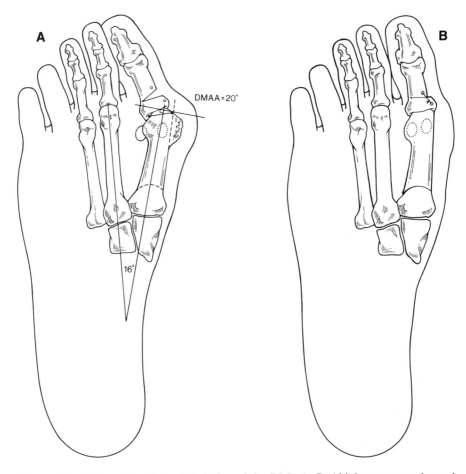

Figure 1 *A,* Example of lateral deviation of the DMAA. *B,* Akin's osteotomy is used to complete hallux valgus correction and to maintain joint congruency.

valgus and a painless bunion. Satisfactory repositioning of the second toe cannot be accomplished unless the hallux is moved out of the way.

PATIENT SELECTION

Considerations in patient selection for Akin's osteotomy should be similar to other bunion procedures. Patients should be good surgical candidates in whom conservative care for bunion symptoms has been unsatisfactory. As an isolated procedure, Akin's osteotomy should be limited to those patients with minimal metatarsal malalignment in whom a mild degree of hallux valgus correction is needed. Under these circumstances, Akin's procedure may be useful in a relatively asymptomatic first toe in which the valgus deformity of the first MP joint causes symptoms or deformity of the second toe.

The procedure most often is performed in combination with other bunion procedures. It has proven to be a useful adjunct to both distal and proximal metatarsal osteotomy techniques. However, it is important not to allow the anticipated correction with the Akin osteotomy to extend the normal indications for the primary bunion operation. Distal metatarsal osteotomies remain limited to those patients with intermetatarsal angles of less than 13° to 14°. Beyond this, a proximal osteotomy is preferable.

Other considerations in selecting the Akin procedure include the degree of hallux pronation associated with the bunion and valgus deformities. When phalangeal osteotomy is indicated, some of the residual rotatory deformity can be corrected at the time of valgus

correction. However, every effort should be made to correct this problem through reorientation of the sesamoid and capsular sling rather than through osteotomy of the proximal phalanx. Attention to the position of the sesamoids is important in Akin's osteotomy planning. Persistent lateral subluxation of the sesamoids may result in a "Z" deformity of the flexor alignment, which predisposes to recurrence of the valgus deformity.

Radiographs should be studied to evaluate the condition of the metatarsal phalangeal joint, as well as the distal metatarsal articular angle (DMAA) of the metatarsal. The DMAA is normally less than 10°. In severe hallux valgus deformity the congruent correction of valgus deviation of the proximal phalanx may be limited by a laterally deviated distal metatarsal articular angle. In patients with a greater than normal DMAA, Akin's osteotomy may be indicated to prevent inadvertent subluxation and resultant incongruency of the articular surfaces during hallux valgus correction. Radiographic review should give some indication of how much correction can be accomplished safely by capsulorrhaphy.

The phalangeal articular angle and degree of hallux valgus interphalangeus also may be determined by measuring the degrees of difference between a perpendicular line drawn among lines parallel to the phalangeal articular surfaces (Fig. 2). Akin's osteotomy corrects approximately 8° of valgus for each 2.5 to 3 mm of medial basilar wedge removed from the phalanx.

The decision to incorporate Akin's proximal phalanx osteotomy with the primary bunion procedure usually is best made at the time of surgery. At the conclusion of the routine bunion procedure, the surgeon can better appreciate whether a satisfactory degree of correction has been achieved. At this time the range of

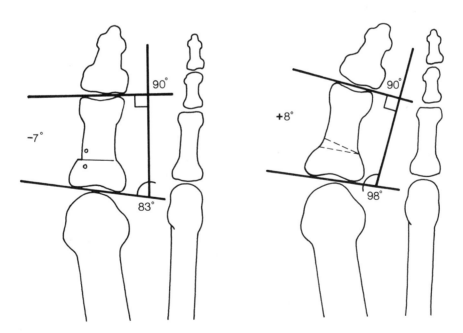

Figure 2 Measurement of the phalangeal articular angle to assess hallux valgus interphalangeus and amount of correction postoperatively.

motion of the MP joint in the corrected position is evaluated. If the joint's movement becomes limited as the alignment is corrected, or if the toe is predisposed to return to a valgus posture despite adequate release of the soft tissues, the joint may be incongruent at the corrected position. Correlation with radiographs and consideration of an Akin procedure are worthwhile under these circumstances.

SURGICAL TECHNIQUE

The procedure typically is performed in an outpatient setting with an ankle block anesthetic and an ankle tourniquet if the latter is believed to be advantageous. A medial longitudinal incision made at the junction of the plantar and dorsal skin is used to expose the medial exostosis and first MP joint. This incision can be readily extended distally at the conclusion of the primary bunion procedure if Akin's osteotomy is indicated.

It is best to wait until all the soft tissue releases and bony corrections have been made before determining the need for Akin's osteotomy. By gently pressing upward against the ball of the forefoot under the first metatarsal head, one can appreciate the degree of valgus orientation of the proximal phalanx relative to the metatarsal head during movement and weight bearing. It is important to determine if other deforming forces, such as the adductor tendon or the lateral capsule, are causing this deviation. In addition, one can compare the relative ease of range of motion of the first MP joint in its resting valgus position and the anticipated corrected position after a capsulorrhaphy. If the toe tends to remain in valgus and resists supple movement in the corrected position, consideration should be given to using Akin's osteotomy to maintain a congruent joint. Other preoperative factors, such as the degree of pronation and its correctability at the time of surgery and the metatarsal articular angle identified on preoperative radiographs, add to this clinical decision.

The Akin procedure is performed by extending the medial incision distally to expose the proximal one-half to two-thirds of the phalanx. The dissection is carried down to bone, and the flaps are elevated dorsally and plantarward with the scalpel and a Freer elevator. Care is taken to preserve the capsular attachments at the base of the proximal phalanx and to avoid stripping of the lateral periosteum, where the primary nutrient arteries to the proximal phalanx enter the bone.

A Freer elevator or small Hohman retractors are used to protect both the flexor and extensor tendons. The flexor tendon is particularly vulnerable near the base of the phalanx, where it is close to the cortical surface. The osteotomy site should be approximately 6 to 8 mm from the joint line located at the junction of the metaphysis and diaphysis. Appreciation of the concave surface of the base of the proximal phalanx prevents inadvertent involvement of the articular surface with the osteotomy. For this reason, the most proximal cut should be made first with attention directed to the orientation of the phalanx and articular surface. An assistant should hold the phalanx in a straight or neutral position to better orient the bone and to facilitate a straight cut relative to the articular surface of the phalanx. This also prevents an inadvertent dorsiflexion or plantar flexion angle of the osteotomy. A thin micro-oscillating saw blade is used to complete the first cut up to, but preferably not completely through, the lateral cortex. This "hinge" stabilizes the bone for the second cut and makes postoperative fixation more secure. The second and distal cut then is made to create a medial wedge that connects laterally with the first cut. It is best to err toward less rather than more bone removal until one assesses the degree of correction. Generally a 3 mm wedge is all that is needed and results in about 8° to 10° of correction. Further correction can be obtained by using the oscillating saw or rasp to remove a little more bone medially on either side of the osteotomy site. Care should be taken to keep the anterior-posterior orientation of the cuts in a vertical direction. Plantar deviation of the proximal phalanx may result in pressure problems at the distal phalanx and interphalangeal joint arthrosis.

Once satisfactory position of the Akin osteotomy site is achieved, some form of fixation is preferable. Options vary from soft tissue suturing to staples or pin fixation. My preference is to use sutures passed through bone. This is accomplished readily by using a 0.045 Kirschner (K-) wire as a drill, producing two sets of parallel holes medially on either side of the osteotomy site. It is helpful for the assistant to hold the toe in a corrected rotatory position to allow proper orientation and placement of the drill hole sites. This is particularly important when correcting pronation, since the holes are not aligned after the hallux is derotated. The K-wire is directed at approximately 45° to 60° to the perpendicular, producing 2 to 3 mm bone bridges on either side of the osteotomy site. The suture is passed through these holes using a UCL needle that is widely available with 2-0 absorbable monofilament PDS suture. This suture has a slight elasticity to it, and excellent compression of the osteotomy site is possible. The sutures are tied to oppose the osteotomy surfaces. This provides excellent fixation and assures maintenance of the corrected position.

Closure is carried out in conjunction with the remaining routine bunion procedure. Capsulorrhaphy is completed to align the toe in a congruent position. Radiographs are useful to confirm satisfactory osteotomy correction of the phalanx and metatarsal. There is little soft tissue over the proximal phalanx medially; however, a 3-0 absorbable suture may be used to approximate the soft tissues before skin closure. Postoperative care is similar to other bunion protocols. Patients are allowed to walk in a protective postoperative shoe with a bulky forefoot dressing that shifts weight posteriorly to the heel. Healing usually is sufficient by 3.5 to 4 weeks to allow active and some passive range of motion of the first MP joint. Radiographs usually are taken within the first week postoperatively and at the 6 week follow-up visit if there is persistent pain or concern about bone healing. The Akin osteotomy site usually is stable clinically within 4 to 6 weeks, but roentgenographic union sometimes is not observed for several months. A nonunion is rare and is reported to occur in less than 1 percent of cases.

SUGGESTED READING

Akin OF. The treatment of hallux valgus: A new operative approach and its results. Med Sentinel 1925; 33:678–679.

Frey C, Jahss M, Kummer FJ. The Akin procedure: An analysis of results. Foot Ankle 1991; 12:1–6.

Goldberg I, Bahar A, Yosipovitch Z. Late results after correction of hallux valgus deformity by basilar phalangeal osteotomy. J Bone Joint Surg 1987; 69A:64–67.

Mitchell LA, Baxter DE. A Chevron-Akin double osteotomy for correction of hallux valgus. Foot Ankle 1991; 12:17–14.

KELLER BUNIONECTOMY

E. GREER RICHARDSON, M.D.
STANLEY C. GRAVES, M.D.

The Keller bunionectomy is a resection hemiarthroplasty of the first metatarsophalangeal (MP) joint combined with removal of the medial eminence of the first metatarsal. The base of the proximal phalanx is removed to decompress the joint and to mobilize the hallux, which allows marked correction of valgus. However, the varus of the first metatarsal is not corrected, and maintaining correction of the valgus of the hallux is difficult. Other complications of the Keller procedure have been emphasized in the literature (with neither the incidence nor the severity of such complications clearly documented) to such an extent that the indications for this procedure have been limited severely. In our experience, however, complications are not frequent when patients are selected carefully. Modifications in the original technique also have allowed expansion of the indications for the Keller bunionectomy.

INDICATIONS

Candidates for the Keller procedure are patients between 55 and 70 years of age with moderate-to-severe hallux valgus (30° to 45°), intermetatarsal angles of 13° or less indicating mild-to-moderate metatarsus primus varus, and pain over the medial eminence with any shoe wear so that variety of shoe wear is severely limited. An incongruous first MP joint caused by lateral subluxation of the phalanx on the metatarsal head, severe lateral displacement of the sesamoids, and any evidence of degenerative cartilage changes in the joint are all radiographic indications for the Keller bunionectomy.

Two modifications in technique, however, can expand these indications to include patients with more severe deformities (Fig. 1), but not to include younger patients; this remains a procedure for mature adults. Patients with 50° or more of valgus of the hallux, 18° to 20° of varus of the first metatarsal, complete lateral dislocation of the sesamoids, marked degenerative changes, and severe pronation of the hallux may benefit substantially both functionally and cosmetically by altering the standard technique.

STANDARD TECHNIQUE

Use of an Esmarch wrap tourniquet is recommended if pedal pulses are good. A forefoot block using 1 percent lidocaine (Xylocaine) and 0.5 percent bupivacaine (Marcaine) in equal proportions within standard dose limits is used. A straight medial incision is begun 1 cm proximal to the interphalangeal joint of the hallux and extended proximally to the junction of the proximal and middle thirds of the first metatarsal. This lengthy incision is suggested to avoid excessive traction tension on the skin in these often elderly patients. The most medial branch of the superficial peroneal nerve is located by blunt dissection at the proximal-dorsal edge of the medial eminence and displaced from harm's way. The incision is taken to the first metatarsal in the midline medially, beginning in the proximal limit of the wound and extending distally across the midline of the medial eminence and along the proximal phalanx to the distal extremity of the wound. The first metatarsal is not exposed over the entire proximal limits of the incision. That portion of the incision, as emphasized earlier, is to avoid excessive tension on the skin during traction for exposure. The deep flap of tissue is raised by sharp dissection dorsally, beginning 1 cm proximal to the medial eminence. The periosteum and capsule are raised dorsally up to one-third to one-half the width of the metatarsal. At the joint the capsular elevation is continued, along with the extensor hallucis brevis insertion, until the proximal third of the proximal phalanx is exposed as far laterally as possible under direct vision. Having an assistant pronate the hallux as the dissection proceeds laterally makes exposure easier. Subperiosteal dissection should expose *only* that portion of the proximal phalanx that is to be removed.

The plantar dissection is just enough to expose the plantar aspect of the medial eminence proximally, the tibial sesamoid in the center of the wound, and the plantar-medial corner of the proximal phalanx. By supinating the proximal phalanx, the plantar corner and proximal third of the shaft are better exposed for the sharp dissection. Then by blunt dissection, the flexor hallucis longus tendon is identified for later retraction plantarward with a small right-angle retractor.

The medial eminence is resected at the sagittal groove, beginning dorsally at its distal edge and directing the 9 mm oscillating blade (or osteotome) plantarward and slightly medially (5° to 10°). Next the base of the proximal phalanx is removed at the metaphyseal-diaphyseal junction, which usually constitutes about the proximal third of the phalanx. Placing a retractor over the bone dorsally and plantarward and rotating the phalanx into view prevents damage to the flexor hallucis longus and the neurovascular bundles. Once the osteotomy has been completed, the basilar fragment is grasped with a small Kocher clamp or towel clip and is rotated while a medial pull is applied to lift it away from its lateral attachments, which are primarily the lateral collateral ligaments and adductor muscle tendinous insertion.

The hallux is brought into a corrected position while the foot is rotated straight up for a preliminary inspection. While the hallux is grasped in one hand and the proximal phalanx remnant is displaced medially, two longitudinal 0.062 inch Kirschner (K-) wires are inserted. The interphalangeal joint must be held straight while the wires are drilled from proximal to distal, emerging a few millimeters plantar to the nail plate. The

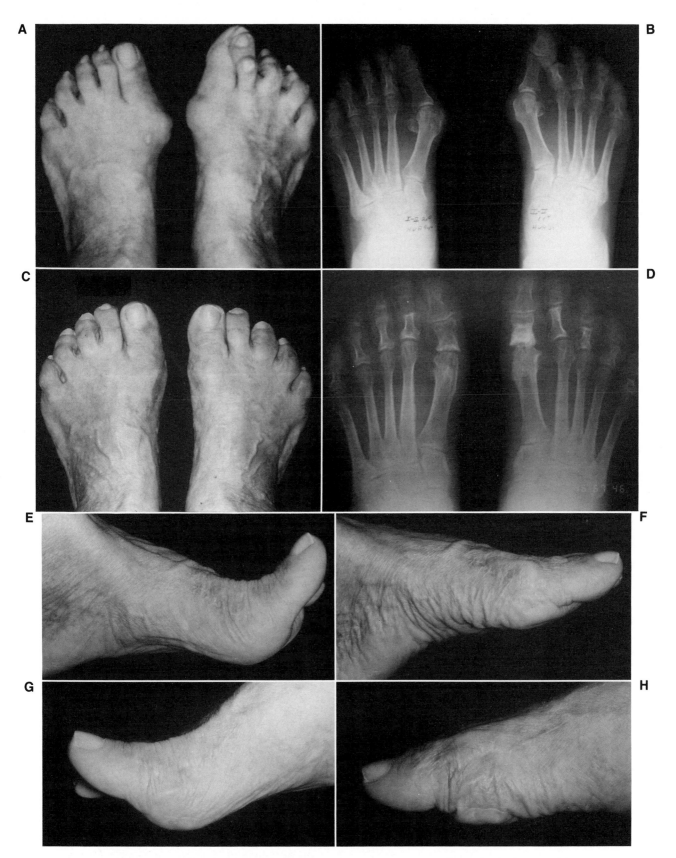

Figure 1 *A* and *B*, Preoperative weight-bearing photograph and radiograph of a 66-year-old female with severe bilateral hallux valgus and varus of the first metatarsal. *C* and *D*, Postoperative weight-bearing photograph and radiograph 1 year after surgery. *E, F, G,* and *H*, Ranges of motion of hallux 1 year after surgery.

foot is returned to the straight-up position, and the wires are drilled through the metatarsal head and out the plantar cortex proximal to the head. The wires should penetrate only 2 to 3 mm past the cortex to avoid tenderness over the pins with weight bearing.

If the K-wires tend to "walk" on the rounded articular surface of the metatarsal head, a small hemostat snugged up against the pin while it is being drilled allows accurate placement. Proper placement of the wires and the desired position of the hallux on the metatarsal may require several attempts. The medial aspect of the proximal phalanx should not rest medial to the medial aspect of the metatarsal head. The hallux is placed straight up in the neutral medial-lateral plane and in 10° of extension. Most of the initial length of the hallux is maintained by the pins. Later collapse occurs once the pins are removed, but improved encapsulation of the hemiarthroplasty by maintaining length for the first few weeks may help maintain a more desirable position long-term. The pins are cut off 2 to 3 mm distal to the skin edge.

The Esmarch wrap tourniquet (if used) is removed, hemostasis is secured, and the capsule is closed with interrupted 2-0 absorbable sutures. A firm, complete capsular closure is imperative. The first stitch should be made distally in the form of a box stitch. Using a swedged needle grasped with a needle driver, the curve of the needle can be increased by bending it manually. Starting plantarward the capsular-periosteal remnant is grasped at the medial aspect of the phalangeal remnant. The needle is passed from outside in and then is moved dorsally for the second pass inside out through any substantive tissue (excluding tendons and nerves) on the dorsal-medial aspect of the phalangeal base. Over the middorsum of the metatarsal head, the needle is passed from outside in through the capsule. If this capsule is redundant, a small amount may be removed, but it is better to leave too much than to remove too much. The final pass is from inside out through the plantar limit of the capsule in line with the dorsal capsular pass. An assistant grasps the ends of the capsule, pulling them together, while the tie is completed. Interrupted sutures are interspersed as needed to complete a firm closure. The skin is closed with nonabsorbable 4-0 sutures, with or without a few interrupted subcutaneous absorbable 4-0 sutures. A compression forefoot dressing is applied, extending just distal to the tarsonavicular tuberosity so that only the toenails are exposed and no loose edges of gauze are raised above the dressing. A snug but nonconstricting, layered, contoured forefoot dressing is vital to reduce edema. The tips of the pins are covered with circular adhesive bandages or commercially available pin balls.

POSTOPERATIVE CARE

A wood-soled shoe is worn and weight bearing is allowed to tolerance, with or without the assistance of crutches or a walker. Bathroom privileges only are allowed in the first 72 hours. The foot is elevated 24 to 36 inches higher than the heart except during meals and bathroom visits. After this period the patient may be up and about as symptoms allow. Taking more pain medication to allow increased activity is discouraged. For 7 to 10 days after surgery, the foot should be propped up when the patient is sitting.

The dressing is changed between 14 and 21 days, and the pins remain in place for 21 to 28 days. If the hallux migrates proximally on the pins, the tips are cut, again 1 to 2 mm distal to the skin edge. Using a medium-sized needle holder longitudinally over the tips of the pins to rotate the pin back and forth gently and to pull with gentle traction allows pin removal without undue discomfort. The foot is elevated for 5 minutes after the pins are removed to prevent excessive bleeding. A good method for elevation is to have the patient be supine with the unoperated knee flexed 90° and the foot flat on the table, and then to place the ankle of the operated foot on the flexed knee. If surgery was performed on both feet, several pillows or a low stool with pillows is required.

A small or medium-sized commercially available toe spacer is worn in the first web for an additional 2 to 3 weeks; this spacer is removed only for bathing. A wide soft shoe is allowed once the pins are removed. Dress footwear is allowed only after most of the edema has resolved, which may take 3 to 4 months.

The expected results are a reasonably well-aligned hallux with 40° to 50° of motion at the MP joint, relief of pain, some improvement in the variety of shoe wear, and a satisfied patient.

MODIFICATIONS OF TECHNIQUE

The following modifications of technique may improve the likelihood of good results and can expand the indications for use with more severe deformities.

Removal of the Fibular Sesamoid

Once the medial eminence and phalangeal base have been excised, the fibular sesamoid is removed as follows. A sturdy two-toothed retractor is placed beneath the metatarsal head, and an assistant lifts it dorsally. Using a Freer elevator, the fibular sesamoid is mobilized. In elderly patients with significant deformity and adherence of the sesamoid to the metatarsal head, this may be difficult. Occasionally a thin, 10 mm wide osteotome is needed. Lifting the metatarsal dorsally for exposure is essential. Once the sesamoid is free and mobile, the flexor hallucis tendon can be identified by flexion and traction on the hallux. The tendon is visible just distal to and in alignment with the sesamoids, which straddle it. Once the flexor hallucis longus is identified, the lateral neurovascular bundle just lateral to the tendon is exposed by blunt dissection. The bundle is retracted out of harm's way, and the intersesamoid ligament is incised longitudinally, with one arm of the scissors under the ligament and on the dorsal side of the flexor hallucis longus and the other arm dorsal to the ligament.

The sesamoid is grasped firmly, the toe is flexed to relax the flexor hallucis longus tendon, and the lateral sesamoid is pulled distally and medially. With the flexor hallucis longus tendon and the lateral neurovascular bundle protected, the attachment of the lateral head of the flexor hallucis brevis is severed sharply. The sesamoid now is detached medially and proximally. Removal is completed by incising the lateral capsular attachments. The flexor hallucis longus and neurovascular bundle are inspected and the pins are placed in standard fashion into the hallux, but not yet into the metatarsal.

Lateral Displacement of the First Metatarsal

The first metatarsal is mobilized by pushing it laterally several times. Occasionally this does not move the metatarsal at all, but some lateral mobiiity usually is present. While standing at the knee side of the foot and looking distally as the patient would view the foot, the surgeon holds the first metatarsal firmly and moves its distal end laterally. Holding the position with one hand, he uses the other hand to place the hallux end on the metatarsal head and out to length. While the first ray is held straight with the foot vertical, an assistant inserts the wires from distal to proximal. Often these wires running through the first metatarsal and hallux hold the first ray surprisingly straight. What is more surprising is that most of this correction is maintained after the wires are removed. The capsular closure is performed as described.

Presumably the laterally displaced fibular sesamoid, when pulled proximally by the relaxed flexor hallucis brevis lateral head, pulls the flexor hallucis longus laterally through the sesamoid apparatus, which encases it and thereby contributes to recurrent valgus and resultant varus of the first metatarsal. In addition, while reoperating a failed Keller procedure, we have seen a strong, linear, fibrous attachment of the fibular sesamoid to the proximal phalangeal remnant (Fig. 2). This, too, pulled the hallux into valgus when tension was applied to it. Whatever the reason, the hallux and first metatarsal maintain better alignment if these two steps are added when the deformity is severe: excision of the fibular sesamoid and displacement of the metatarsal laterally toward the second metatarsal while the pins are drilled across the "joint."

COMPLICATIONS

Cock-up Hallux

Complications of the Keller procedure have been related to the intrinsic muscle attachments to the phalangeal base. Without the intrinsic muscles flexing the hallux, an extension deformity or contracture may

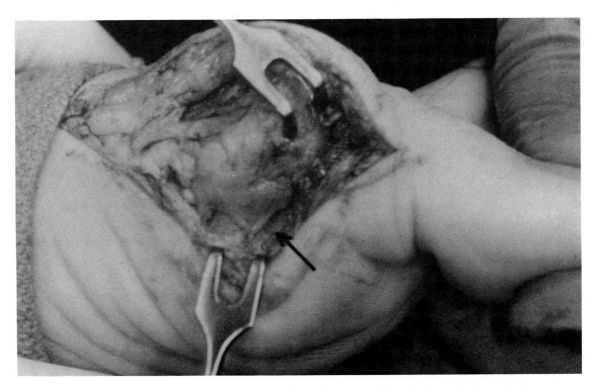

Figure 2 Firm fibrous band connecting the fibular sesamoid to the base of the proximal phalanx *(arrow)*. Traction on the band pulled the hallux into valgus. Removing the fibular sesamoid and holding the hallux straight for 4 weeks improved the result.

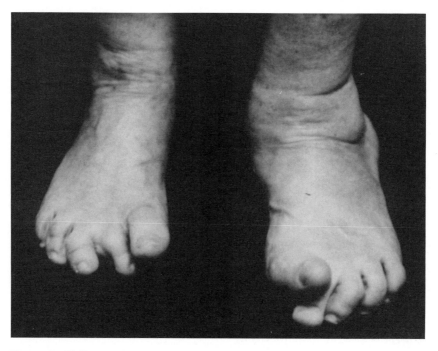

Figure 3 Hallux extensus on the right foot; hallux extensus and recurrent valgus on the left foot. These complications should be preventable when suggested techniques are used.

develop at the first MP joint with a concomitant flexion deformity at the interphalangeal joint. If a callus develops at the dorsum of the interphalangeal joint of the hallux, this is best treated by arthrodesis of the joint, lengthening of the extensor hallucis longus, and extensive dorsal capsulotomy. The corrected position must be maintained with K-wires for 6 weeks, and a short-leg walking cast extending distal to the toes is recommended during this time.

The severity of the cock-up hallux deformity and the shortening of the hallux, or a combination of deformities (Fig. 3), may require an interposition corticocancellous bone graft for correction of the deformity. This is a most tedious procedure with a long recuperative period, and failure of the arthrodesis to unite is not uncommon.

Metatarsalgia

Metatarsalgia present before surgery may be exacerbated by the Keller procedure. Because of unloading of the medial column by extreme varus of the first metatarsal, painful callosities may develop beneath one or more metatarsal heads. Realigning the first ray should increase its work load and reduce the lesser metatarsal load. We have found this to be true more often than the reverse; however, some workers have listed transfer metatarsalgia as a complication of the Keller bunionectomy. We tell our patients that the pain beneath the lesser metatarsal heads may not improve after the Keller procedure and possibly could worsen, but that has not been our experience.

Stress Fractures of the Lesser Metatarsal

Uncommonly, stress fractures may occur in the second, the third, or rarely the fourth metatarsal. The patient in whom this occurs usually is a postmenopausal female. Attempting to reduce weight on the first ray may overload the lesser metatarsals and cause a stress fracture. Protected weight bearing, a wood-soled shoe, or even skillful neglect usually is sufficient to relieve symptoms within 3 to 4 weeks. Occasionally, however, a stress fracture angulates, so some sort of protection is preferable.

SUGGESTED READING

Cleveland M, Winant EM. An end-result study of the Keller operation. J Bone Joint Surg 1950; 32(A):163.

Coughlin MJ, Mann RA. Arthrodesis of the first metatarsophalangeal joint as a salvage for the failed Keller procedure. J Bone Joint Surg 1987; 69(A):68.

Dhanendran M, Pollard J, Hutton W. Mechanics of the hallux valgus foot and the effect of Keller's operation. Acta Orthop Scand 1980; 51:1007.

Keller W. The surgical treatment for bunions and hallux valgus. N Y Med J 1904; 80:741.

Love TR, Whynot AA, Farine I, et al. Keller arthroplasty: A prospective review. Foot Ankle 1987; 8:46.

METATARSOCUNEIFORM ARTHRODESIS FOR HALLUX VALGUS AND METATARSUS PRIMUS VARUS

MARK MYERSON, M.D.

Paul Lapidus popularized the closing-wedge arthrodesis of the first metatarsocuneiform joint for the correction of hallux valgus associated with metatarsus primus varus. The premise of this operation is based on atavism and metatarsus primus varus in the development of hallux valgus, as well as the orientation of the metatarsocuneiform joint, which has changed from one facing medially in the primate foot to one directed more anteriorly in humans. Nevertheless, even in the human the plane of the first metatarsocuneiform joint is not necessarily perpendicular to the long axis of the foot and is angulated slightly medially. This type of foot probably never developed fully, retaining some of the features normally present in lower primates. The metatarsocuneiform arthrodesis for management of hallux valgus associated with metatarsus primus varus evolved accordingly.

In addition to the benefit of stabilizing the metatarsocuneiform articulation, the arthrodesis is performed at the apex of the deformity. Of course, the more proximally realignment is performed along the metatarsal, the greater the potential correction. This simultaneously stabilizes the articulation and prevents recurrent deformity. Metatarsus primus varus often is associated with a hypermobile first ray, characterized by an increased mobility of the metatarsal in both the horizontal and sagittal planes. In the sagittal plane, this excessive mobility is characterized by dorsal elevation or by dorsal prominence of the first metatarsal. Hindfoot valgus, midfoot and forefoot pronation, and hallux valgus with transfer to the second metatarsal and second metatarsal overload also may be associated with this hypermobility. This is easily visible radiographically, with increased cortical hypertrophy along the medial border of the second metatarsal shaft. Callosity under the second metatarsal head also may be present. The instability at the metatarsocuneiform joint usually is multiplanar, and although this usually is an isolated finding in the foot, it often is associated with generalized ligamentous laxity. Although it is easy to demonstrate this excessive motion clinically, neither concepts of hypermobility of the first ray nor what constitutes abnormal motion is defined clearly.

PREOPERATIVE ASSESSMENT

In addition to parameters such as the size, shape, and function of the foot, the range of motion of the entire foot and ankle as well as the medial longitudinal arch in weight bearing are assessed. Hypermobility of the first ray is evaluated by grasping the patient's right foot with the examiner's left hand and then manipulating the first metatarsal with the right thumb and forefinger. Particular attention is paid to the increased arc of motion in the dorsal direction, because this excess causes loss of stability of the medial border of the foot in weight bearing.

Weight-bearing radiographs should be obtained. Measurements of the first-second intermetatarsal angle, the first metatarsocuneiform and hallux valgus angles, and the metatarsus adductus are obtained. The lengths of the first and second metatarsals and the congruity of the hallux metatarsophalangeal (MP) joint are noted. The indications for this operation are as follows:

1. Severe metatarsus primus varus
2. Hypermobility of the first ray
3. Generalized ligamentous laxity
4. Metatarsocuneiform arthritis
5. The adolescent bunion with moderate-to-severe deformity associated with hypermobility
6. Selected cases of revision surgery for failed bunionectomy

Contraindications to this operation are as follows:

1. A short first metatarsal
2. Moderate deformity in the absence of first ray hypermobility
3. If better alternatives to correction exist
4. In the adolescent with open epiphyses

The goals of this operation are to correct and stabilize the first metatarsal at the apex of the deformity, particularly in the presence of a hypermobile first ray. This operation is appropriate in the adolescent provided the physis is closed, particularly since recurrent deformity following adolescent bunionectomy is such a common problem. I have found that in some adolescents with a hypermobile first ray, the operative procedure can be accomplished with the closing-wedge arthrodesis without resecting the medial eminence or releasing the adductor tendon (Fig. 1). My results in adolescents have been stable over time, supporting the concept that the primary deforming force is at the metatarsocuneiform joint.

It is important that patients understand the nature of the operation, as well as the various alternatives to conservative and surgical care. This operation involves potential problems unique to the arthrodesis. Patients need to be aware of the potential for complications including prolonged recovery time, pseudoarthrosis, and malunion, particularly dorsal tilting of the metatarsal. I have found that these patients clearly have more discomfort and swelling postoperatively when compared with other similar procedures for severe hallux valgus and metatarsus primus varus. Problems with wound healing, incisional neuromas, and hardware removal are otherwise the same as for any bunion operation.

A

B

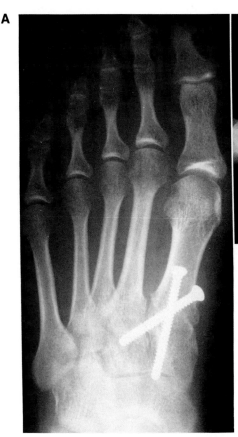

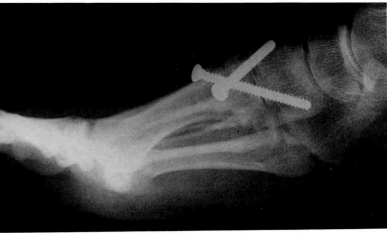

Figure 1 *A* and *B,* Complete correction of metatarsus primus varus in this adolescent was obtained at the metatarsocuneiform joint alone. A distal soft tissue release and exostectomy were not performed, and the alignment is well maintained.

SURGICAL TECHNIQUE

Bilateral procedures are not performed simultaneously. Surgery is performed with the patient under regional ankle block anesthetic. No tourniquet is used, and hemostasis is controlled and bleeding minimized with small hemostat clamps. A medial-longitudinal incision is made over the hallux MP joint at the junction of the dorsal and plantar skin. The capsular incision I prefer, and one I credit to Dr. Michael Coughlin, is L-shaped, with the apex dorsal and proximal (Fig. 2). The capsule is dissected subperiosteally off the metatarsal neck, exposing the entire medial eminence (Fig. 3). The advantage of this flap is the broad exposure of the medial eminence and later ease of capsular closure under the appropriate amount of tension, simultaneously controlling pronation of the hallux. If little or poor soft tissue is observed along the dorsal-medial aspect of the metatarsal neck to reattach the capsule, a small hole is made with a 0.062 Kirschner (K-) wire to attach the capsule.

A soft tissue release, including an adductor tenotomy with partial lateral capsulotomy, is performed through a separate dorsal incision over the distal first-second intermetatarsal space. In some adolescents with marked hypermobility of the first ray, the adductor release may not be necessary. I do not attempt to reattach the adductor to the metatarsal neck. Instead,

the adductor is freed up off the flexor brevis tendon, and an incision is made dorsal to the sesamoid, between it and the metatarsal head and neck. It is important to restore fully the sesamoid mechanism with this operation, which is possible provided the sesamoids are able to glide under the metatarsal head. Remember that the fibular sesamoid rotates vertically in the first web space associated with metatarsus primus varus and hallux valgus. Unless the sesamoid is freed completely from its scarred attachments in the web space, accurate repositioning of the sesamoid mechanism is not possible. If the deformity is severe, part of the lateral head of the flexor brevis tendon must be cut to relax the contracture. Following perforation of the lateral capsule with a #15 knife blade, the hallux is pushed passively over into varus to ensure smooth range of motion of the hallux in the corrected position.

A third incision is made proximally, medial to the extensor hallucis longus tendon to expose the metatarsocuneiform joint. In earlier descriptions of this procedure, I recommended using a saw to remove a biplanar wedge from the joint. The wedge was removed with the base lateral and plantar to ensure plantar flexion of the metatarsal. Despite the attempt to remove minimal articular surface to prevent shortening of the metatarsal, the articulation often was unstable and difficult to fuse. There also was a tendency to remove insufficient bone from the plantar-apical joint surface, and a thin rongeur

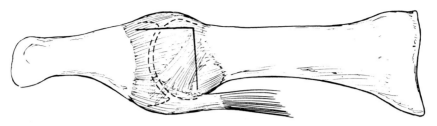

Figure 2 The capsular flap is an inverted L with the apex dorsal and proximal.

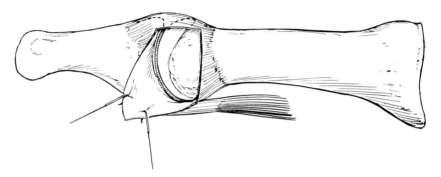

Figure 3 With the flap peeled, plantar and distal exposure of the medial eminence is easy. This flap either can be resutured or attached to the neck of the metatarsal with a drill hole.

was used to remove bone from the depths of the joint. Although this biplanar wedge resection still is probably integral to this operation, the key is to remove as little bone as possible. I often experienced difficulty with the fixation and was dissatisfied with the potential for shortening and malunion of the metatarsal. Recognizing the anatomic variations of the metatarsocuneiform joint and the base of the first metatarsal, I felt that a biplanar wedge resection of the joint as described previously was not necessary for all patients. I now believe that the metatarsal may be repositioned with little if any bone resection. Because of the concave-convex shape of the metatarsocuneiform articulation, this is accomplished easily with a more natural movement of adduction, plantar flexion, and slight internal rotation of the first metatarsal (Fig. 4). The articular cartilage only is removed lateral and plantar, leaving the medial aspect of the joint intact. It is important to plantarflex as well as adduct the first metatarsal; however, because of the anatomy of the joint this is not accomplished easily.

The articular surfaces of the metatarsocuneiform joint are not always flat, but occasionally saddle- or bean-shaped. Numerous configurations of the joint surface are encountered, some of which enhance and some of which block the repositioning of the metatarsal. Occasionally two separate facets are observed on the base of the metatarsal. The plane of this concavity is toward the second cuneiform, and the convexity faces medially. The base of the articular surface is extremely

deep and sometimes difficult to reach, even with a long curette.

When resecting any bone from this articulation, there is a tendency to remove insufficient bone from the deeper plantar base of the metatarsal and cuneiform. This can be accomplished only by careful repeated inspection and removal of the deeper part of the metatarsal with a long rongeur or thin chisel. An osteotome does not work well in this location because of the depth of the joint. A chisel blade has a single beveled edge, and a more precise cut of the metatarsal can be made by reversing the chisel so that the sharper edge cuts into the plantar base of the metatarsal.

As I stated earlier, however, the idea is to slide the metatarsal, not move it by too large a wedge resection from the joint. Care is taken not to overcorrect the first metatarsal, because a hallux varus deformity may result if a negative intermetatarsal angle is created. I emphasize this point, because it is easy to remove too large a wedge at the tarsometatarsal joint, producing varus instability (Fig. 5). The metatarsal is held in adduction and plantar flexion and secured with a K-wire for temporary fixation. Following radiographic evaluation, permanent fixation is performed using 3.5 mm cortical screws. The first screw is introduced dorsal to plantar from the medial cuneiform proximally into the first metatarsal distally, using a lag screw technique. When I introduced the screw from distal to proximal, there were too many problems associated with insertion of the

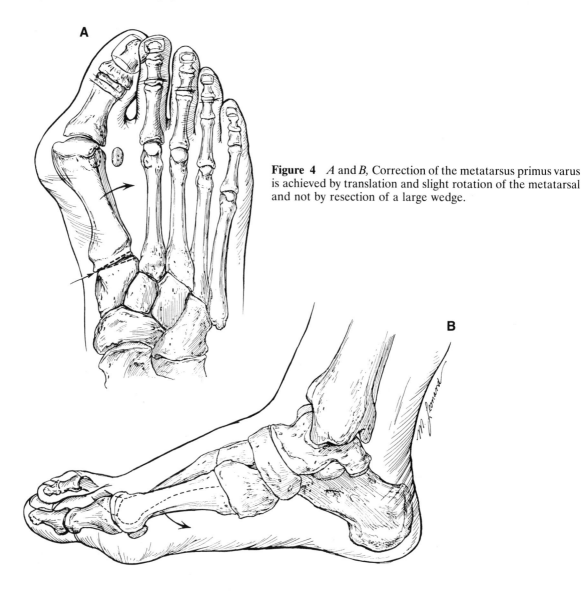

Figure 4 *A* and *B,* Correction of the metatarsus primus varus is achieved by translation and slight rotation of the metatarsal and not by resection of a large wedge.

screw, and I believe that this modification, which was brought to my attention by Dr. Kenneth Johnson, is far preferable. The second screw is introduced medially from the first metatarsal into the second metatarsal base from slightly plantar to dorsal, avoiding the middle cuneiform (Fig. 6). This second screw is not introduced with a lag technique and is used to control rotation of the joint only (Fig. 7). A burr is used to create two or three small troughs across the joint both dorsally and medially, and local bone graft is used to fill these defects.

Once the metatarsal has been stabilized, attention again is directed to the distal alignment. The congruity of the MP joint again is evaluated. If any potential for medial impingement and incongruity exists, the range of motion of the MP joint decreases in the corrected position. It then is preferable to leave the hallux in a slight valgus position and perform a closing-wedge osteotomy at the base of the proximal phalanx (Fig. 8). The hallux finally should rest in a neutral position and

closure made without relying on the capsulorrhaphy to straighten it. The capsulorrhaphy is performed as described earlier, using the L-shaped flap and attachment with a K-wire hole into the metatarsal neck if necessary.

Postoperatively, patients use crutches until comfortable followed by weight bearing as tolerated in either a short-leg cast or a stiff surgical shoe. If the patient is highly active, I recommend a cast. Generally the cast may be removed by the sixth week and progress to a surgical shoe until comfortable, usually a few more weeks. A soft bunion splint to maintain the hallux in neutral alignment at nighttime is used for another 4 weeks. At 8 to 10 weeks, patients are allowed to walk in a comfortable sneaker, and by 4 months shoe wear is unrestricted. Nevertheless, most patients find that the foot is still swollen at 3 months and are unable to return to the shoes they had worn preoperatively up until approximately 4 to 6 months. Some swelling, stiffness, and aching persist up

Figure 5 Good correction was achieved in this patient with slight shortening of the metatarsal. The screw position shown here is not ideal since the proximal-oblique screw crosses a partly mobile articulation.

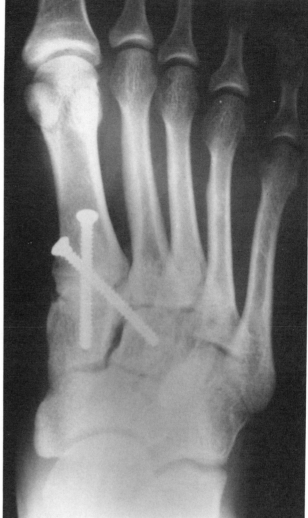

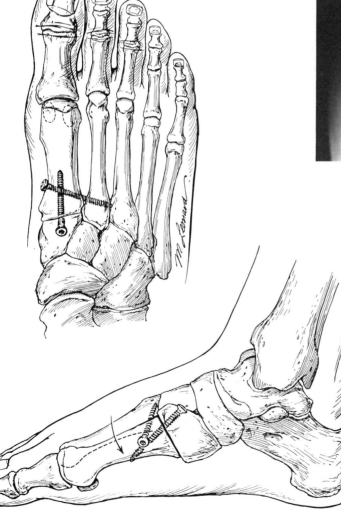

Figure 6 *A* and *B,* The screw position I prefer is illustrated. The metatarsocuneiform screw is inserted from proximal and dorsal to distal and plantar in a lag fashion. The medial derotation screw is inserted just dorsal to this screw in the midshaft of the first metatarsal and enters the second metatarsal. This need not be inserted in a lag fashion.

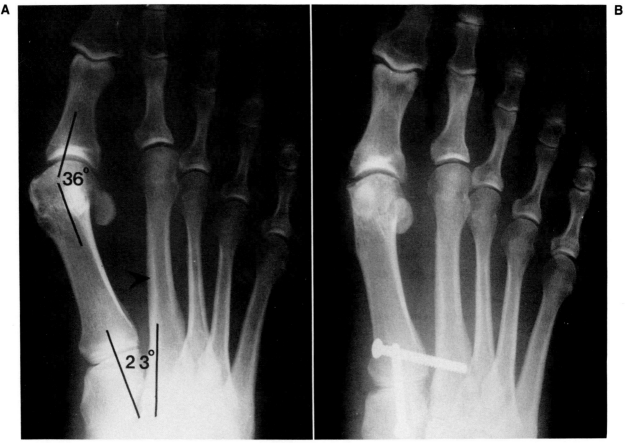

Figure 7 *A* and *B,* The screw fixation is illustrated (in this patient) with a 23° intermetatarsal angle (*A,* corrected postoperative to 9°; *B,* note hypertrophy of the medial shaft of the second metatarsal.)

to 6 months. During this rehabilitation phase, patients are encouraged to ambulate and obtain physical therapy to improve their activities of daily living.

COMPLICATIONS

Pseudoarthrosis, stiffness, and dorsal elevation of the first metatarsal definitely are potential problems with this procedure. Although nonunion is a problem, I have reduced the incidence of this problem over the past few years by different screw techniques and careful attention to immobilization postoperatively. Nonunion typically is associated with persistent swelling, aching, and intermittent pain. However, symptoms do not persist in all patients, and with further follow-up, most become asymptomatic. A dorsal bunion may develop in association with elevation and malunion of the first metatarsal. Although most are asymptomatic, decreased range of motion of the hallux MP joint may be present and is treated either with cheilectomy or revision of the arthrodesis.

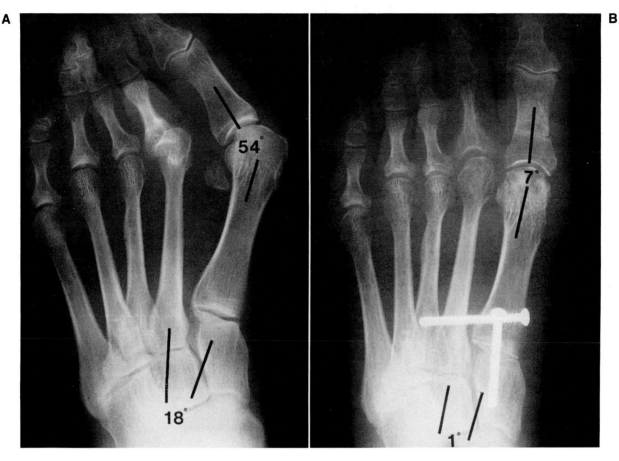

Figure 8 *A* and *B,* Correction in this patient was obtained with both the metatarsocuneiform arthrodesis and a closing-wedge osteotomy of the base of the proximal phalanx of the hallux to preserve motion at the MP joint.

SUGGESTED READING

Clarke HR, Veith RG, Hansen ST. Adolescent bunions treated by the modified Lapidus procedure. Bull Hosp Jt Dis 1987; 47:109–122.

Lapidus PW. The author's bunion operation from 1931 to 1959. Clin Orthop 1960; 16:119–135.

Lapidus PW. Discussion following McBride's paper. JAMA 1935; 105:1068.

Lapidus PW. The operative correction of the metatarsus varus primus in hallux valgus. Surg Gynecol Obstet 1934; 58:183–191.

Lapidus PW. A quarter of a century of experience with the operative correction of the metatarsus varus in hallux valgus. Bull Hosp Jt Dis 1956; 17:404–421.

Myerson MS. Metatarsocuneiform arthrodesis for treatment of hallux valgus and metatarsus primus varus. Orthopedics 1990; 13: 1025–1031.

Myerson MS, Allon S, McGarvey W. Metatarsocuneiform arthrodesis for treatment of hallux valgus. Foot Ankle 1992; 13:107–115.

HALLUX VARUS

MARK MYERSON, M.D.

Surgical management of hallux varus is determined by the magnitude of the deformity and the presence of degenerative changes of the metatarsophalangeal (MP) joint. The age and activity level of the patient and shoe wear requirements are taken into account in planning surgery.

The causes for hallux varus are as follows:

1. After bunionectomy:
   Excessive lateral soft tissue release
   Fibular sesamoidectomy
   Excessive medial capsulorrhaphy
   Overcorrection following a first metatarsal osteotomy (distal or proximal)
   Excessive resection of the medial eminence
   Malunion from a hallux phalangeal osteotomy
2. Inflammatory synovitis and arthritis
3. After trauma

In each of these conditions, the underlying etiology is addressed, and wherever possible the anatomy is restored. The exact treatment depends on the underlying cause of the varus deformity, but wherever possible attempt is made to restore the dynamic motion of the hallux at the MP joint. In most cases this can be achieved through a soft tissue corrective procedure. Where degenerative changes of the MP joint are present, an arthroplasty or arthrodesis procedure is preferred. For a younger, more active individual I prefer an arthrodesis. This stabilizes the joint and improves both push off and distribution of weight under the metatarsal heads and toes. For a more sedentary or elderly individual, a resection arthroplasty is an option. Somewhere in between is a doubled-stemmed implant arthroplasty. Although implant arthroplasty is not my preferred method of treatment, it is an option in a middle-aged sedentary individual. In both arthroplasty procedures, it is imperative to balance tension of the soft tissues on the lateral and medial aspects of the MP joint. One cannot expect to resect the joint and hope that the soft tissue imbalance corrects itself.

After resection arthroplasty (the Keller procedure), the hallux must rest in a neutral position. This may require division of the abductor hallucis tendon, complete medial capsular release, and lateral soft tissue plication with the attachment of the lateral head of the flexor brevis tendon. I secure the joint with temporary internal fixation using one or two threaded $7/64$ inch Steinmann pins for approximately 4 weeks to maintain the alignment.

In some severe and advanced cases of hallux varus, in addition to the medial deviation, the hallux is extended at the MP and flexed at the interphalangeal (IP) joints. This fixed flexion contracture is difficult to treat without an arthrodesis of the IP joint (Fig. 1). In some patients, once the hallux is realigned—whether by soft tissue correction, arthroplasty, or arthrodesis—this clawed hallux slowly corrects itself. This results from rebalancing the sesamoid apparatus under the metatarsal head.

In some instances I prefer to treat this with an arthrodesis of the IP joint and either a soft tissue corrective procedure or arthroplasty at the MP joint. I prefer not to end up with an arthrodesis of both the IP and MP joints, although these patients seem to do reasonably well despite the rigidity of the hallux.

SOFT TISSUE CORRECTION FOR HALLUX VARUS

This procedure is based on the description of hallux varus correction by Johnson in 1984, using the extensor hallucis longus tendon. The indications for this procedure are hallux varus, with no degenerative changes in the MP joint, and no incongruity of the MP joint after correction. The extensor hallucis longus tendon is split and passed underneath the deep transverse metatarsal ligament and through the base of the proximal phalanx to create a dynamic stabilizing effect at the MP joint. In the presence of a rigid flexed IP joint, the entire extensor hallucis longus tendon may be harvested and the soft tissue procedure combined with IP joint arthrodesis. It is important to balance the soft tissues correctly after this procedure and not to rely on the tendon transfer itself to pull the hallux into neutral. For this reason, adequate medial soft tissue release, including release of the capsule and abductor tendon, should be performed.

A longitudinal incision is made along the dorsolateral aspect of the extensor hallucis longus tendon (Fig. 2) or using a previous dorsal incision from the original bunionectomy. The procedure cannot be performed through a medial bunion incision. The incision is deepened through subcutaneous tissue, and the sheath of the extensor hallucis tendon opened. Care must be exercised to preserve the attachment of the extensor hallucis brevis tendon. Since the entire extensor hallucis longus tendon may be required, dysfunctional extension of the hallux occurs if the brevis tendon is disrupted. The soft tissues are dissected free on the medial aspect of the MP joint, preserving the dorsomedial cutaneous nerve. A vertical capsulotomy is made extending slightly plantarward so as to release the abductor hallucis tendon. At the completion of this capsular release, one should be able to push the hallux manually into a valgus position without undue resistance or tension.

The extensor hallucis longus now is used to function as a dynamic stabilizer to hold the hallux in this corrected position. On the lateral aspect of the MP joint, the soft tissues are dissected superficially into the first web space. The deep transverse metatarsal ligament is identified as is the adductor hallucis tendon, if still

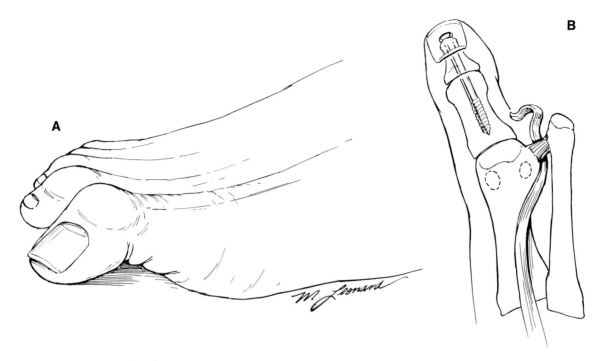

Figure 1 If a fixed IP joint contracture is present *(A)*, an arthrodesis is performed and the entire tendon may be used *(B)*.

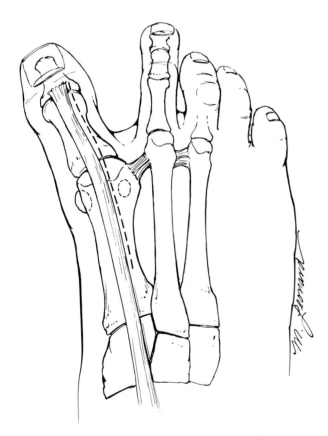

Figure 2 Hallux varus deformity. An anteroposterior view, noting the skin incision. Note the medial shift of the tibial sesamoid.

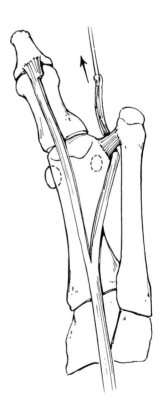

Figure 3 The extensor hallucis longus tendon is split longitudinally and passed under the deep transverse metatarsal ligament.

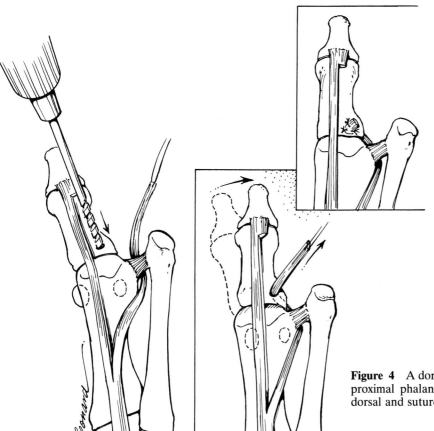

Figure 4 A dorsoplantar 3.2 mm drill hole is made in the proximal phalanx; the tendon is passed from plantar to dorsal and sutured to the capsule (inset).

present. The extensor hallucis longus tendon now is split longitudinally in half from its point of attachment at the distal phalanx and then proximally for a length of 4 inches. It is important to split the tendon for at least 2 inches proximal to the MP joint, otherwise excessive pull from the tendon transfer leads to weakness in dorsiflexion. The split tendon now is secured with a suture and then passed underneath the deep transverse metatarsal ligament (Fig. 3). A hemostat clamp can be passed from distal to proximal under this ligament and the suture grasped and then pulled distally. I find it helpful to insert a toothed lamina spreader into the first web space to facilitate exposure.

The base of the proximal phalanx now is exposed with subperiosteal dissection from lateral to medial. A 3.2 mm drill hole now is made from dorsal to plantar in the lateral half of the base of the proximal phalanx (Fig. 4). This should be made at the metaphyseal flare, approximately 6 mm from the articular surface.

The tendon now is passed from plantar to dorsal through the drill hole. It is best to pass this using a suture passer, making sure that the tendon does not bunch up at the plantar-lateral hole margin. The tendon should be appropriately tensioned before suturing it down. This is done with the ankle in the neutral position and mild tension placed on the tendon. It should pull the hallux into 5° to 10° of valgus. If the tendon is pulled too tightly, the remaining portion of the extensor hallucis longus, which is attached to the distal phalanx, becomes slack. If necessary, this can be addressed by inserting a weaving-type suture through the tendon to tighten it. The tendon is sutured back down onto the periosteal tissue of the dorsomedial aspect of the hallux and to the attachment of the extensor hallucis brevis tendon.

It is important to hold the hallux in the corrected position postoperatively. This can be done with a Kirschner (K-) wire introduced percutaneously across the MP joint for approximately 3 weeks. Alternatively the hallux should be bandaged and splinted into a neutral position for the first 6 to 8 weeks postoperatively. Patients are allowed to weight bear in a stiff surgical shoe to tolerance immediately postoperatively. At 4 weeks active and passive range-of-motion exercises are begun. The motion at the MP joint rarely is normal postoperatively, but usually is sufficient for functional activities.

The tendon transfer may not be required if the

hallux varus was caused by overplication of the medial capsulorrhaphy after bunionectomy. In these patients a simple release of the capsule and the abductor tendon is sufficient, with attention to bandaging and early motion postoperatively.

Hallux varus caused by an overcorrected metatarsal osteotomy is difficult to correct with this soft tissue procedure without revising the metatarsal osteotomy. This should be done at the apex of the deformity, whether or not this was a proximal or distal osteotomy. I use a dome saw introduced with the concave surface facing proximally and the cut made from dorsal to plantar at 90° with respect to the metataral shaft. The osteotomy is secured with two or three 0.045 inch K-wires. Careful attention to soft tissue balancing also is important with this procedure, and a medial soft tissue release with or without repair of the adductor complex also should be performed.

SUGGESTED READING

Jahss MH. Disorders of the hallux and the first ray. In: Jahss MH, ed. Disorders of the foot and ankle. 2nd ed. Philadelphia: WB Saunders, 1992.

Johnson KA, Spiegel PV. Extensor hallux longus transfer for hallux varus deformity. J Bone Joint Surg 1984; 66A:681–686.

HALLUX RIGIDUS: TREATMENT BY CHEILECTOMY

STANLEY C. GRAVES, M.D.

Hallux rigidus is a condition involving the first metatarsophalangeal (MP) joint that is characterized by diminished range of motion and degenerative arthritis. The condition first was described in 1887 by Davies-Colley and called hallux flexus. The term *hallux rigidus* was coined by Cotterill in 1888. Several other names used for this condition include metatarsus primus elevatus, dorsal bunion, and hallux equinus. Early arthritic changes and a mild limitation of motion occasionally are referred to as hallux limitus; however, the most commonly used term is hallux rigidus.

The etiology for hallux rigidus is unknown, but several authors have proposed theories. Nilsonne, Bonney, and McNab have suggested that a long first metatarsal is responsible for the development of hallux rigidus. Morton coined the term *index-plus foot,* in which the first metatarsal is longer than the second. Morton thought that this index-plus condition increased the pressure in the first MP joint, predisposing the patient to hallux rigidus. Dorsiflexion of the first metatarsal also has been suggested as a possible etiologic factor. If the first metatarsal is elevated, dorsiflexion may be limited and cause impingement dorsally on the metatarsal head and subsequent degenerative changes. Several case reports have noted previous trauma to the first MP joint, with possible contusion to the cartilage of the joint and later degenerative changes as a possible etiology. Some workers have implicated the metatarsal sesamoid articulation; however, in my experience this rarely is involved in hallux rigidus. Systemic arthritic processes and joint infections also must be considered.

CLINICAL EVALUATION

Patients present initially with complaints of pain and swelling around the MP joint and may have limited dorsiflexion as the condition progresses. Both dorsiflexion and plantarflexion often are painful. This pain is caused by impingement of the dorsal osteophytes during dorsiflexion and stretching of the capsule across the same osteophytes during plantarflexion. Some patients complain of tingling and numbness, particularly in the lateral aspect of the hallux. These sensory changes are caused by pressure on the dorsomedial cutaneous nerve by frequently present lateral osteophytes. Physical examination reveals various degrees of swelling around the first MP joint, and many patients have tenderness over the dorsal osteophyte. Patients also may have tenderness in the first web space secondary to a prominent exostosis on the lateral joint line. Decreased range of motion and pain during dorsiflexion and plantarflexion often are present. A significant degree of hallux valgus is unusual with this condition.

Radiographic evaluation reveals varying degrees of degenerative arthritis of the MP joint. The anteroposterior (AP) view reveals narrowing of the joint space with an often prominent lateral osteophyte. The lateral view reveals a dorsal osteophyte and joint space narrowing, often worse on the dorsal half of the joint. The sesamoid complex rarely is involved.

THERAPEUTIC ALTERNATIVES

Conservative management of hallux rigidus may be successful in the early stages of this process. Some patients have difficulty with shoe wear secondary to the large dorsal osteophyte, and an extra-depth or soft-top shoe such as a jogging shoe may improve function. Anti-inflammatories and intra-articular steroid injections may be helpful. Otherwise the goal of conservative care is to limit painful motion at the MP joint. A stiff-soled shoe or a full-length orthotic that limits MP joint motion during activity may decrease pain. These orthotics occupy space in the shoe, and the toe box must have sufficient room to accommodate the dorsal osteophyte.

Several surgical options have been described for the treatment of hallux rigidus, and successful results have been reported. I find that cheilectomy, arthrodesis, or a Keller procedure are the easiest and most reasonable options for handling this problem. Implant arthroplasty, although sometimes successful in an inactive patient, is fraught with hazards that are difficult to salvage. A dorsiflexion osteotomy of the proximal phalanx also has been described (Moberg's osteotomy) but this rarely is necessary.

CHEILECTOMY

A cheilectomy is a debridement of the osteophytes around the joint by removing the dorsal third of the metatarsal head. This procedure relieves impingement dorsally and decreases the stretch of the capsule across the osteophytes with plantarflexion. Another advantage of the cheilectomy is that an unsatisfactory result can be salvaged with an arthrodesis.

My experience with cheilectomy has met with moderate success; however, patients with less severe joint space narrowing and fewer complaints of pain from the dorsal osteophyte have done well. A young patient with a significant hallux rigidus likely would do well with an arthrodesis, but often rejects the idea of "a stiff toe." In this case a cheilectomy can be performed. However, the patient must be informed that if the cheilectomy is unsuccessful, future arthrodesis is indicated. Patients also should be told that they will continue to have some joint pain after cheilectomy. Although Mann and Clanton showed a slight increase in range of motion after cheilectomy, my experience shows little improvement in motion. Satisfaction with cheilectomy is more likely if the patient and the physician have reasonable expectations regarding outcome. Clearly the results following chei-lectomy depend on careful patient selection. Although increased motion is desirable, this often is not achieved. Pain relief is, however, a realistic goal, provided the disease process is not too advanced.

A cheilectomy is performed most easily through a dorsal incision centered over the first MP joint. The extensor hallucis longus tendon is exposed, and a plane between the extensor hood mechanism and the capsule is developed medially and laterally. Dissection in this plane protects the superficial nerves. The collateral ligaments on the medial aspect of the joint are not divided. Similarly, excessive stripping of the capsule medially should be avoided because both may result in iatrogenic hallux valgus. A synovectomy then is per-formed, and the osteophytes are observed easily by plantarflexing the toe. Frequently one-third to one-half of the dorsal articular cartilage is absent and subchon-dral bone is exposed. Involvement of the phalangeal cartilage also may be present; however, this degenera-tion usually is less severe. Significant involvement of the sesamoid apparatus is uncommon.

Once the metatarsal head is exposed and inspected,

the dorsal osteophyte is removed. The technique is performed using a small osteotome, starting distally on the metatarsal head and ending just proximal to the origin of the osteophyte. Commonly, the metatarsal head resection is started immediately dorsal to the normal articular cartilage. The amount of bone removed is proportional to the severity of the case. Bone should be removed aggressively as demonstrated in Fig. 1. The dorsum of the metatarsal then is contoured in a curvilinear fashion with a rongeur rather than cutting it straight with the osteotome. The lateral osteophytes then are exposed and removed flush with the metatarsal shaft. At times a large osteophyte is present on the dorsum of the proximal phalanx and should be removed. If large and prominent, osteophytes on the medial and lateral edges of the proximal phalanx also may be removed, but this step usually is not necessary.

At completion of the procedure, the toe should dorsiflex to 70° or 80° without impingement. The wound is irrigated, and bone wax may be used on the raw surfaces. The extensor hood is reapproximated over the bone surfaces, and the skin is closed. A snug compres-sion dressing is applied. This dressing should be changed in 1 week when the sutures are removed. A compression dressing should be applied for at least 2 weeks to prevent

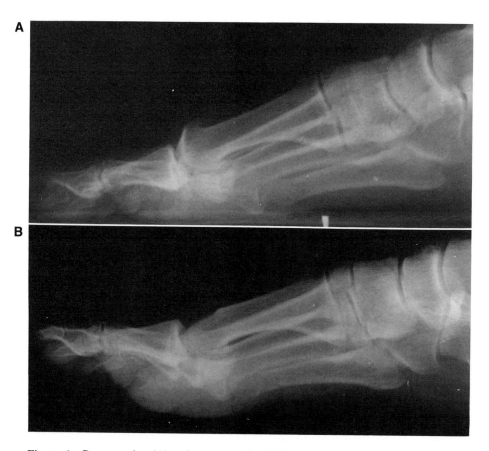

Figure 1 Preoperative *(A)* and postoperative *(B)* lateral radiographs demonstrating the amount of bone removed from the dorsum of the metatarsal head when performing a cheilectomy.

the wound from splitting open from swelling. A range-of-motion program is started at 2 weeks. The patient wears a postoperative wooden shoe for the first 2 weeks, and then is encouraged to wear a supportive shoe as tolerated. Patients should be informed that thickening around the MP joint may be present for up to 6 months after surgery.

SUGGESTED READING

Hattrup SJ, Johnson KA. Subjective results of hallux rigidus following treatment with cheilectomy. Clin Orthop 1988; 226:182–191.

Mann RA. Hallux rigidus. In: Greene WB, ed. Instructional course lectures. 1990:15.

Mann, RA, Clanton TO. Hallux rigidus: Treatment by cheilectomy. J Bone Joint Surg 1988; 70-A:400–406.

DOUBLE-STEM SILICONE IMPLANT ARTHROPLASTY OF THE FIRST METATARSOPHALANGEAL JOINT

GEORGE J. LIAN, M.D.

Implant arthroplasty has enjoyed a prominent place in the orthopedic treatment of arthritic joints. Although the proximal joints of the lower extremity are replaced routinely with a high degree of success, the application of these principles to the joints of the foot and ankle has not been accepted widely. Still, implant arthroplasty offers the best possibility of maintaining motion and function in the arthritic joint.

The use of implant arthroplasty to treat pathology of the first metatarsophalangeal (MP) joint began with a metallic prosthesis for the first metatarsal head in 1952. In 1962 Swanson began to use a single-stem silicone implant to replace the resected base of the proximal phalynx. Next, a double-stem silicone implant was developed to reconstruct MP joints with articular destruction of both the phalanx and metatarsal and for problems with malalignment.

The Silastic flexible-hinge toe implant is made of silicone elastomer, and its design is based on the flexible-hinged finger implant. The midsection is thicker and wider than the finger implant, and the flexor concavity of the hinge is designed to be placed dorsally to allow for greater dorsiflexion than plantarflexion. The stems have a rectangular cross-section that provides rotational stability within the medullary canals. A recent improvement has been the addition of titanium grommets that protect the shoulders of the implants from abrasion against bone edges and decrease the possibility of implant fracture. The silicone implant acts as a spacer and a substrate for the formation of a fibrous pseudocapsule. This allows for functional motion, and when the soft tissues have been balanced appropriately, it keeps the toe stable and properly aligned.

Double-stem silicone implants have been used to treat all types of pathology of the first MP joint including hallux valgus, hallux rigidus, and arthritis (posttraumatic, degenerative, or inflammatory). Over the past decade, reports of implant fracture and foreign-body reactions to silicone particles, requiring implant removal and further reconstructive surgery, have tempered the early enthusiasm for this procedure. However, it still should be included in the foot surgeon's repertoire for properly selected patients.

THERAPEUTIC ALTERNATIVES

The alternatives to treatment by implant arthroplasty include the more traditional methods of dealing with problems of the first MP joint. Modification of shoe wear usually is tried first. For patients with significant hallux valgus and bunions, this usually means an accommodative shoe. Those with hallux rigidus may benefit from a stiff sole with a rocker bottom to decrease the stress on the joint and allow for a near-normal gait. Arthritis may be treated with a combination of these modifications, depending on the particular circumstances; occasionally metatarsal pads or other inserts may be indicated.

When conservative treatments do not prove satisfactory, various surgical interventions are available for each of the general types of first MP joint pathology. When hallux valgus occurs without arthritis, the proper treatment is a bunion procedure, the choice of which is dictated by the significance of the patient's deformity and other factors including age and activity level. Hallux rigidus often is treated by cheilectomy when the condition is not too severe. Arthrodesis is useful in treating more significant hallux rigidus, as well as severe hallux valgus and arthritic MP joints. It also can be used in the salvage of failed previous surgery on this joint.

An arthrodesis provides pain relief by eliminating the diseased joint and yields a stable medial ray for walking, but at the expense of MP motion. This lack of motion may make other gait patterns impossible and limits the patient's selection of shoe wear. Recovery from arthrodesis typically is prolonged relative to implant arthroplasty and to other procedures described.

Resection arthroplasty may be used for patients with low demands who have painful arthritis or hallux valgus. They usually are left with limited function of the first ray.

PATIENT SELECTION

Several well-established and successful techniques are available to treat first MP joint pathology. Double-stem silicone implant arthroplasty should be reserved for a rather narrow group of patients. The ideal patient is young, with inflammatory arthritis, and with no more than moderate hallux valgus. A patient who is too debilitated or elderly will not benefit from the functional advantage of this procedure. Resection arthroplasty may be more appropriate in this setting. More severe hallux valgus deformities make balancing the soft tissues difficult, which may lead to recurrent deformity and failure of the procedure. Arthrodesis should be performed for these patients, and also for those who are highly active because they may place excessive stress on the implant, which could cause it to fracture or fragment. Generally those with inflammatory disease do not place high demands on their prostheses and thus are better candidates for implant arthroplasty.

The procedure should not be used in patients with

previous infection in the MP joint or in patients with a history of sensitivity to silicone implants.

SURGICAL TECHNIQUE

Preoperative antibiotics are given routinely, and a thigh tourniquet is applied. A medial or dorsal-medial longitudinal incision is made over the MP joint and the capsule exposed. The capsulotomy is made in an L shape, with the long arm longitudinal in the dorsal third of the joint (Fig. 1). The short arm, directed from dorsal to plantar, is made just posterior to the medial eminence. The flap then is reflected plantar and distal and the dorsal capsule retracted laterally to expose the joint. The medial eminence is removed if it is excessive.

The amount of bone to be resected from the base of the proximal phalanx and metatarsal head depends on the relative length of the great toe and the lesser toes and

on the ability to position the toe. The phalangeal cut is made first and should be perpendicular to its long axis. A minimal amount of bone is resected. It is important to retain full function of the flexor hallucis brevis, which will be compromised if the phalangeal cut is excessive. Should its attachment be lost, a pair of drill holes must be made in the plantar aspect of the phalangeal base and the tendons reattached with a nonabsorbable suture before the implant is placed. A cock-up deformity results if this is neglected.

The metatarsal cut then is made in the midportion of the head, with approximately 10° of angulation proximal-laterally to impart a gentle valgus orientation relative to the long axis of the metatarsal shaft. The distal third of the sesamoids usually is exposed by a proper cut in the metatarsal head.

The soft tissues are balanced next, first by releasing any contracture on the lateral side of the joint. If the adductor hallucis is deforming the toe, it is released. The

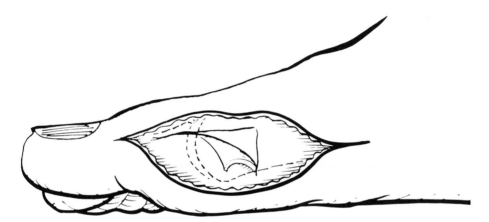

Figure 1 L-shaped medial capsule flap is reflected plantar and distal to expose the MP joint.

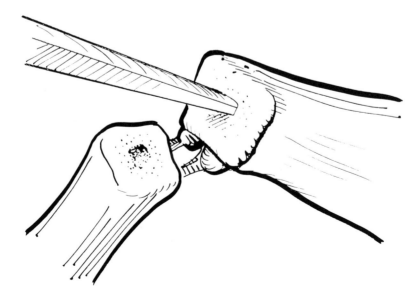

Figure 2 A small broach is passed down the canal to prepare it for the implant.

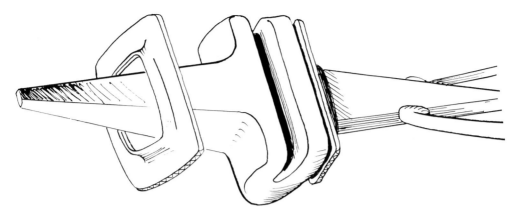

Figure 3 Titanium grommets fit over the two stems and rest against the shoulders of the hinge.

lateral capsule is incised if it is tight. The sesamoids are assessed: they must be free and lying in their proper grooves under the metatarsal head at the completion of this part of the procedure. If they are dislocated laterally, they must be freed both laterally and proximally to ensure that they are located properly. The extensor hallucis longus tendon is Z-lengthened routinely at this point.

The medullary canals then are prepared, first by passing a small broach down each canal (Fig. 2). If the bone is hard, a small power burr can be used to widen the canal. It also is useful to provide final contouring of the bone ends as needed.

A reduction then is performed with the largest trial implant that fits. If the implant is too small, adequate stability is not provided at the joint, and an implant that is too large is bulky and inhibits motion. The rotational and angular position of the toe is assessed and any final bone or soft tissue adjustments made.

The trial implant then is removed, and a small drill hole is made in the medial metatarsal shaft for reattachment of the capsule. If the short flexors were released previously, they also are reattached at this time through drill holes in the plantar base of the proximal phalanx. The proper prosthesis and corresponding titanium grommets are chosen and placed in an antibiotic solution. The canals also are irrigated with this antibiotic solution. With careful "no-touch" technique, the grommets are placed over the two medullary stems and the implant inserted first into the metatarsal canal and then into the phalangeal canal (Fig. 3). The grommets should fit snugly against both the bone ends and the shoulders of the implant.

The L-shaped medial capsule flap then is trimmed to remove any excess and securely reattached to the medial metatarsal with an absorbable suture (0 Vicryl). The capsule is closed carefully and securely and the extensor hallucis longus tendon repaired. It is imperative that the toe now sits in the proper alignment, or the final result will be unsatisfactory (Fig. 4). It must be remembered that this is a soft tissue balancing procedure. The implant

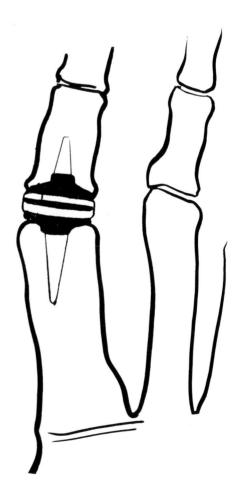

Figure 4 Implant is shown in place with the toe properly aligned.

is designed to be a spacer and should not be expected to provide stability if the soft tissues are not balanced.

The skin incision is closed with nylon or Prolene sutures, and a flat silicone drain is inserted between the stitches into the wound. Dressings are applied and the toe wrapped to provide support. The patient is kept non–weight bearing until the first postoperative day when the dressings are changed and the drain removed. Weight bearing then is allowed in a postoperative shoe. The dressings are changed weekly for 4 to 6 weeks and the skin sutures routinely removed at the third week. The patient advances to an athletic-type shoe at 4 to 6 weeks.

Implant arthroplasty of the first MP joint often is combined with other reconstructive procedures of the lesser toes. When used in combination with other procedures, it is best to begin with the great toe, doing the appropriate soft tissue releases and the bone cuts on the first MP joint, and then addressing the lesser toes. After finishing with the lesser toes, the canals should be prepared and the implant sized and placed.

COMPLICATIONS

Significant complications fortunately are rare, but include infection, implant fracture, and silicone synovitis (an inflammatory reaction to small fragmentation particles). An implant that fractures without evidence of infection or synovitis may be treated by a direct exchange. If infection or synovitis is suspected, the implant must be removed, the bone and soft tissue debrided, and specimens sent for culture and pathologic examination. This is sufficient treatment for synovitis, but if infection is found, appropriate antibiotic therapy must be undertaken. Salvage options for these problems include leaving the toe with essentially a resection arthroplasty or conversion to an arthrodesis.

SUGGESTED READING

Cracchiolo A III, Swanson A, DeGroot Swanson G. The arthritic great toe metatarsophalangeal joint: A review of flexible silicone implant arthroplasty from two medical centers. Clin Orthop 1981; 157:64–69.

Swanson AB, Lumsden RM II, DeGroot Swanson G. Silicone implant arthroplasty of the great toe: A review of single stem and flexible hinge implants. Clin Orthop 1979; 142:30–43.

Wilson DW. Hallux valgus and rigidus. In: Helal B, Wilson D, eds. The foot. New York: Churchill Livingstone, 1988:411.

ARTHRODESIS

ARTHRODESIS OF THE METATARSOPHALANGEAL AND INTERPHALANGEAL JOINTS OF THE HALLUX

IAN J. ALEXANDER, M.D., FRCSC

This chapter focuses on arthrodesis of the interphalangeal (IP) and metatarsophalangeal (MP) joints of the hallux, with primary emphasis on surgical techniques to achieve a satisfactory outcome. Indications for distal first ray fusions at both the IP and MP joints include painful degenerative, inflammatory, or post-traumatic arthritis; deformity (e.g., severe hallux valgus [HV], claw hallux); and rarely chronic instability. Arthrodesis in many cases is the optimal means of salvaging failed first MP joint surgery (i.e., bunionectomy, cheilectomy). When disease (e.g., rheumatoid arthritis) or previous surgery (e.g., a Keller resection arthroplasty or implant arthroplasty) has created a bony defect at the first MP joint, a solid arthrodesis with a well-positioned hallux of reasonable length may be achieved with one of a variety of interposition bone graft techniques.

ARTHRODESIS OF THE HALLUX INTERPHALANGEAL JOINT

IP joint shape, with flattening of the phalangeal head relative to the base, limits surface preparation for arthrodesis of this joint to either straight cutting or simply denuding the articular surfaces. This is best accomplished through a dorsal transverse incision across the joint with terminal curves (Fig. 1A). After removing the articular surfaces, the distal phalanx is drilled retrograde, exiting the toe tip just below the nail. The joint surfaces then are apposed and position and contact are checked. Then with the drill bit entering the terminal phalanx distally through the previously drilled tract, the proximal phalanx is drilled. Fixation is achieved with a 4.0 mm cancellous lag screw that compresses the fusion site, a technique described by Shives and Johnson. Lack

of rotational control provided by the screw alone has in a few of my patients led to nonunion despite excellent initial screw fixation. To prevent this rotation, an obliquely placed 0.45 or smaller Kirschner (K-) wire currently is used to transfix the joint (Fig. 1B). Two plane intraoperative radiographs are advisable to assess bone contact at the fusion site and screw position. Both the screw and the wire are removed at 3 months if the fusion is solid. Lacking back-cutting threads, late screw removal can be difficult. With the supplemental oblique K-wire, success rate and patient satisfaction with the outcome of this procedure have been excellent.

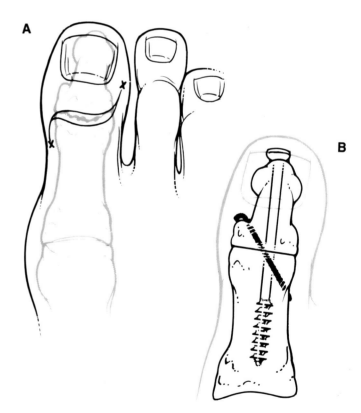

Figure 1 *A,* Incision for interphalangeal arthrodesis of the great toe. (© Ian Alexander, M.D.) *B,* Fixation for interphalangeal arthrodesis of the great toe. (© Ian Alexander, M.D.)

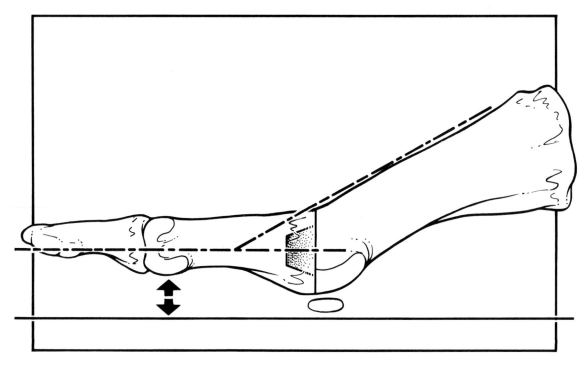

Figure 2 Positioning of the proximal phalanx parallel to the floor to allow clearance for roll off. (Reprinted with permission from Biomet, Inc., Warsaw, Indiana.)

ARTHRODESIS OF THE FIRST METATARSOPHALANGEAL JOINT

Although many surgeons are reluctant to consider arthrodesis as a treatment option for disorders of the first MP joint, their concerns often are unjustified. Unquestionably, arthrodesis of the first MP joint has an adverse effect on foot mechanics; however, in situations in which first MP mechanics already are abnormal, fusion of the joint to eliminate pain or severe deformity actually may improve foot function. Alternatives to first MP arthrodesis include resection or implant arthroplasty. These procedures definitely have a place and retain some first MP motion, but are not without potential problems including flail hallux, recurrent deformity, and implant failure. Often the only salvage for these complications is a technically more difficult fusion. Successful arthrodesis depends on achieving a solid fusion with a hailux in optimal position. This chapter focuses on achieving these objectives in relatively routine cases, as well as examining the role of arthrodesis in complex reconstructive problems of the distal first ray.

PREOPERATIVE PLANNING

It is critical that the most desirable position of the hallux is known before operative intervention is initiated. Optimal hallux position should be considered preoperatively in the three primary planes.

Sagittal Plane

Failure to position the hallux well in the sagittal plane is the most frequent positioning error. Excessive hallux extension results in dorsal toe irritation at the IP joint, related to shoe wear, and reduced hallux function that may predispose development of the second metatarsalgia. Excessive plantar flexion may result in hallux overload and painful plantar callosities at the IP joint, particularly when a sesamoid lies in the flexor hallucis longus just proximal to its insertion. Sagittal position seems to be optimal in most cases when the sagittal axis of the proximal phalanx is parallel to the floor with the foot plantigrade. With the sesamoids elevating the first metatarsal head and the normal sigmoid curvature of the plantar surface of the proximal phalanx, the head of a proximal phalanx that is fused parallel to the floor clears the floor by 5 to 10 mm (Fig. 2). This clearance allows for relatively normal roll off without hallux overload, and dorsally toe irritation rarely is a problem.

The sagittal arthrodesis angle (SAA) widely quoted to achieve optimal position is 25° to 30° (see Fig. 2). This usually is correct, because in most "normal" cases the metatarsal inclination angle (MIA) to the floor usually measures between 25° to 30° (Fig. 3). In the case of pes planus and pes cavus, however, routinely fusing the hallux at 25° to 30° results in malposition. For example, if the MIA is 15° (pes planus) and SAA is 30°, the hallux fuses at 15° of dorsiflexion and dorsal toe irritation ensues. On the other hand, if the MIA is 45° (pes cavus) and the SAA is 30°, the hallux is plantar flexed 15° and

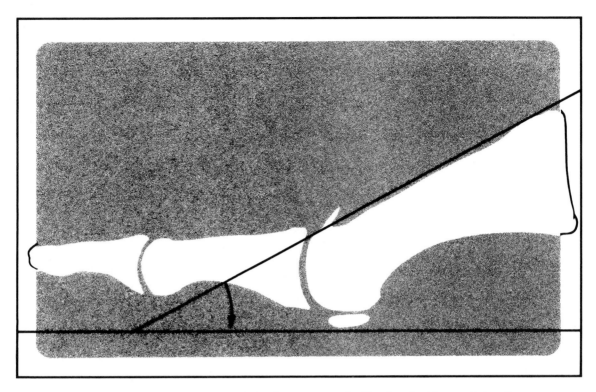

Figure 3 Angle of inclination of the first metatarsal. (Reprinted with permission from Biomet, Inc., Warsaw, Indiana.)

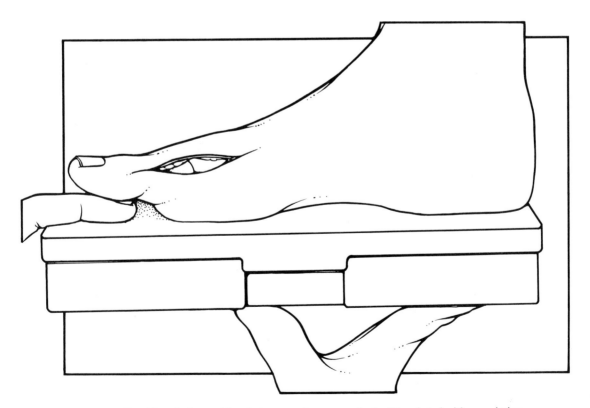

Figure 4 Checking phalangeal head clearance intraoperatively. (Reprinted with permission from Biomet, Inc., Warsaw, Indiana.)

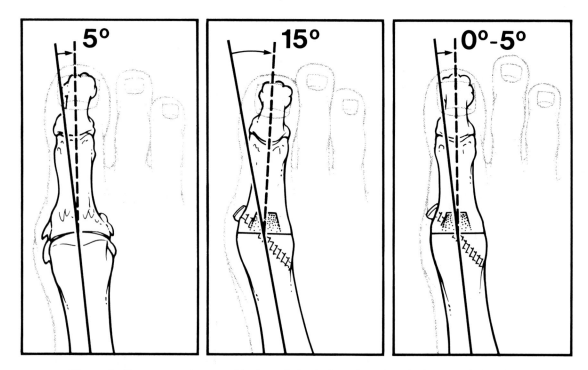

Figure 5 Transverse plane positioning of the hallux. (Reprinted with permission from Biomet, Inc., Warsaw, Indiana.)

overload may result. To achieve a hallux that is parallel to the floor, the SAA should equal the MIA. The MIA can be determined easily from the preoperative standing lateral radiograph by measuring the angle between the floor and a line intersecting the top of the head and the base of the first metatarsal (see Fig. 3). To assess sagittal plane position intraoperatively, pressure is applied to the plantar aspect of the foot with a flat rigid surface (Fig. 4). With this load-bearing simulation, the proximal phalangeal head should clear the surface by 5 to 10 mm. If the head rests against the surface, plantar flexion is excessive. If the operator's index fingertip passes easily under the phalangeal head, extension likely is excessive. Lateral observation should show that the hallux is parallel to the rigid surface.

Transverse Plane

Two clinical problems result from transverse plane malposition: excessive valgus results in painful great toe–second toe impingement, and excessive varus may lead to IP joint degeneration. Again, recommending a specific HV angle (15° to 20° often is recommended) as optimal is a fallacy. The best example of this is first MP arthrodesis for hallux rigidus. In many hallux rigidus patients, the HV angle is 0° to 5°, and the second toe is parallel to and resting against the hallux. If the hallux in this case is fused at 15° to 20° of valgus, painful great toe–second toe impingement and crossover predictably occurs (Fig. 5). In this instance the optimal transverse plane fusion angle is the same as the preoperative HV

angle. It is difficult to understand why the incidence of IP joint arthritis would increase when the toe is lying in its usual transverse plane position rather than 15° to 20° as has been recommended. The best rule therefore is to fuse the great toe in a transverse plane position to prevent second toe impingement if the preoperative HV angle is less than 15°. If the HV angle exceeds 15°, the hallux is best fused at approximately 15° of HV. Correction of a malaligned second toe also may be necessary to prevent impingement problems if preoperatively it is deviated medially.

To be sure that impingement is not a problem postoperatively, a small gap should be present between the great and second toe during the load-bearing simulation intraoperatively.

Frontal (Coronal) Plane

Frontal plane rotation, often referred to as pronation or supination of the hallux, also influences outcome but is not as critical as the other primary planes. The most frequent problem in this plane is excessive pronation, which usually is encountered when severe hallux valgus has been corrected with an arthrodesis. The lateral capsule contracture associated with the primary pathology resists hallux derotation. The consequence of a pronated fused hallux is that terminal push off occurs on the plantar-medial aspect of the hallux at the IP joint rather than on the fleshy pulp of the great toe, potentially causing a painful callus at the IP joint. In addition, with hallux malrotation, IP flexion and exten-

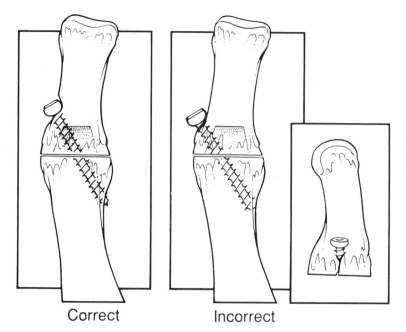

Correct   Incorrect

Figure 6 Fixation of an MP arthrodesis—importance of countersinking to avoid splitting the phalangeal cortex. (Reprinted with permission from Biomet, Inc., Warsaw, Indiana.)

sion occur at an angle oblique to the normal sagittal plane. Proper hallux rotation intraoperatively is checked by observing symmetry of nail alignment and being sure that IP flexion and extension occur in the sagittal plane.

SURGICAL TECHNIQUE

In addition to optimizing position, obtaining a solid arthrodesis also is important in achieving a successful outcome, although it is not altogether essential because at least half of patients with a nonunion are asymptomatic. The following contribute to rapid reliable healing of first MP fusions: (1) extensive cancellous bone contact, (2) inherent stability of the fusion configuration, and (3) rigid mechanically sound fixation.

Maximal cancellous bone contact and greatest inherent stability are provided by techniques that prepare the phalangeal base and the metatarsal head into interlocking conical or truncated cone shapes. With these techniques cancellous bone contact is maximized and inherent stability is sufficient that fixation with a single small-fragment screw usually provides excellent positional control (Fig. 6). Dome and straight-cut surfaces provide little inherent stability and are therefore more dependent on internal fixation devices. To attempt to provide better control in these situations, a number of methods have been tried including (1) longitudinal heavy threaded pins that transfix the IP joint and may contribute to late IP joint arthritis; (2) dorsal plate and screws, which are prone to mechanical failure, being located on the compression surface; and (3) multiple small K-wires that require removal. Optimal fixation with planar or dome surfaces or in the presence of osteoporotic bone is provided by crossed small-fragment screws (Fig. 7).

Preparing Conical Surfaces

Three methods of preparing inherently stable conical surfaces that provide extensive cancellous contact are (1) manual surface preparation with a rongeur, (2) the Marin Reamer System, and (3) the Truncated Cone Reamer System.

It is possible to prepare the joint surfaces with a rongeur, but this process is tedious and extremely time-consuming if the bone is dense. Obtaining an accurate stable fit often is difficult. The greatest advantage of this method is that no special instrumentation is required.

The Marin reamers are manual reamers that help improve the fit provided by the rongeur technique. The Marin reamers taper the surface to a pointed cone after initial surface shaping with a rongeur. Problems encountered with this method include significant shortening of the hallux and difficult surface preparation if the bone is dense.

The Truncated Cone Reamer System is designed to use power instrumentation to prepare the articular surface quickly and easily in a reproducible manner based on measurements taken from preoperative radiographs. In addition, cancellous apposition and inherent stability are maximized by the accurately machined Morse taper configuration of the prepared surfaces. Shortening is limited when using a truncated cone versus a full cone. The system consists of guides, templates, and a series of K-wire–guided reamers (Fig. 8A and B) that facilitate accurate positioning and surface preparation. In my hands this system has provided a reliable reproducible means of achieving a well-positioned solid arthrodesis. Fusion failures with this technique were the result of early unprotected loading of the hallux in two elderly osteoporotic females. Malposition is a result of inadequate attention to the intraoperative assessment of

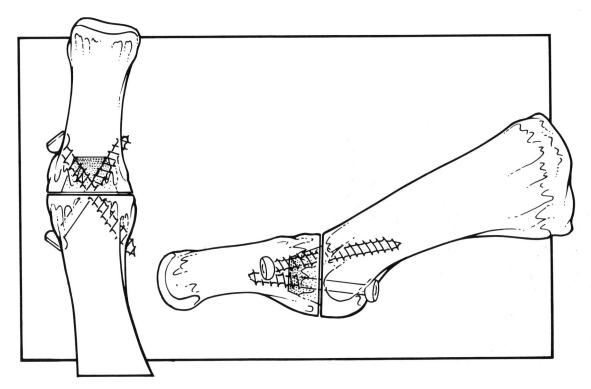

Figure 7 Crossed screw fixation for osteopenic bone or inherently unstable arthrodesis. (Reprinted with permission from Biomet, Inc., Warsaw, Indiana.)

sagittal position with simulated weight bearing or neglected great toe–second toe impingement present at the time of surgery.

Interposition Bone Graft Techniques

When pain, deformity, or instability at the first MP joint is associated with bone deficiency caused by erosive arthritis or previous surgery involving bone resection, apposition of existing bone to obtain a stable, well-aligned, and pain-free hallux may result in an unacceptable degree of first ray shortening. Under these circumstances, filling the defect with autogenous iliac crest bone graft often allows the surgeon to meet the objective of the arthrodesis while restoring first ray length and more normal foot geometry. The basic structural component of the interposition bone graft is a tricortical block of iliac crest. This block is fashioned to fit the size, shape, and cortical deficiency of the defect to be filled (Fig. 9). The surgical approach to the joint in these individuals usually is dictated by previous surgical incisions. Frequently there are multiple previous surgical approaches to the first MP joint and neuromas of the dorsal proper digital nerve and medial-plantar hallucal nerve, which were identified preoperatively on physical examination and should be dealt with to avoid these potential sources of persistent postoperative pain. Fibrous and other soft tissues filling the bone defects should be excised, and initially all bone attached solidly

to the metatarsal or phalanx should be left intact even if only a relatively thin cortical shell. Efforts should be made to preserve periosteal blood supply whenever possible. If the defect is asymmetric (e.g., primarily dorsal cortical erosion with a double-stem Silastic implant), it may be possible to appose the residual cortices and still maintain length. Trimming these surfaces and apposing them provides a bridge that may improve stability and healing. The graft then is fashioned to fill the defect. Cortex should be removed from the graft to provide cancellous contact with existing bone, but whenever possible, cortex should be left on the interposition graft surface where it will be bridging cortical defects or windows. Failure to provide this cortical strut makes structural support dependent on cancellous bone, predisposing to collapse or late stress fracture. Fixation of these fusions depends on the size and shape of the interposition graft. Cross-threaded K-wires and/or screws may provide excellent stabilization if the interposition graft is short, but plates and screws frequently are necessary for longer segmental grafts. These plates on the dorsal surface are under mechanical compression and are prone to failure when subjected to bending loads. In routine first MP fusions, load is transferred to the healed bone usually before plate fracture occurs, but in the case of interposition grafts, incorporation is a much longer process. As a result, avoidance of weight bearing is essential, at least until solid healing is obvious radiographically.

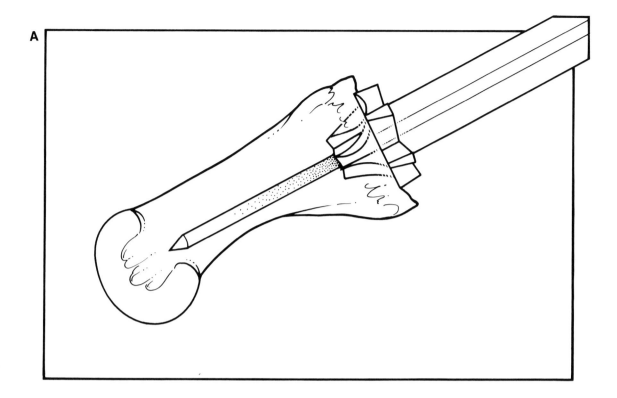

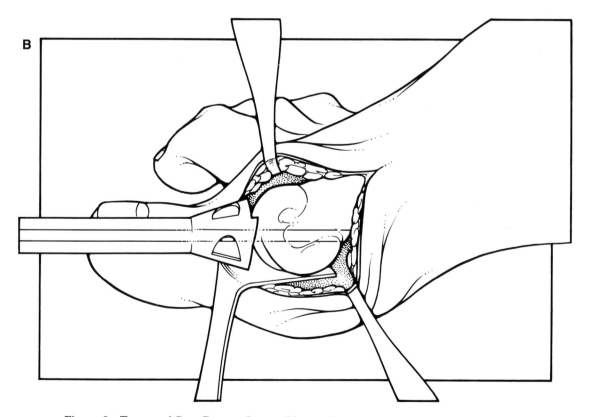

Figure 8 Truncated Cone Reamer System, Biomet, Inc. *A,* Phalangeal reamer. *B,* Metatarsal reamer. (Reprinted with permission from Biomet, Inc., Warsaw, Indiana.)

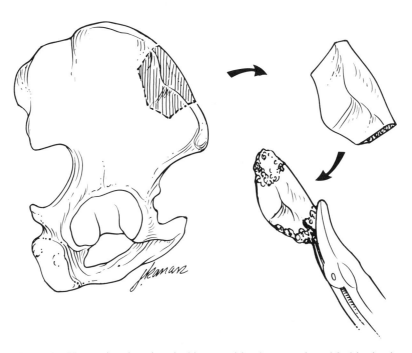

Figure 9 Harvesting the tricortical interposition bone graft and fashioning it with a rongeur. (© Ian Alexander, M.D.)

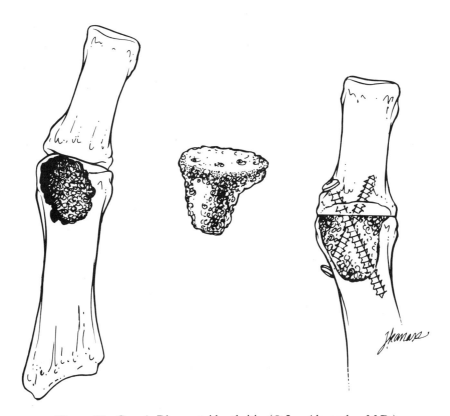

Figure 10 Case 1: Rheumatoid arthritis. (© Ian Alexander, M.D.)

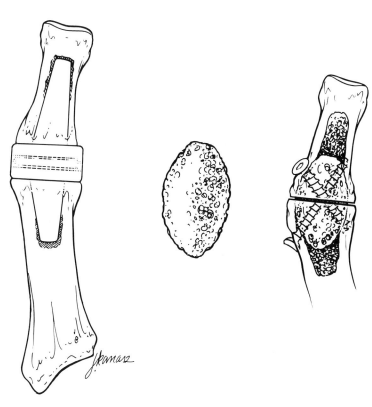

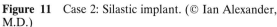

Figure 11   Case 2: Silastic implant. (© Ian Alexander, M.D.)

The following illustrated case histories probably best demonstrate the variability in graft design and fixation.

Case 1.   A woman with rheumatoid arthritis presented with pain in the first MP joint. Radiographs showed a large lytic defect in the first metatarsal head with a thin cortical shell (Fig. 10). At surgery the cyst was curetted, and the articular surface and subchondral bone of the base of the phalanx and the remaining metatarsal head were removed. An entirely cancellous graft was fashioned to fill the defect, and stable fixation was provided by cross screws.

Case 2.   This patient presented with a painful MP joint after a double-stem Silastic implant (Fig. 11). At surgery almost the entire cortical rim was intact circumferentially, but no cancellous bone remained in either the phalangeal base or the distal metatarsal. The bone ends were planed with a saw to provide flat apposing surfaces, and a football-shaped totally cancellous graft was fashioned to fill the defect. Chips of cancellous bone were placed proximal and distal to the interposition graft to fill the defect, and cross screws provided excellent fixation.

Case 3.   A woman with a painful nonfunctional great toe presented after previous bunion surgery (Fig. 12). Although the shape of the phalangeal base was unusual, this patient apparently had undergone a previous Keller resection arthroplasty. To maintain hallux length a full tricortical graft with cancellous surfaces facing proximally, distally, and medially was interposed and fixed with longitudinal threaded K-wires using a technique described by Coughlin and Mann.

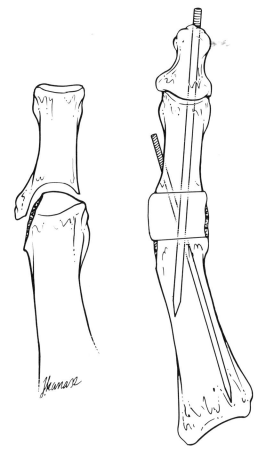

Figure 12   Case 3: Previous bunion surgery. (© Ian Alexander, M.D.)

A

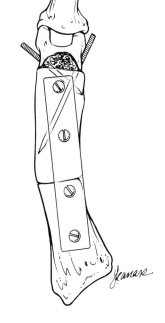

B

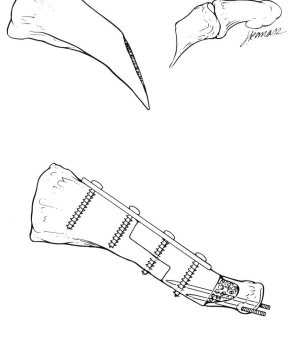

Figure 13 *A* and *B,* Case 4: Silastic implant. (© Ian Alexander, M.D.)

Case 4. A woman presented with a flail, malpositioned, and painful great toe after removal of a double-stem Silastic implant that had caused extensive dorsal bone destruction and perforation of the IP joint (Fig. 13*A* and *B*). At surgery the residual phalangeal condyles surprisingly had intact articular cartilage. An extensive tricortical graft was fashioned to fill a defect, and at its distal end cortical bone was removed and a dome of cancellous bone was fashioned to fit the proximal surface of the remaining phalanx. Proximal fixation was obtained with a dorsal plate, and distally two cross-threaded K-wires were placed to hold the phalanx to the interposition graft.

In my follow-up of these and other interposition graft patients, I found an excellent subjective outcome in terms of patient satisfaction with position, stability, and pain relief, but dynamic foot pressure analysis in almost all cases showed little or no significant hallux function.

DISCUSSION

Arthrodesis is an excellent means of dealing with pain, deformity, and instability of distal articulations of the first ray. Techniques that most reliably lead to a solid arthrodesis and critical intraoperative evaluation of position result in optimal outcomes.

SUGGESTED READING

Coughlin MJ, Mann RA. Arthrodesis of the first metatarsophalangeal joint as salvage for the failed Keller procedure. J Bone Joint Surg 1987; 69A:68–75.

Marin GA. Arthrodesis of the first metatarsophalangeal joint for hallux valgus and hallux rigidus. Int Surg 1968; 50:174–178.

Shives TC, Johnson KA. Arthrodesis of the interphalangeal joint of the great toe: An improved technique. Foot Ankle 1980; 26–29.

TONGUE AND TROUGH METATARSOPHALANGEAL FUSION

CARROLL A. LAURIN, M.D., FRCSC

The appeal of any surgical technique is based on its simplicity, efficacy, and ease of postoperative management. The tongue and trough (T&T) metatarsophalangeal (MP) fusion is such a technique, since a fusion can be achieved reliably and yet internal fixation, plaster cast immobilization, and specific postoperative care are unnecessary.

INDICATIONS

Obvious factors influencing the choice of operative procedure on the MP joint are the age and activity of the patient, the severity of the pathology, the status of adjoining joints, the surgeon's preference, and the demands of the postoperative regimen (i.e., postoperative cast immobilization, period of non–weight bearing, implant retrieval).

The main indications for an MP fusion are severe MP arthritis and gross hallux valgus. Arthrodesis also is useful in the correction of iatrogenic deformity and instability of the hallux MP joint.

When performed for MP osteoarthritis, the alternatives to an MP fusion are an excisional arthroplasty (the Keller arthroplasty) or an implant arthroplasty. The age of the patient, a high level of activity, and symptomatic plantar calluses are considerations that may argue in favor of an arthrodesis rather than an arthroplasty.

The indications to fuse the MP joint for gross hallux valgus admittedly are less widely accepted. The reasons possibly are related to the historical use of internal fixation and postoperative plaster cast immobilization when performing a fusion. However, if the postoperative course following an MP fusion essentially is comparable to that of a Keller arthroplasty, the arguments favoring an MP fusion for severe hallux valgus become more appealing, particularly in the presence of transfer lesions to other parts of the foot (e.g., plantar calluses) or secondary toe deformities such as an overriding second toe (ORST). See Table 1 for clinical classification of hallux valgus.

SURGICAL TECHNIQUE

Through a curved, dorsal, midline skin incision (Fig. 1), a transverse, dorsal-medial MP arthrotomy (Fig. 2) is performed 5 mm proximal to the phalanx, extending from the extensor hallucis brevis to the tibial sesamoid. The extensor hallucis brevis then is cut 1 cm proximal to its phalangeal insertion; the stump of the extensor hallucis brevis then is retracted distally (Fig. 3), exposing the side-to-side midpoint of the articulating surface of the proximal phalanx, where a notch is made with a rongeur. During this maneuver the lateral MP capsule and the adductor hallucis *must* be left intact.

When the bursa is dissected over the medial eminence, it is vital to maintain its continuity with the abductor hallucis (Figs. 3, 4); the medial exostectomy is mostly distal and should be limited to the medial eminence, maintaining the periosteum over the metatarsal shaft in continuity with the medial MP capsular flap and with the abductor hallucis (Fig. 4).

Table 1 Clinical Classification of Hallux Valgus

Grade I	Angular, valgus deformity of the MP joint only
Grade II	Grade I +
	Pronation deformity of the first phalanx (usually with callus on the medial-plantar aspect of the big toe)
Grade III	Grade II +
	Splay foot (wide foot with gross varus of the first metatarsal ray)
Grade IV	Grade III +
	Transfer plantar lesions, e.g., plantar calluses
Grade V	Grade IV +
	Overriding second toe (ORST)

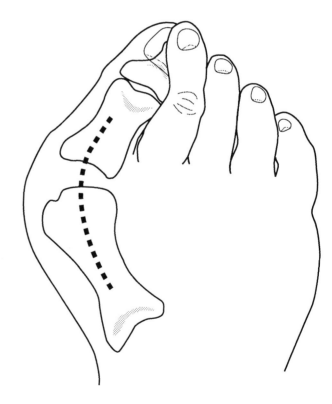

Figure 1 Grade V hallux valgus in a 60-year-old patient, an ideal candidate for a T&T MP fusion, through a curved, dorsal, midline incision.

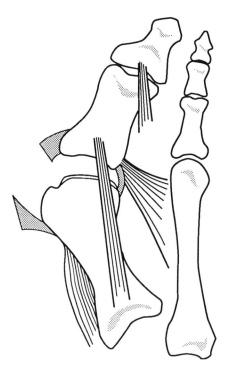

Figure 2 Transverse dorsal-medial MP capsulotomy extending from the tibial sesamoid to the extensor hallucis brevis, leaving the lateral capsule and adductor hallucis intact.

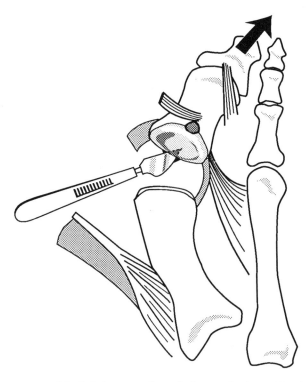

Figure 4 Medial bursa reflected in continuity with the abductor hallucis and removal of the medial eminence. While traction is applied to the toe, the plantar phalangeal attachment of the MP capsule is incised at its midpoint, in line with the dorsal notch (see Fig. 3). Note that the lateral capsule and adductor hallucis are left intact.

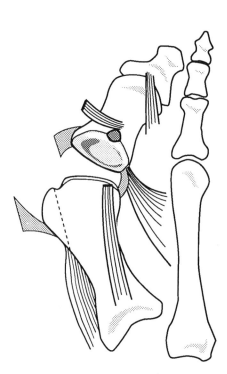

Figure 3 Extensor hallucis brevis transected and reflected distally to expose the midpoint of the proximal phalanx, where a notch is made while the MP joint is flexed and the valgus deformity is exaggerated. The medial bursa is reflected proximally to expose the medial eminence; it also is reflected in a plantar direction toward the abductor hallucis.

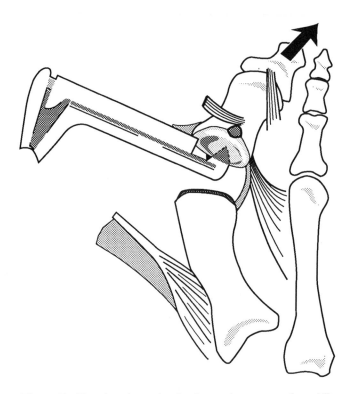

Figure 5 Traction is maintained on the toe, and a 45° Kerrison rongeur is inserted in the plantar capsular breach (see Fig. 4) to make a notch in the midpoint of the undersurface of the articulating surface of the phalanx, in line with the dorsal notch (see Fig. 3).

The valgus deformity at the MP joint then is exaggerated by pulling on the toe to visualize the plantar phalangeal attachment of the MP capsule, which then is sectioned at its midportion (see Fig. 4); the blade should be parallel to, and close to, the undersurface of the phalanx, so as to spare the underlying flexor hallucis brevis and flexor hallucis longus. This breach in the plantar and phalangeal attachment of the MP capsule allows the insertion of an angled Kerrison rongeur (45°) (Fig. 5) to cut a plantar notch in the articulating surface of the proximal phalanx. This may be the most important step of the procedure, since the position of this notch determines the site and orientation of the trough in the phalanx. While positioning the Kerrison rongeur, the surgeon must pull on the toe and maintain the toenail precisely parallel to the ground, thus correcting the valgus and pronation deformity of the hallux (Fig. 6). The trough should be cut in a manner such that the toe eventually fuses in a position of neutral rotation and minimal valgus; for that reason, the trough should begin at the plantar notch, a few millimeters lateral to the midpoint of the proximal-articular surface of the phalanx. A point of reference for this midpoint of the articular surface is the dorsal notch that was cut at the top of the phalanx under the phalangeal attachment of the extensor hallucis brevis (see Fig. 3).

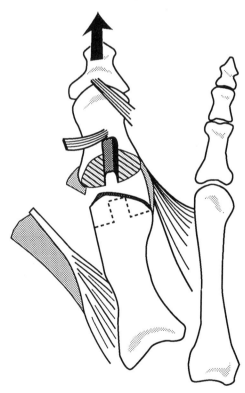

Figure 6 A 90° Kerrison rongeur is used to connect the plantar and dorsal notches in the phalanx to make a sagittal groove in the proximal phalanx. Phalangeal articular cartilage then is removed on either side of the trough. The metatarsal head then is shaped into a vertical tongue that is slightly wider than the groove, but of equal length. Note again that the lateral MP capsule and the adductor hallucis are always left intact.

Once the plantar notch has been made in the plantar cortex of the proximal phalanx with the 45° Kerrison rongeur, the surgeon changes to a 90° Kerrison rongeur to complete the trough, which should extend sagitally from the plantar notch to the dorsal notch (see Fig. 6), i.e., from the dorsal to the plantar cortices of the proximal phalanx; the trough should measure 0.5 cm in width (corresponding to the width of the Kerrison rongeur) and 0.75 cm in depth. A burr may be used to make this trough, but I prefer Kerrison rongeurs.

Using a small regular rongeur or a curette, the surgeon removes the articular cartilage on either side of the phalangeal trough (see Fig. 6). Visualization and cartilage removal are facilitated by pulling on the toe. The surgeon should use great care to spare the medial and lateral capsular attachments to the phalanx, particularly the lateral MP capsule.

Once the trough is completed, the metatarsal head then must be contoured in the form of a vertical tongue, or ridge, extending from the top to the bottom of the metatarsal head (see Fig. 6). The trough in the phalanx should be completed before reshaping the metatarsal head into a vertical ridge. If the order is reversed and the metatarsal head tongue is made first, the latter may be broken inadvertently while attention is directed to the preparation of the phalangeal trough. Except for the medial exostectomy, the only surgery that should be performed on the metatarsal head before preparation of a trough in the proximal phalanx is removal of articular cartilage over the apex of the metatarsal head (see Fig. 5). The main reason for doing this, at this particular time, is that otherwise the Kerrison rongeur tends to slip, or slide, on either side of the slippery, mucin-covered, metatarsal head as one attempts to position the Kerrison rongeur under the midpoint of the proximal phalanx. Once the cartilage has been removed from the metatarsal head, the latter has a more irregular surface, and positioning the Kerrison rongeur is easier. When reshaping the metatarsal head in the form of a vertical or sagittal tongue, it is better to start removing bone from the lateral side of the head. The reason for this sequence is that the bone is much denser on the lateral side of the metatarsal head, particularly in cases of severe and long-standing hallux valgus, whereas it is rather soft and spongy on the medial side. If the sequence is reversed and the medial third of the metatarsal head is excised first, the ridge may be fractured at the base, as one then removes bone from the dense lateral side of the metatarsal head. Therefore it is safer to start on the lateral side of the metatarsal head.

During this first phase of the procedure, at which time the lateral and medial sides of the metatarsal head are excised with a rongeur, it is important to keep in mind the position and orientation of the trough in the phalanx as the toe is held in the corrected position by the surgeon (see Fig. 6). If the phalangeal trough is not in the correct position, this can be compensated for by mild adjustments in the position and orientation of the metatarsal tongue.

A finer rongeur then is used to make the final

adjustments and shape the metatarsal tongue so that it is slightly wider, but not longer, than the trough. The length of the tongue should correspond exactly to the depth of the trough so that the shoulders of the metatarsal head abut and contact perfectly with the denuded phalangeal bone on either side of the phalanx, once the tongue is impacted in the trough (Fig. 7). If the tongue and trough have been prepared correctly, a mild compression force suffices to impact the metatarsal tongue into the phalangeal trough. The insertion of the tongue into the trough begins on the plantar side of the fusion site while the toe is held in 30° of flexion; as the tongue is impacted firmly, it is dorsiflexed to neutral (and no more). Immediate stability should be observed at the fusion site.

Unless the tongue does not penetrate completely into the trough, it is best not to separate them once they are impacted. If bony contact between the tongue and the trough is not satisfactory, one should consider and correct one or all of the following:

1. The sesamoids sometimes are adherent to the undersurface of the metatarsal head, thus impairing penetration of the metatarsal tongue into the phalangeal trough. Using a rongeur, cartilage then should be removed from the undersurface of the metatarsal head and the superior surface of the sesamoids. This not only frees the sesamoids, it also may increase the fusion mass by facilitating a fusion between the sesamoids and the MP fusion site.

2. One also should verify the parallelism between the bone on either side of the phalangeal trough and the bone on either side of the metatarsal tongue. Bone may have to be removed from one or more of these areas so that they are parallel to one another.

3. The last adjustment is to make the phalangeal trough wider or the metatarsal tongue thinner. The former is preferable, although it may not be possible, particularly in small patients, since one or both sides of the trough may be broken as the trough is enlarged. Unless the surgeon is careful and experienced with this technique, it is possible to fracture the shoulders of the phalangeal trough accidentally while deepening the trough with a Kerrison rongeur. For that reason, the surgeon must avoid a side-to-side motion of the Kerrison rongeur when trying to free bone that has been grasped by the instrument. Rather, the instrument should be mobilized along the sagittal axis of the phalanx, thus avoiding "inside-outside" pressure to either side of the trough.

If the metatarsal tongue is to be made thinner, it is best to use fine osteotomes rather than rongeurs. Osteotomes should not be used earlier, except possibly to mark the position and orientation of the tongue on the metatarsal head cartilage at the beginning of the procedure. An early use of osteotomes, rather than rongeurs, when starting to reshape the metatarsal head may fracture the base of the tongue accidentally.

Once the foregoing three adjustments have been made, it should be relatively easy to impact the fusion site firmly and note immediate stability (see Fig. 7). If there is insufficient stability, usually because the trough is too wide or the tongue is too thin, stability is achieved by crossed Kirschner (K-) wires; plaster cast immobilization rarely is necessary.

The stability of the fusion site is enhanced considerably by the capsular closure, particularly in instances of surgery for severe hallux valgus, with a retracted, tight, lateral MP capsule. Because the valgus malalignment has been corrected, there is redundant medial bursa capsule, which now must be resected (usually 1 cm), usually from the proximal flap (see Fig. 7). Since the lateral MP capsule has been left intact, closure of the medial capsule is like closing a book, and further stability immediately is noted following capsular closure, particularly if the tendon of the abductor hallucis has been mobilized dorsal-medially and has been firmly sutured to the phalangeal capsular flap (Fig. 8). The closure is completed by suturing the distally attached stub of the extensor hallucis brevis to the metatarsal flap, preferably to the tendon of the abductor hallucis, with resultant further stability.

It then is possible to flex and extend the distal

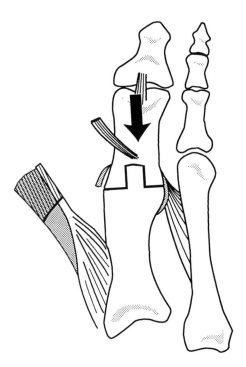

Figure 7   The phalangeal trough is impacted firmly onto the metatarsal tongue; note the correction of the metatarsus varus as the adductor hallucis now pulls laterally on the metatarsal bone rather than on the phalanx. Because of this correction of the metatarsus varus, there is minimal shortening of the big toe. The "bursa-abductor hallucis" flap now is too long, and excess tissue is resected distally.

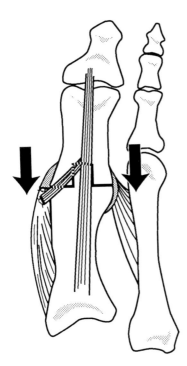

Figure 8 Medial capsular closure, including the abductor hallucis and the distal stub of the extensor hallucis brevis, provides immediate stability. Further compression of the fusion site is exerted by the abductor hallucis medially, the adductor hallucis laterally, as well as the relocated flexor and extensor tendons.

interphalangeal joint passively without inducing motion at the fusion site. One may even grasp the distal phalanx of the big toe and shake it vigorously without noting any motion at the MP site, which is already highly stable.

Because of this immediate stability, these patients are managed postoperatively as though they had a Keller procedure. No internal fixation is used, and no plaster cast is applied. The operation is performed as an outpatient procedure; crutches are used for a few days, and immediate full weight bearing is possible. Patients are instructed to walk mostly on their heels on a postoperative dressing that is protected by commercially available orthopedic boots. At 2 weeks the sutures are removed and patients walk in regular postoperative boots until they can get into their former shoes, usually a month after the operation.

RESULTS

The relatively high fusion rate with this technique is not only a result of the immediate postoperative stability, it also results from the increased surface area of bone contact at the fusion site provided by the T&T configuration (see Fig. 7). I suspect that the muscles on the four sides of the joint (the flexors on the plantar side, the extensors dorsally, the abductor hallucis medially, and the adductor hallucis laterally) compress the fusion site,

thus providing a compression type of arthrodesis (see Fig. 8).

POSITION OF FUSION

I was concerned initially that fusing the MP joint in patients with a gross metatarsus varus, in instances of severe hallux valgus, might result in a postoperative hallux varus deformity. This complication may occur if the MP joint is fused accidentally in a few degrees of varus, hence the recommendation to fuse the joint in minimal valgus. When the MP joint is fused in 0° of varus or valgus, a postoperative varus deformity never develops, in spite of obvious preoperative metatarsus varus. The explanation is that the lateral capsule and phalangeal attachment of the adductor hallucis are left intact. Once the MP site is stabilized, the metatarsus varus regresses as the tight adductor hallucis exerts its passive and active action on the metatarsal bone rather than on the phalanx. This can be documented consistently by immediate postoperative radiographs, which confirm that the intermetatarsal angle always is decreased by fusion of the MP joint in patients with hallux valgus.

In the past I fused the MP joint in 20° to 30° of dorsiflexion. Patients, particularly males, who eventually fused in 30° of dorsiflexion, frequently were unhappy with their toe "sticking in the air" when walking barefoot. For that reason, I now fuse the hallux in a neutral position with respect to the floor without any dorsiflexion; patients can walk barefoot more comfortably and still may wear shoes with normal heels. This undoubtedly is caused by the mobility at the tarsometatarsal joint and, to a lesser degree, at the interphalangeal joint. If the tarsometatarsal and interphalangeal joints are noted preoperatively to be particularly rigid, these patients are warned that they may be restricted in their choice of heel height or, if they prefer, they are fused in 20° of dorsiflexion.

Since patients are allowed immediate weight bearing without plaster cast immobilization, it may be that patients themselves position their MP joint in a position of slight dorsiflexion compatible with their life-style and their preferred heel height. However, postoperative radiographs and clinical assessments have shown that most MP joints were fused in 0° of extension, a more functional and more esthetically pleasing position.

COMPLICATIONS

In spite of the occasional, painless pseudoarthrosis, which is seen in 6 percent of patients and only when the fusion had been performed for hallux valgus, all fusions were stable clinically with no recurrence of the hallux valgus deformity. Only one patient reported pain at the pseudoarthrosis site, and none were revised surgically. All patients noted regression, usually complete, of their plantar calluses.

Supplementary K-wires were used in 10 percent of my original patients, and almost never in the last 10 years.

Radiographic and clinical evidence of osteoarthritis of the interphalangeal joint of the big toe was noted in 20 percent of patients, but only one patient required a fusion of the interphalangeal joint. In retrospect, this particular patient had preoperative radiographic signs of mild interphalangeal joint involvement, an obvious contraindication to an MP fusion.

SUGGESTED READING

Humbert JL, Bourbonniere C, Laurin CA. Metatarsophalangeal fusion for hallux valgus: Indications and effect on the first metatarsal ray. CAM J 1979: 120.

Marin GA. Arthrodesis of the metatarso-phalangeal joint of the big toe for hallux valgus and hallux rigidus: A new method. Int Surg 1968; 50:175.

McKeever DC. Arthrodesis of first metatarso-phalangeal joint for hallux valgus, hallux rigidus and metatarsus primus varus. J Bone Joint Surg 1952; 34A:129.

Moynhan FJ. Arthrodesis of the metatarso-phalangeal joint of the great toe. J Bone Joint Surg 1967; 49B:544.

Nicod L. Etiologie du hallux valgus. Rev Chir Orthop 1976; 62:161.

TARSOMETATARSAL ARTHRODESIS

MARK MYERSON, M.D.

Arthrodesis of the tarsometatarsal joint is indicated for the following:

1. Post-traumatic arthritis
2. Degenerative osteoarthritis
3. Neuroarthropathy (see the chapter *Arthrodesis for Diabetic Neuroarthropathy*)
4. Truncated wedge arthrodesis for forefoot cavus deformity
5. As part of the Lapidus bunionectomy

Conservative treatment for painful arthritis is initiated with nonsteroidal anti-inflammatory medication, accommodative orthoses, and shoe wear modifications. Rigid orthoses are not well tolerated, because they abut under the painful plantar-medial surface of the foot. A shoe with a ¼ inch tapered rocker-bottom sole also may help. In patients who are refractory to conservative treatment, and in whom operative treatment is not an option, a polypropylene ankle-foot orthosis alleviates the pain, albeit temporarily.

ARTHRODESIS FOR POST-TRAUMATIC ARTHRITIS

The injury to the tarsometatarsal joint complex may be subtle, and the initial trauma often may go undetected. Subtle shifts of the tarsus result in painful collapse of the midfoot and a post-traumatic flatfoot deformity. The appearance of the foot often is clinically worse than observed on radiographs. This is a result of elongation, tearing, or attenuation of the tendinous and ligamentous support of the midfoot. In severe cases the posterior tibial tendon is elongated, and attenuation of the anterior tibial tendon occurs. Elongation of the short and long plantar ligaments and tearing of the ligamentous support around the tarsometatarsal joint complex occur. Functional loss therefore may be far greater than the discomfort from the post-traumatic arthritis.

Preoperative Planning

In planning surgical correction, it is important to realign the foot and anatomy by recreating the medial-longitudinal arch and adducting the forefoot. This is accomplished by a lateral soft tissue release, resection of joint fibrosis, adduction of the forefoot, and plantar flexion of the first and second metatarsals.

Preoperative planning is important. It is extremely useful to draw an overlay template of the normal foot on an anteroposterior radiograph of the abnormal foot. The talometatarsal angle, and the position of the cuneiforms with respect to the metatarsals, are marked out and compared with the abnormal foot. It is only after this radiographic comparison that the significance of the deformity truly is appreciated, and this now can be used to plan the realignment.

It is well worth anticipating potential complications preoperatively. Neuromas of the deep and superficial peroneal nerve, nonunion, malunion, and problems with wound healing occur, all of which should be prevented through careful dissection and correct operative technique.

Surgical Approach

The operative approach depends on the pattern of dislocation. Generally three types of deformity require correction. The first involves the medial column only, in which the first metatarsal and/or cuneiform are dislocated. The second pattern includes the central column and involves the second and third metatarsals. This is the most common pattern of deformity, and it is rare that the second metatarsal does not need to be included in the arthrodesis. Usually the third metatarsal follows the second metatarsal because of its attachments through the deep transverse metatarsal ligament on the plantar base of the metatarsal. The third pattern of dislocation involves the entire midfoot. Although the second through fifth metatarsals are obviously involved radiographically, the change affecting the first metatarsal is more subtle. The first metatarsal always is displaced and should be included in the arthrodesis. Usually the arthrosis of the lesser metatarsocuneiform joints is obvious, but the articular surface of the first metatarsocuneiform joint may appear intact. Nevertheless, this medial joint rarely is congruent, and careful comparison with the normal foot confirms this deviation.

For the medial column deformity, a single dorsomedial incision is used, placed between the insertion of the anterior and posterior tibial tendons. For the central column deformity, a lengthy incision is placed between the second and third metatarsals extending from the metatarsal neck distally to the talus proximally. The longer this incision, the less the soft tissue retraction required for exposure. This is important particularly in fusions following crush injuries, in which the potential for skin necrosis is high. Where the entire foot is involved, three longitudinal incisions are used: one dorsomedial, which is directly anterior or slightly lateral to the anterior tibial tendon; the second between the second and third metatarsals; and the third along the length of the fifth metatarsal cuboid joint.

In the medial column dislocation, the medial cuneiform frequently is rotated and subluxed medially and plantarward (Fig. 1). In this pattern of injury, the fusion must include the naviculocuneiform joint, the medial middle cuneiform, and if necessary the first metatarsocuneiform if this also is involved (Fig. 2). For middle column injury, the base of the second metatarsal must be

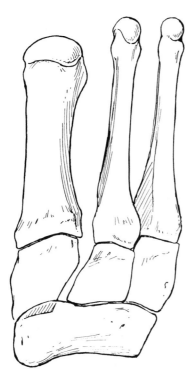

Figure 1 Medial column dislocation with plantar subluxation and rotation of the medial cuneiform is shown.

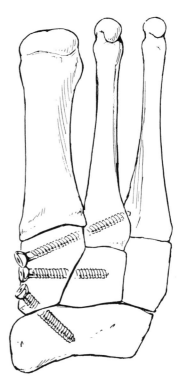

Figure 2 Arthrodesis is accomplished with lag screw fixation through the medial cuneiform into the second metatarsal, the middle cuneiform, and occasionally into the navicular.

included in the arthrodesis. The incision is deepened in through subcutaneous tissue, the branch of the superficial nerve identified and retracted laterally, and the incision deepened directly onto the second metatarsal. If you have inadvertently made the incision too far medially, it is imperative to look for the neurovascular bundle, which lies directly underneath the extensor hallucis brevis tendon. I prefer to identify the bundle and retract it out of the way rather than work around it. Damage to the perforating branch of the dorsalis pedis artery may occur in the first web space, and it is worth exposing and tying off this vessel before dissecting in this location.

Once the base of the second metatarsocuneiform joint is identified, I work subperiosteally to raise the entire flap without subcutaneous dissection. The flap should be extended both medially and laterally, depending on the pattern of arthrodesis. One should be able to include the second and third metatarsal base in the fusion through this incision without any undue tissue retraction. The metatarsocuneiform joint now is debrided, care being taken to remove cartilage but minimal bone. If the articulation is freed with minimal cartilage and bone excision, bone graft is not necessary. It is important to use sharp osteotomes or chisels. There usually is a tendency to remove excessive amounts of cartilage and bone dorsally, leaving the apical plantar surface of the joint intact. This automatically dorsiflexes

the metatarsal in the fusion, causing a malunion with ultimate transfer metatarsalgia.

When the entire tarsometatarsal articulation is to be fused, the third incision is made laterally between the fourth and fifth metatarsals toward the cuboid (Fig. 3). If the pre-existing deformity is severe, this joint is difficult to reduce. The soft tissue attachments have to be freed, and the insertion of the peroneus brevis onto the base of the fifth metatarsal elevated or the peroneus brevis tendon lengthened. Occasionally an osteotomy through the base of the fifth metatarsal reduces the tension laterally. This preserves the peroneus brevis tendon attachment. Generally, however, I free the soft tissue attachments and slide the fourth and fifth metatarsals over medially. These are secured with two 0.062 inch Kirschner (K-) wires introduced through the base of the fifth metatarsal into the cuboid. These K-wires are left in place for approximately 12 to 14 weeks and then removed once a stable arthrofibrosis has been achieved (Fig. 4). It rarely is necessary to fuse the metatarsocuboid articulation. Despite radiographic arthrosis, this joint does well provided the alignment is corrected.

For complete forefoot column correction, the first metatarsal should be realigned first. The second metatarsal then is keyed into the mortise, and once adducted and plantar flexed it should be held temporarily with a 0.062 or 0.045 inch K-wire. Anteroposterior and lateral

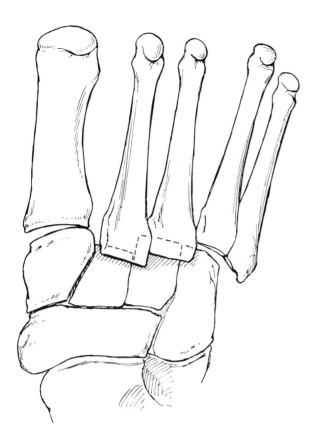

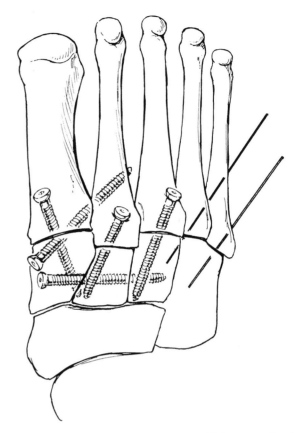

Figure 3 Dislocation of the entire tarsometatarsal joint always involves the first metatarsal, although this may be subtle.

Figure 4 Arthrodesis is accomplished with lag screw fixation into the medial and middle columns and percutaneous pin fixation of the lateral column.

radiographs are obtained and the position of the forefoot checked. Generally one underestimates the amount of correction required to adduct the foot. Not infrequently the K-wires need to be removed and the metatarsals repositioned in either more adduction or plantar flexion.

When the surgeon is satisfied with the position, screws are inserted for definitive fixation. The 3.5 mm cortical screws are inserted in a lag fashion; 4.0 mm cancellous screws are not strong enough to stabilize this articulation. It is important to countersink the screw to prevent splitting the metatarsals between the screw hole and the cuneiform. Once stable fixation has been achieved, a high-speed 4 mm burr is used to denude the remaining cortical surface between the cuneiforms and metatarsals. Cancellous bone chips now are packed into this denuded space. It usually is necessary to use bone graft, although in some more isolated fusions this can be avoided if the metatarsals are carefully repositioned with minimal bone loss.

Postoperative Care

Patients are immobilized in a cast for 3 weeks postoperatively, until sutures are removed, and then commence early range-of-motion exercises. Patients remain non–weight bearing for 12 weeks. At 12 weeks partial weight bearing is commenced, and the metatarsocuboid pins are removed. Physical therapy modalities are a useful adjunct to recovery, and patients benefit from softer accommodative orthoses.

SUGGESTED READING

Johnson J, Johnson KA. Dowel arthrodesis for degenerative arthritis of the tarsometatarsal joints. Foot Ankle 1986; 6:243–253.

Myerson MS. The diagnosis and treatment of injuries to the Lisfranc joint complex. Orthop Clin North Am 1989; 20:655–664.

Sangeorzan BJ, Veith R, Hansen ST. Salvage of Lisfranc's tarsometatarsal joint by arthrodesis. Foot Ankle 1990; 10:193–200.

SUBTALAR ARTHRODESIS

GEORGE E. QUILL, JR., M.D.

The single-axis subtalar joint is a hinge joining the talus and calcaneus. This joint allows the human foot to adapt readily to uneven terrain, modifies the forces of ambulation imposed on the rest of the skeleton, and influences the performance of the more distal foot articulations as well. When the structure and function of this joint are altered by arthritis, trauma, instability, or tarsal coalition, subtalar arthrodesis may prove to be a most gratifying procedure in treating the patient's resultant disability.

THERAPEUTIC ALTERNATIVES

In cases of rheumatoid arthritis or osteoarthritis affecting the subtalar joint, oral anti-inflammatory medication or judicious use of intra-articular corticosteroid injection through a lateral sinus tarsi approach may be indicated. Selected patients may have arthritic subtalar symptoms alleviated by shoe wear modifications or by wearing orthoses of a semirigid, UCBL, or short-leg variety. Even a trial of therapeutic casting may be indicated in patients whose hindfoot symptoms are both mechanical and inflammatory.

Patients with significant instability of the hindfoot of a post-traumatic,* neuromuscular, or developmental nature also may benefit from orthotic management.

For select patients with talocalcaneal tarsal coalition, resection of the bar with or without interposition arthroplasty may be indicated, potentially allowing the patient to retain subtalar motion.

Arthroereisis of the subtalar joint, a procedure used to correct valgus of the hindfoot by reducing, but not eliminating, motion — usually by means of interposing bone, methacrylate, polyethylene, or a staple in the sinus tarsi — recently has gained popularity in the podiatric literature. The body of existing orthopedic literature, however, does not offer convincing evidence that this procedure reproducibly corrects pes planovalgus deformity and eliminates its symptoms.

Patients presenting with clinically significant subtalar pain and/or instability refractory to nonoperative care should be considered for subtalar arthrodesis.

Children 4 to 12 years of age with paralytic equinovalgus hindfoot deformity classically have been managed with the Grice and Green extra-articular subtalar arthrodesis, since there is little interference with future growth of the foot using this procedure. Except in practices heavily weighted toward pediatric orthopedic surgery or those located where poliomyelitis

still is endemic, this procedure rarely is indicated. Many other extra-articular techniques for subtalar arthrodesis have been described, but I prefer intra-articular procedures because of the ease with which they allow the surgeon to address the joint pathology directly and optimize correction of deformity and fixation.

PREFERRED APPROACH

The vast majority of hindfoot pathology requiring subtalar arthrodesis may be divided into feet with significant hindfoot deformity and those feet in which there is relatively good maintenance of the normal hindfoot architecture. The most common hindfoot deformities addressed with subtalar arthrodesis are diminished heel height and increased heel width, usually as a result of rheumatoid deformity or more commonly occurring after fracture of the talus or joint depression –type calcaneus fractures.

Heel height may be best assessed preoperatively on a standing lateral radiograph of the affected foot by measuring the distance in millimeters from the plane of support to the most cephalad portion of the talar dome and comparing this value to the contralateral, unaffected foot. Alternatively one may measure the talar declination angle on a standing lateral radiograph of the foot. This angle is formed by the longitudinal axis of the talus and the plane of support and is a measure of the "horizontal attitude" assumed by the talus. Patients with a talar declination angle of less than 20° and those with more than an 8 mm loss of heel height consistently demonstrate anterior tibiotalar impingement, diminished ankle range of motion, and difficult shoe wear.

A subtalar distraction bone block arthrodesis, as described by Carr and co-workers, may be indicated for patients with disabling subtalar arthritis, a loss of heel height greater than 8 mm on the affected side, and a talar declination angle of 20° or less. An in situ subtalar arthrodesis with compression screw fixation and iliac crest bone grafting may be performed for patients with disabling arthritis of the subtalar joint in the presence of more normal heel height and tibiotalar alignment.

In Situ Subtalar Arthrodesis

In situ subtalar arthrodesis is performed with the patient in the lateral decubitus position with the affected extremity up and with the patient under a satisfactory general or spinal anesthetic. Care is taken to pad all bony prominences, an axillary roll is used in the "down" axilla, and the patient usually is fastened securely to the table with beanbag and chest braces. A pneumatic tourniquet is placed about the thigh. The affected lower extremity is prepped and draped in the usual sterile and free fashion. Simultaneously the ipsilateral iliac crest also is prepped and draped in a separate field. An in situ arthrodesis usually is best accomplished through an incision made parallel to Langer skin lines and beginning no more than 15 mm distal to the anterolateral tip of the

---

*Recall that the calcaneofibular ligament normally stabilizes both the tibiotalar and talocalcaneal joints.

fibula. This incision is made on the anterolateral surface of the foot overlying the sinus tarsi and is carried carefully into the subcutaneous layer, where superficial veins are ligated carefully and cuticular nerves preserved where possible. The wound should extend from the lateral border of the peroneus tertius without opening its tendon sheath to the most cephalad anterior border of the peroneal tendon sheath, taking care to identify, protect, and retract the sural nerve. The deep fascia of the foot is incised, leaving a readily identifiable layer for closure at the end of the procedure. The contents of the sinus tarsi are excised sharply with a knife and rongeur. The plane of dissection need not expose the calcaneocuboid or talonavicular joints, and the proximal origin of the intrinsic extensors is reflected only a short distance as a distally based flap. I prefer to use sharp interchangeable chisel blades to remove the remaining articular cartilage on all facet surfaces of the talar and calcaneal side of the subtalar joint. These chisels also may be used carefully to resect any wedges necessary for making planar apposable surfaces and correcting preoperative deformity.

I find it helpful to use a small lamina spreader in the posterior facet to afford better exposure of the middle and anterior facets. Alternatively, when I wish to expose the posterior surfaces of the talus and calcaneus, I place the lamina spreader more anteriorly in the arthrodesis site. Division of the calcaneofibular ligament and retraction of the peroneus brevis and longus posteriorly also aids in this exposure.

Once the reduction of the arthrodesis site is deemed congruous, with the intended position of subtalar arthrodesis being approximately 3° to 5° of valgus, the tourniquet may be deflated while the surgeon harvests autogenous iliac bone graft.

For the severely valgus hindfoot with a normal ankle and a supple forefoot, the position of choice is indeed 5° of valgus, leaving the entire foot plantigrade and using cancellous and corticocancellous bone graft to fill the void within the subtalar arthrodesis site created when the os calcis is brought out of its severe valgus preoperative position. Conversely, if the hindfoot was in a varus position preoperatively, resection of the appropriate subtalar bone and division of the ligamentous tissues still allow the hindfoot to be brought over into a more normal 5° of valgus, even with this lateral approach.

Once the iliac graft has been harvested and that wound closed, the surgeon should irrigate the foot wound and reinflate the tourniquet if necessary after exsanguination by gravity. Cancellous graft is placed and the hindfoot held in the appropriate position, and then internal fixation added. I prefer the 7.0 mm cannulated screw system for fixing the talocalcaneal arthrodesis site. The guidewire can be inserted in a dorsal-plantar direction through the talar neck across the arthrodesis site and into the tuberosity of the os calcis, or the threaded guidewire may be passed percutaneously through the posterior-inferior os calcis across the arthrodesis site, engaging subchondral bone of the talar

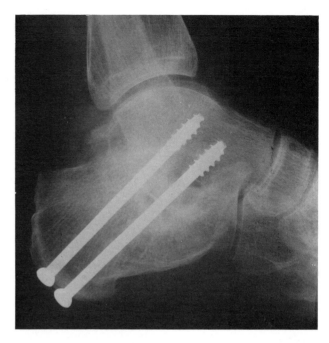

Figure 1 Subtalar arthrodesis using 7.0 mm cannulated screws with a 16 mm thread.

dome. Intra-operative radiographs may be necessary to ascertain the appropriate screw length. If a screw with a short thread (16 mm) is chosen and inserted in the appropriate fashion, rigid fixation and compression across the arthrodesis site may be obtained with as few as one and certainly no more than two screws (Fig. 1). The wound usually is closed over a drain, and a nonadherent, bulky, slightly compressive dressing incorporating plaster coaptation splints applied.

Subtalar Distraction Bone Block Arthrodesis

The technique for subtalar distraction bone block arthrodesis recently was described by Carr and coworkers, modifying an earlier procedure described by Gallie in 1943. The patient is positioned and the iliac crest and lower extremity draped as described earlier. For this procedure I prefer a longitudinal incision, paralleling and just posterior to the fibula, because intraoperative distraction of the hindfoot can affect closure of a more transverse wound adversely. Again, one must identify and protect the sural nerve and the lesser saphenous vein. After debriding and preparing the subtalar arthrodesis site, a tricortical wedge of iliac crest is taken and contoured into the shape of a trapezoid, cutting the graft 2 to 3 mm higher on the intended medial side so that the subtalar joint is held distracted into slight valgus and not overcorrected into varus. This is best accomplished with the use of a large lamina spreader, and one may obtain intraoperative radiographs to measure the amount of distraction and determine the appropriate width for the graft (Fig. 2). Also, to prevent tilting the heel into varus with insertion of the graft, a

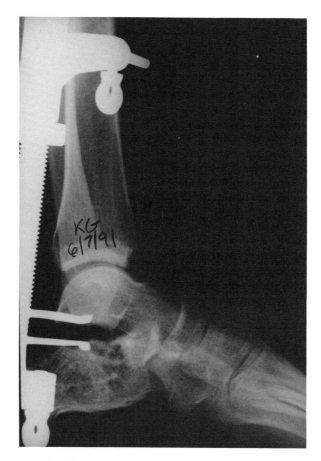

Figure 2   Distraction for a subtalar bone block arthrodesis is performed with a large lamina spreader. A unilateral distractor is applied medially to prevent varus tilt.

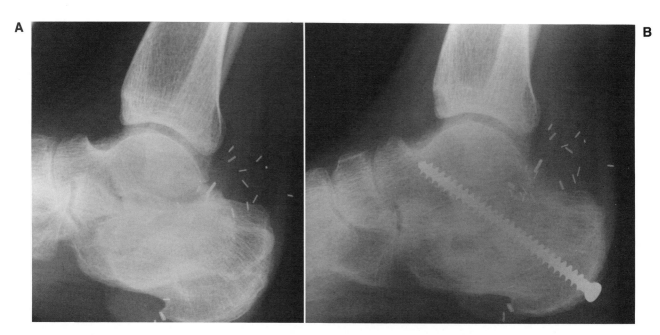

Figure 3   *A,* Loss of heel height and decrease in the talar declination angle and tibiotalar impingement is present. *B,* This was corrected with a bone block fusion.

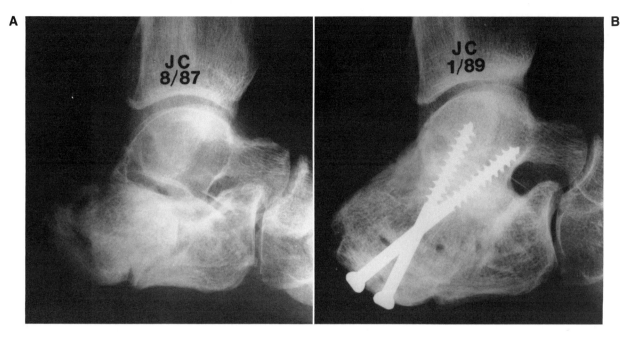

Figure 4 *A,* Loss of heel height and tibiotalar impingement. *B,* This was corrected with a bone block fusion.

medially applied femoral distractor may be inserted with one pin in the calcaneus and one in the tibia. Thus the subtalar joint is distracted and simultaneously tilted into valgus while the graft is inserted. Wound closure and dressing are performed in the standard fashion after the graft has been inserted and fixed with a fully threaded 6.5 mm cancellous screw or one that has threads measuring at least 32 mm in length, helping to maintain the distraction (Figs. 3 and 4). The compression dressing usually is changed to a lightweight, non–weight-bearing cast within the first postoperative week. A full 6 weeks of non–weight-bearing activities usually are required for proper healing, followed by 4 to 6 weeks of weight bearing as tolerated in a walking cast. Clinical and radiographic union usually are apparent by 10 to 12 weeks.

Complications of subtalar arthrodesis include delayed union or nonunion, but because the patient usually is allowed to weight bear across this relatively transverse arthrodesis site, these complications rarely are encountered. A meticulous operative approach should be employed to prevent postsurgical neuromata and an inordinate amount of postoperative edema. Correct alignment can be difficult to judge during bone block distraction arthrodesis with the patient in a lateral decubitus position. Further, insertion of the graft may cause the heel to tilt into varus. If problems do occur, they can be corrected satisfactorily with a closing-wedge valgus osteotomy of the calcaneus.

Patients must be told to expect some difficulty, but little pain, while walking on uneven terrain as a result of the loss of normal subtalar motion after this procedure and transmission of those forces to the ankle, a hinged

joint whose plane of motion does not accept those stresses readily.

PROS AND CONS OF SUBTALAR ARTHRODESIS

Subtalar arthrodesis through the lateral approach described earlier is applicable to both varus or valgus preoperative hindfoot deformities, provides a large surface area at the arthrodesis site, and is readily fixed internally. This procedure has a low incidence of delayed union or nonunion, with immobilization time averaging 10 to 12 weeks. This procedure offers advantages over triple arthrodesis in that the transverse tarsal joints are preserved, heel height is maintained, and abnormal heel width may be addressed by calcaneal ostectomy through the same incision.

Complications are infrequent, and one rarely sees degenerative changes in the transverse tarsal joints. In actuality, these joints usually increase their normal range of motion, as does the ankle, in a compensatory fashion after subtalar arthrodesis. Screw removal may be indicated for patients who have persistent discomfort under the tuberosity of the os calcis or in whom the distal threaded end of the screws may be close to the ankle joint or talofibular recess.

Despite these potential problems, subtalar arthrodesis in situ and the posterior distraction bone block arthrodesis techniques readily restore the length of the gastrocnemius-soleus complex, the normal talocalcaneal and tibiotalar relationships, and facilitate decompression of the peroneal tendons and subfibular recess through one wound.

SUGGESTED READING

Carr JB, Hansen ST, Benirschke SK. Subtalar distraction bone block fusion for late complications of os calcis fractures. Foot Ankle 1988; 9:81–86.

Close JR, Inman VT. The action of the subtalar joint. University of California Prosthetic Devices Res Rep Ser II. Issue 24, 1953.

Gallie WE. Subastragalar arthrodesis in fractures of the os calcis. J Bone Joint Surg 1943; 25:731–736.

Grice DS. An extra-articular arthrodesis of the subastragalar joint for correction of paralytic flatfeet in children. J Bone Joint Surg 1952; 34A:927.

ANKLE ARTHRODESIS

TYE J. OUZOUNIAN, M.D.

Severe end-stage degeneration of the ankle is relatively rare compared with other major weight-bearing joints. The most common causes include post-traumatic arthritis, primary osteoarthritis, rheumatoid arthritis, and avascular necrosis of the talus. When end-stage degeneration occurs, operative options are limited. Immobilization of the ankle in a polypropylene AFO allows increased activity. Although ankle replacement may be considered in rheumatoid arthritis, the majority of patients generally are too active to consider an ankle replacement. The most frequently accepted operative procedure for the treatment of end-stage ankle degeneration is an ankle arthrodesis. A combined intra- and extra-articular technique of ankle arthrodesis using rigid internal compression is described.

PATIENT SELECTION

The most important factor in patient selection is to establish the exact location and cause of pain. The differentiation between ankle and subtalar symptoms may not be obvious immediately (Fig. 1). Severe valgus deformity of the hindfoot actually may be caused by an angulation of the talus within the ankle mortise, and the subtalar joint may be normal (Fig. 2A and B). In other situations there may be involvement of both the ankle and subtalar joints. Selective diagnostic injections with lidocaine and bupivacaine help to identify the most symptomatic articulation. Once the symptoms are correlated with the involved articulation, the appropriate procedure may be considered.

A variety of surgical techniques have been described for performing an ankle arthrodesis. Popular techniques include both intra- and extra-articular procedures. Most successful clinical series have incorporated the concept of compression arthrodesis, as initially described by Sir John Charnley. The technique described here incorporates a combination of both an intra- and extra-articular arthrodesis, along with rigid internal fixation.

SURGICAL PROCEDURE

The operative procedure is performed with the patient supine on the operating table. A bolster is placed under the ipsilateral buttock. Perioperative antibiotics are administered; general or spinal anesthetic is preferred. The procedure may be performed with or without a proximal thigh tourniquet, although it is easier to perform the initial exposure and cartilage removal in a bloodless field. The leg should be prepped and draped above the knee to optimize visualization of the relationship between the foot and leg.

The lateral ankle is approached through a 6 inch incision over the distal aspect of the fibula, curving gently anteriorly at its tip. The superficial peroneal nerve may be in the operative field and is protected during the remainder of the procedure. By subperiosteal dissection, the distal 4 inches of the fibula is exposed. The fibula is osteotomized approximately 4 inches from its distal end, and the distal fragment is reflected off the interosseous membrane. If possible, retain the most distal attachments of the ankle ligaments. Strip the periosteum off the anterior and posterior aspects of the ankle joint and insert a blunt Hohmann-type retractor to protect the adjacent structures. A lamina spreader is useful to improve visualization of the lateral aspect of the ankle mortise. Remove all the articular cartilage from the distal aspect of the tibia and the talar body, preserving the contours of each. This may be accomplished using osteotomes, gouges, and a power burr.

The medial aspect of the ankle always is approached and performed through a separate 2 inch incision over the medial malleolus; the dissection is carried down to

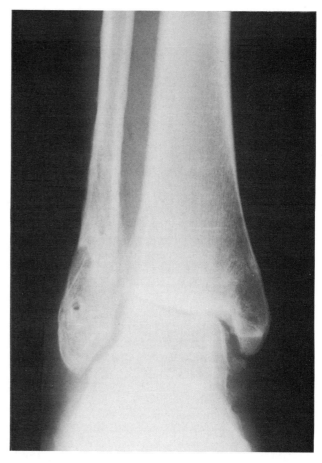

Figure 1 Preoperative weight-bearing anteroposterior (AP) radiograph demonstrating narrowing of the tibiotalar joint.

A

B

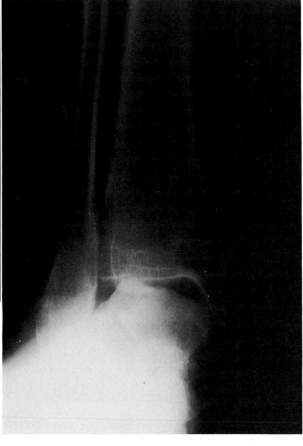

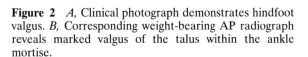

Figure 2 *A,* Clinical photograph demonstrates hindfoot valgus. *B,* Corresponding weight-bearing AP radiograph reveals marked valgus of the talus within the ankle mortise.

bone. All remaining articular cartilage is removed, again preserving the contours of the osseous structures. The malleolus is not removed, functioning as a buttress medially and increasing the surface area of the fusion. After all articular cartilage is removed, small drill holes are placed into the subchondral bone to promote bleeding if the subchondral bone surfaces are sclerotic.

Attention now is directed toward positioning of the ankle for arthrodesis and application of the internal fixation. Buttress the talus against the medial malleolus and place the ankle into the desired position of neutral dorsiflexion, 5° of heel valgus and 10° to 15° of external rotation relative to the knee. The foot also should be translated slightly posteriorly under the tibia. In difficult cases a large smooth Steinmann pin may be inserted retrograde through the calcaneus into the tibia to maintain the desired position temporarily. Since this pin crosses the subtalar joint, it is preferable to avoid using it. In most patients the ankle may be positioned manually as the guide pins are inserted.

The 7.0 mm AO cannulated screw set has proven useful, although other similar systems are available. Noncannulated screws also may be used, although they are technically more difficult to position. Two guide pins are inserted, one from the medial aspect of the tibia into the talar body and one from the posterior-lateral tibia directed toward the talar neck. Pin position is verified using fluoroscopy. After determining the desired screw length, advance the guide pin an additional 1 to 2 cm. This prevents the guide pin from becoming dislodged as the remainder of the cannulated instruments are used. The pilot holes are drilled and tapped, and the cannulated screws are inserted. After the screws are inserted, the talus should be fixed firmly to the distal aspect of the tibia, with the foot in the desired position. Screw position is verified using fluoroscopy or plain radiographs.

This completes the intra-articular portion of the arthrodesis. The addition of an extra-articular, tibiofibulotalar arthrodesis adds stability and provides additional means for fusion to occur. Returning to the lateral incision, the fibula is split longitudinally in the sagittal plane using an oscillating saw. The inner portion is morcellized and retained for use as autogenous bone graft. The outer fragment is used as an onlay graft. The lateral aspect of the tibia is roughened using a burr, and any remaining articular cartilage is removed from the lateral aspect of the talus. The fibula is contoured to match the surface of the tibia and talus. The fibular graft then is secured to the tibia and talus, using a 4.5 mm cortical screw to the tibia and an 4.0 mm malleolar screw to the talus. A 1 cm section of the proximal aspect of the distal fibula may be removed, leaving a gap between the proximal segment and the distal fragment to prevent the formation of a painful fibrous union. Permanent radiographs are obtained to document final hardware position.

If the tourniquet has not already been deflated, it is released before inserting the morcellized graft. The morcellized fibular graft is packed into any remaining gaps. Generally graft is used in the medial gutter and laterally at the tibiofibulotalar area. Suction drains are inserted, and the wounds are closed in layers. A short-leg, posterior, molded splint is applied.

Occasionally minor variations in this technique are necessary. If there is a prominence of the medial malleolus, the malleolus may impinge on the shoe counter. In this situation contour the medial malleolus by osteotomizing its distal portion and use this fragment as additional cancellous bone graft. The described technique allows for correction of moderate equinus deformities. Mild amounts of varus or valgus may be corrected by removing appropriate wedges of bone from the distal aspect of the tibia or the talar body. More severe deformities may require additional wedge resections and may not be suitable for this technique.

POSTOPERATIVE COURSE

The immediate postoperative splint remains in place for 2 weeks. The splint and sutures are removed at 2 weeks and a short-leg cast is applied. The patient remains non–weight bearing for an additional 4 weeks. If healing is demonstrated radiographically, a weight-bearing cast is applied at 6 weeks. A walking heel is placed directly in line with the long axis of the tibia, allowing weight bearing with a direct axial load across the ankle. Progressive weight bearing is encouraged for an additional 6 weeks. The cast is removed when adequate healing is demonstrated radiographically, usually between 3 and 4 months (Fig. 3). Progressive activities then are permitted.

Patients demonstrate improvement for 3 to 4 months following cast removal and generally plateau after 6 to 12 months. Following arthrodesis, the extremity is shortened 0.5 to 1.5 cm. Approximately 30° of plantar flexion is retained, which occurs primarily through the subtalar and transverse tarsal joints (Fig. 4*A* and *B*). Approximately 25 to 50 percent of hindfoot motion is lost postoperatively. Most patients tolerate normal shoe wear. Women note that there is limitation in the available heel heights. Shoe modifications most frequently are required following a combined ankle and subtalar or pantalar fusion. If patients do not tolerate normal shoe wear, a shoe incorporating a SACH heel and rocker bottom usually relieves their symptoms.

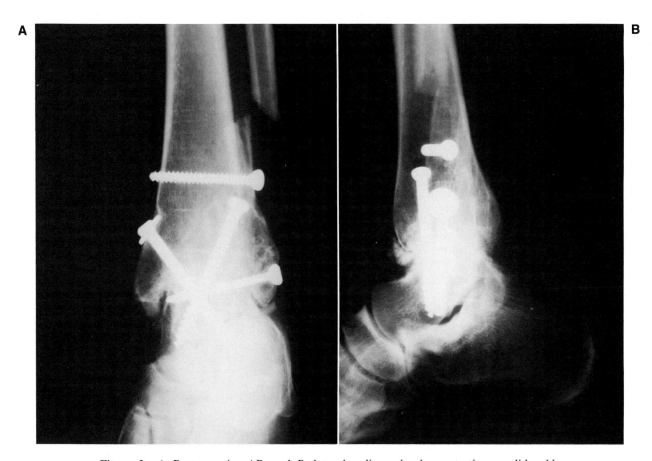

A   B

Figure 3 *A,* Postoperative AP, and *B,* lateral radiographs demonstrating a solid ankle arthrodesis.

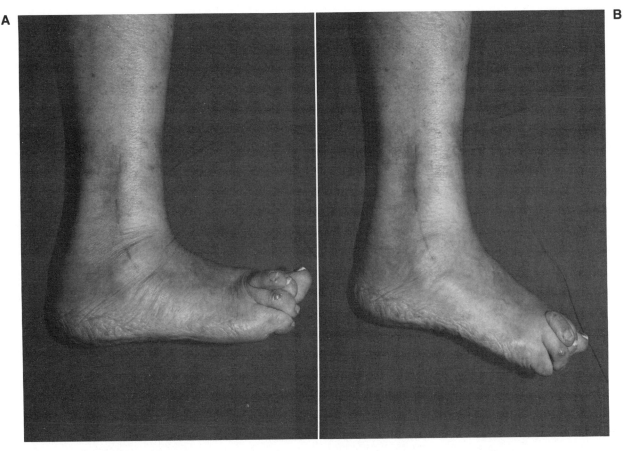

Figure 4 Clinical photographs taken after solid ankle arthrodesis documenting residual dorsiflexion *(A)* and plantar flexion *(B),* occurring through the hindfoot.

COMPLICATIONS AND SEQUELAE AND THEIR TREATMENT

Few complications are unique to an ankle fusion. The most common complications include malunion, delayed union, and nonunion. Minor malunions may be accommodated by shoe modifications and are reasonably well tolerated. Extreme equinus is tolerated poorly, and a secondary osteotomy may be necessary to produce a plantigrade foot. Delayed unions may responded to prolonged cast immobilization or a bone stimulator. Established nonunions require additional operative intervention with rigid compression arthrodesis and bone grafting with autogenous cancellous graft.

SUGGESTED READING

Cracchiolo AC. Methods and follow-up statistics on ankle arthrodesis. Clin Ortho 1991; 268:2–111.

Mann RA. Major surgical procedures for disorders of the ankle, tarsus, and midtarsus. In: Mann RA, ed. Surgery of the foot. 5th ed. St. Louis: Mosby–Year Book, 1986.

Ouzounian TJ, Kleiger B. Arthrodesing procedures. In: Jahss MH, ed. Disorders of the foot and ankle: Medical and surgical management. 2nd ed. Philadelphia: WB Saunders, 1991.

ANKLE ARTHRITIS

CECIL A. CASS, F.R.C.S.

When established arthritis causes painful impairment of function at work, during leisure activity, together with nocturnal rest pain, and there is no consistent improvement with adequate conservative measures, surgical intervention is indicated.

In some patients debridement of the joint surfaces and margins either by arthrotomy or arthroscopy can be effective initially. Long-term improved function with debridement is related directly to the degree of arthritic change, mechanical stability, and work load placed on the ankle joint by occupation and sporting activities. Following arthroscopic debridement in the active middle-aged patient, a return of the symptoms is common and unfortunately occurs in a relatively short time.

The alternatives of arthroplasty and fusion offer better long-term improvement, although arthroplasty of the ankle does not have results as consistently effective as in the knee and hip. The arthroplasty of choice must not remove excessive cancellous bone from the tibial plafond or talus, because this can cause technical difficulties if arthrodesis is necessary at a later stage.

Where excessive bone loss occurs, particularly from the talus, a tibiocalcaneal fusion is required with iliac bone graft to make up the loss of good bone stock at the fusion site.

ANKLE FUSION

I use a modification of the method described by Goldthwaite. It combines intra- and extra-articular fusion, allowing correction of malalignment and bone loss with ready use of AO fixation for stability.

The recent work of Thordarson and co-workers confirms the value of using the fibula as a lateral fixation strut graft in ankle fusion, in addition to tibiotalar screw fixation.

Any skin or soft tissue deficiency must be treated initially, so there is no tissue tension with risk to primary healing of the ankle. Similarly, any infection of the ankle must be eradicated before fusion is undertaken. If infection is combined with osteomyelitis, it is reasonable to consider alternative techniques.

Preoperative Assessment

Preoperation assessment includes recent ankle radiographs; complete blood cell count and erythrocyte sedimentation rate (ESR); a computed tomographic (CT) scan; and peripheral vascular assessment (in patients over 45 years of age). A CT scan is helpful particularly in patients with combined ankle and subtalar joint pathology. In these patients differential intra-articular block with lidocaine and bupivacaine adds useful information about the contribution of the subtalar joint to the hindfoot and ankle pain.

Operation Method

With the patient supine and the leg under tourniquet control, an anterolateral incision exposes the distal

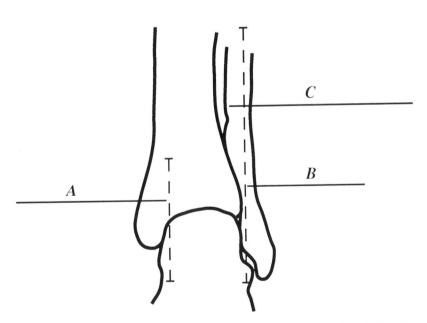

Figure 1 *A,* Anteromedial incision. *B,* Anterolateral incision. *C,* Level of fibular osteotomy.

10 cm of the fibula. It is divided and rotated externally on a posterolateral soft tissue hinge to expose the lateral side of the ankle joint. The medial side of the rotated fibula is cleaned of ligament and soft tissue at the inferior tibiofibular joint, and the bone surface is roughened with a gouge or burr from the tip of the fibula to 3 cm above the ankle joint.

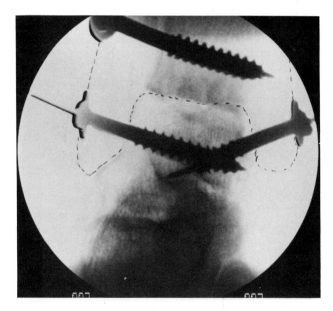

Figure 2 Cannulated 6.5 mm AO screws over guidewires.

The ankle joint surface is debrided to cancellous bone over more than half of both exposed surfaces. A smaller anteromedial incision (Fig. 1) exposes the remainder of the joint surfaces for cartilage debridement, including the articular surface of the medial malleolus. The cancellous surfaces then are carefully shaped to give good bone apposition in the required alignment. The talus is placed in the middle of the plafond surface to ensure more normal weight load transfer to the subtalar joint and the correct heel prominence recommended by Charnley. This position is held by three Kirschner (K-) wires, the first from the medial malleolus directed downward and forward 20° to 30° into the anterior body of the talus near the neck of the talus. This K-wire is inserted with the talus firmly apposed to the prepared medial malleolus and plafond and the ankle in the plantigrade position.

Firm stable fixation to the medial malleolus with the convex body of the talus located in the middle of the concave plafond surface gives virtual anatomic alignment in both anteroposterior (AP) and lateral planes. The plafond surface and width give ample scope to correct severe malalignment by bone preparation and narrowing if required.

The fibula is used as a stabilizing compression strut graft to make the fixation soundly rigid and stable. It is rotated into the prepared osseous bed in the lateral side of the plafond, firmly abutting the tibia and the prepared lateral side of the talus. The fibula is held by two K-wires, one above the ankle joint and another in the posterior half of the body of the talus, utilizing the obliquity of the

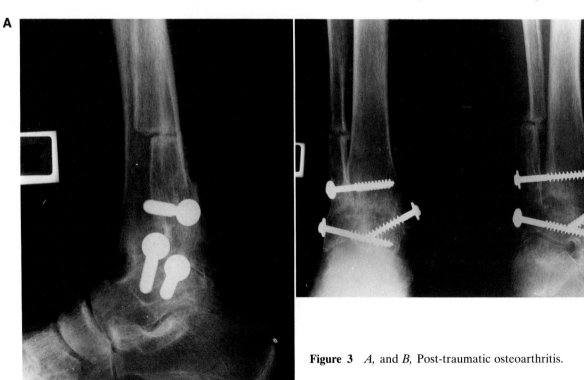

Figure 3 *A,* and *B,* Post-traumatic osteoarthritis.

malleolar axis for the placement of this wire. The position of all three wires is checked with the image intensifier.

If the position of the three K-wires is satisfactory, a cannulated AO drill is passed over the guidewires to the required depth, and the cannulated AO 7.0 mm screws are inserted over the guide pins. The medial malleolus is secured first, the fibular plafond next, and last the fibulotalar screw and washer are inserted to complete the fixation (Figs. 2 and 3). Any space in the fusion site is filled with cancellous bone graft usually obtained locally. The operative site is drained for 24 hours.

The use of cannulated AO screws over the initial stabilizing K-wires facilitates the screw and washer fixation. The preferred angle for fusion of the ankle is neutral dorsoplantar flexion, the heel in 3° to 5° of valgus, and comparable external rotation.

Postoperative Management

The postoperative immobilization is an incomplete three-slab below-knee cast until the swelling settles, and then a definitive below-knee cast for 3 months. Partial weight bearing commences after 2 months when radiographs confirm bone union is progressing satisfactorily.

Results

This method of ankle fusion gives reliable results when care is taken to prepare bone surfaces adequately and place fixation screws properly. Postoperative cast immobilization with graduated weight bearing up until 3 months is necessary.

SUGGESTED READING

Charnley J. Compression arthrodesis of the ankle and shoulder. J Bone Joint Surg 1951; 33B:180.

Cierny G, et al. Ankle arthrodesis in presence of ongoing sepsis. Orthop Clin North Am 1989; 20:709–721.

Goldthwaite JE. An operation for stiffening of the ankle joint in infantile paralysis. Am J Orth Surg 1908; 5:271.

Schwartz RP. Arthrodesis of subtalus and mid tarsal joints of the foot: Historical review, preoperative determinations and operative procedure. Surgery 1946; 20:619.

Stuart MJ, Morrey BF. Arthrodesis of the diabetic neuropathic ankle. Clin Orthop 1990; 253:209–211.

Thordarson DB, et al. Arthrodesis of the ankle with cancellous bone screws and fibular strut graft. J Bone Joint Surg 1990; 72A: 1359–1363.

Wagner H, Puck HG. Die Vershraubungs-arthrodese de Sprunggelerke. Unfallheilkunde 1982; 85:280.

EXTENDED ARTHRODESIS OF THE ANKLE AND HINDFOOT FOR POST-TRAUMATIC ARTHROSIS

JOHN A. PAPA, M.D.

The treatment of patients with post-traumatic arthrosis is difficult when both the subtalar and ankle joints have been refractory to nonoperative modalities. In addition to debilitating pain, these patients frequently have diffuse stiffness of their entire foot and ankle secondary to former injuries, prolonged immobilization, and previous operations. Further, associated vascular or neurologic compromise may significantly influence the outcome of any salvage procedure. Operative treatment options are limited to either an extended fusion procedure or a Syme or below-knee amputation. Although amputation generally is associated with resolution of pain in the affected extremity and offers patients the ability to walk with only a limited increase in energy expenditure compared to normal, it is not without shortcomings. A prosthesis must be worn for most walking after a Syme amputation and for any ambulation after below-knee amputation. In addition, cosmetic and psychological factors must be considered.

The expected outcome following extended arthrodesis procedures is not well established. Most reports of extended arthrodeses focus on the treatment of paralytic extremities. Reviews that deal with patients with post-traumatic arthrosis are few and generally include only a limited number of such patients. A variety of technical factors regarding extended arthrodesis procedures remain controversial including the benefits of staging, operative approach, type of fixation, and the need for bone graft.

To better define the associated morbidity, and the expected functional results and limitations following extended ankle and hindfoot arthrodesis, a retrospective review was conducted at Union Memorial Hospital. This included 21 patients who had undergone an extended ankle and subtalar arthrodesis between 1986 and 1989 using a standard surgical technique by a single surgeon.

PREFERRED TECHNIQUE

Extended arthrodesis procedures should be reserved for patients who have failed nonoperative management for painful disabling arthrosis and/or deformity involving both the ankle and subtalar joints. Patients who lack protective plantar sensation should not be considered candidates for extended ankle and hindfoot arthrodesis. Physical examination and plain radiographs are the primary determinants in the selection of which joints to include in the fusion. Diagnostic sequential blocks with a local anesthetic, computed tomography, and technetium bone scanning also can be helpful in making this determination.

The operation is performed with the patient in the supine position with a bolster positioned under the ipsilateral buttock. A pneumatic thigh tourniquet is employed, and both the iliac crest and involved extremity are prepped and draped. The extremity is draped free above the knee to allow good visualization for accurate intraoperative assessment of alignment. An extended lateral approach is used, starting proximally in line with the distal fibula and curving distally over the sinus tarsi. If a previous incision exists laterally, this is used. Otherwise, an attempt is made to maintain adequate skin bridges and avoid crossing previous incisions at a right angle. Full-thickness flaps are created. The distal fibula is exposed subperiosteally, osteotomized approximately 7 cm proximal to its tip in an oblique fashion with an oscillating saw, and removed. A second incision is made medially. This is placed directly over the medial malleolus when a tibiotalocalcaneal fusion is to be performed, and just anterior to the medial malleolus and extended dorsally over the talonavicular joint when a pantalar arthrodesis is to be performed. The medial malleolus is osteotomized obliquely with a chisel and removed. The remaining articular surfaces of the tibial plafond and talar dome are removed with an oscillating saw held perpendicular to the long axis of the tibia. Irrigation is used to minimize thermal necrosis, and an effort is made to preserve as much bone stock as possible. Sharp chisels are employed to remove remaining articular cartilage from the subtalar, and when appropriate, calcaneocuboid and talonavicular joints. It should be noted that it is rare to perform an in situ arthrodesis, since the majority of patients requiring this type of operation have significant underlying deformity. Wedges are removed as necessary to allow correction of existing deformities so that a plantigrade foot can be achieved. Equinovarus deformities are managed with a dorsal-lateral biplanar wedge resection from the apex of the deformity, which usually is at the level of the subtalar joint. The final alignment sought is 0° to 5° of hindfoot valgus, 0° to 5° of calcaneus, external rotation equal to the contralateral side, and 0.5 to 1 cm of posterior translation of the talus under the tibia. The position of the midfoot and forefoot are monitored closely regarding the effects of hindfoot wedge resections. In the presence of a rigid midfoot and forefoot, rotational correction and fusion at the level of the transverse tarsal joint usually accompany the correction of hindfoot deformities.

A variety of fixation techniques can be employed. My preference is the 7.0 ml partially threaded, cannulated, cancellous screw system. Alignment and potential screw placement location are verified with intraoperative radiographs after temporary fixation is achieved with 2.0 ml guide pins. Autogenous cancellous bone graft is employed in all cases. The previously removed malleoli usually provide an adequate source of bone graft.

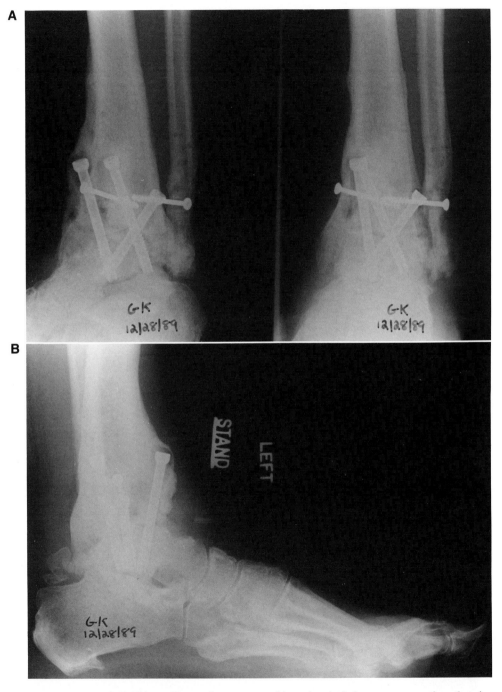

Figure 1 *A* and *B,* This patient underwent an ankle arthrodesis for post-traumatic arthrosis. A pseudoarthrosis is present with collapse and migration of the screws into the subtalar joint.

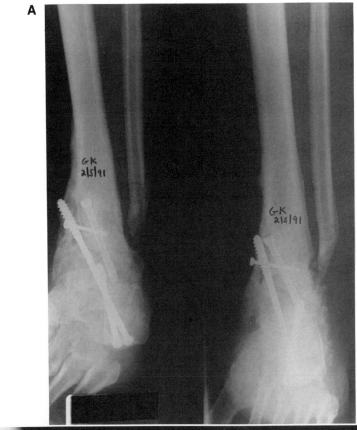

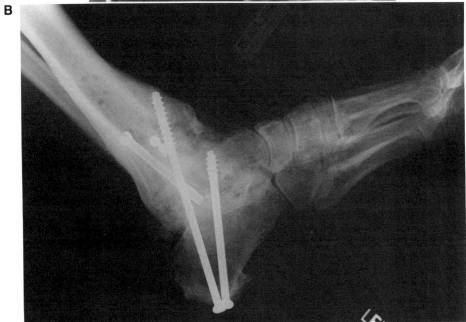

Figure 2 *A* and *B*, Post-traumatic arthrosis was successfully corrected with a tibiotalo-calcaneal arthrodesis.

However, when felt to be insufficient, additional cancellous bone is obtained from the anterior iliac crest. Optimal screw placement is thought to be achieved when screws are directed proximally from the posterior-inferior calcaneus through the body of the talus and into the distal tibia. Purchase on the anterior tibial cortex with at least one screw is sought. Excellent compression generally is achieved across both the tibiotalar and talocalcaneal arthrodesis sites with this technique. Occasionally an additional screw is placed from the distal tibia across the talus into the calcaneus. When performing a pantalar arthrodesis, screw or power staple fixation of the talonavicular and calcaneocuboid arthrodesis sites also is performed.

Wounds are drained and closed in layers. A bulky dressing and plaster splints are applied. Patients are placed in a non–weight-bearing below-knee fiberglass cast 10 to 14 days postoperatively. Weight bearing is begun in a below-knee cast 6 weeks following surgery.

Clinical evaluation, cast changes, and radiographic examinations are repeated at approximately 3 to 4 week intervals until union is noted. Successful fusion is indicated by bony trabeculation across the arthrodesis sites. Walking then is allowed in a shoe with a cushioned heel and rocker sole. Compensation for leg length inequality is provided by a shoe lift selected so that the operated extremity remains approximately 0.5 cm shorter than the contralateral side.

RESULTS OF TREATMENT

Patient satisfaction after an extended arthrodesis usually is high, although few patients are pain-free. Walking and standing endurance generally improve dramatically, and patients rarely require a cane, crutches, or a walker. Many are able to return to occupations requiring standing.

A variety of arthrodesis techniques undoubtedly exist that are capable of producing acceptable results. The single-stage, transfibular, extended lateral approach described, using rigid internal fixation and autogenous bone graft, has proven effective and versatile. Avascular necrosis has not been noted with this technique despite significant soft tissue stripping from the talus. The use of cancellous lag screws crossing both the talocalcaneal and tibiotalar joints has provided rigid fixation and a nonunion rate of less than 15 percent. By engaging the anterior tibial cortex, the compression achieved with screw fixation is enhanced greatly (Figs. 1 and 2).

The technical demands of an extended arthrodesis procedure performed in a single stage should not be underestimated. In contrast to isolated hindfoot or ankle arthrodeses, all local compensatory motion is eliminated by extending the arthrodesis to include both the ankle and hindfoot, except for the small residual present in the midfoot and forefoot. Final alignment therefore is critical. Equinus position is associated with increased forefoot loading, which frequently results in metatarsalgia. In addition, equinus alignment may be associated with the development of genu recurvatum. Therefore no attempt should be made to compensate for leg length inequality by placing the foot in equinus. Equalization of leg length can best be achieved with the use of a shoe lift. Mild calcaneus of up to 5° in these patients is well tolerated without the development of significant heel pain. Varus malunion generally is not well tolerated, particularly in the case of a pantalar fusion, where compensatory pronation at the transverse tarsal joint is not possible. Malunion in varus leads to excess weight bearing on the lateral aspect of the foot, which frequently is associated with callus formation and pain. In the case of tibiotalocalcaneal fusions, varus alignment is associated with increased rigidity at the transverse tarsal joint.

Gait is optimized by mild posterior subluxation of the talus on the tibia and the avoidance of internal rotation. The transverse tarsal joint probably should be spared fusion when possible. The small amount of motion provided at this joint appears to provide an important compensatory function following combined tibiotalar and talocalcaneal fusion. The early development of degenerative arthritis at the talonavicular and calcaneocuboid joints has not been seen after tibiotalocalcaneal fusion.

In summary, an extended ankle and hindfoot arthrodesis is an effective salvage procedure for post-traumatic arthrosis in properly selected patients. Precise final alignment is essential if optimal results are to be achieved following this technically demanding operation.

SUGGESTED READING

Barrett GR, Meyer LC, Bray EW III, et al. Pantalar arthrodesis: A long-term follow-up. Foot Ankle 1981; 1:279–283.

Ouzounian TJ, Kleiger B. Arthrodesis in the foot and ankle. In: Jahss MH, ed. Disorders of the foot and ankle: Medical and surgical management. 2nd ed. Vol. 3. Philadelphia: WB Saunders, 1991:2614.

Papa J, Myerson M. Pantalar and tibiotalocalcaneal arthrodesis for post-traumatic osteoarthrosis of the ankle and hindfoot. J Bone Joint Surg; 74A:1042–1044.

Russotti GM, Johnson KA, Cass JR. Tibiotalocalcaneal arthrodesis for arthritis and deformity of the hind part of the foot. J Bone Joint Surg 1988; 70:1304–1307.

Waugh TR, Wagner J, Stinchfield FE. An evaluation of pantalar arthrodesis: A follow-up study of one hundred and sixteen operations. J Bone Joint Surg 1965; 47:1315–1322.

ARTHRODESIS FOR DIABETIC NEUROARTHROPATHY

MARK MYERSON, M.D.

Neuroarthropathy goes through three predictable stages, and treatment of the extremity depends to a large extent on the phase of activity of the disease. During the initial stages of this disease process, the foot typically is warm and swollen. It is not uncommon for these patients to be treated for cellulitis or even to undergo surgical drainage for presumed deeper infection during this acute inflammatory phase. Although diagnosis of acute neuroarthropathy can be difficult, it is made on the basis of painless swelling associated with warmth of the affected area and various radiographic changes. There is no correlation between the severity or control of the diabetes and the extent of neuropathy and neuroarthropathy. Therefore, in the absence of an obvious source of infection, all patients with or without diabetes who present with a warm, swollen, painless foot should be treated presumptively for a neuroarthropathic process. Radiographs often are helpful, but the typical changes of neuroarthropathy, such as fragmentation and new bone formation, often are not present during the acute stage. Radiographs therefore can be misleading, since little other than soft tissue swelling or subtle subluxation may be seen during this acute stage. It is particularly important to obtain weight-bearing radiographs of the foot and ankle, since those obtained without bearing weight may not identify the extent of the articular disruption.

The pathologic process of neuroarthropathy is not well understood. Clearly the fracture is not always associated with significant trauma, and often a history of even minor trauma is not forthcoming. It is most likely that a combination of events is associated with the onset of acute neuroarthropathy. It is my belief that the basic process may not even be a fracture, but a disruption of the periarticular ligamentous support. This is followed

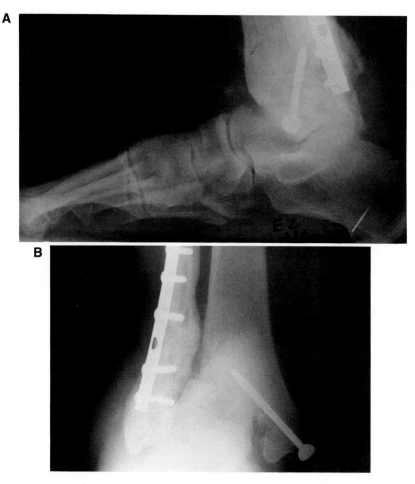

Figure 1 *A* and *B,* This patient began to walk prematurely after open reduction and internal fixation for a bimalleolar ankle fracture.

Continued.

by minor disruption, culminating in the gross fracture or dislocation perpetuated by continued weight bearing. This pathologic sequence is most typical for the tarsometatarsal joints and the midfoot.

The patient with acute neuroarthropathy is at significant risk. Most patients are extremely noncompliant, and without a careful program of education bear weight and complicate the fracture management further. During this initial acute phase, I recommend that the foot be immobilized and the patient kept non–weight bearing for approximately 8 to 12 weeks. Restricted activities and ambulation in these patients is difficult to enforce, because many patients with diabetes are noncompliant and have pre-existing problems with ambulation and balance. Nevertheless, strict non–weight bearing with elevation should be encouraged during the acute inflammatory phase. Ambulation may begin when swelling and warmth subside, best detected by skin thermometers or thermistors.

Once ambulation begins, I use a total-contact cast to control the swelling and keep the patient ambulatory. It is imperative to change the cast frequently during the initial stages of ambulation, since the edema rapidly dissipates with protected ambulation. If the foot is swollen, the first cast change is performed between 2 and 5 days, followed by regular cast changes at 1 to 2 week intervals thereafter. The duration of casting is determined to some extent by the nature and site of the deformity in the foot and ankle, but I prefer to prolong this for approximately 9 to 12 months, following the acute episode. Immobilization is continued until the disease process is quiescent, determined by the absence

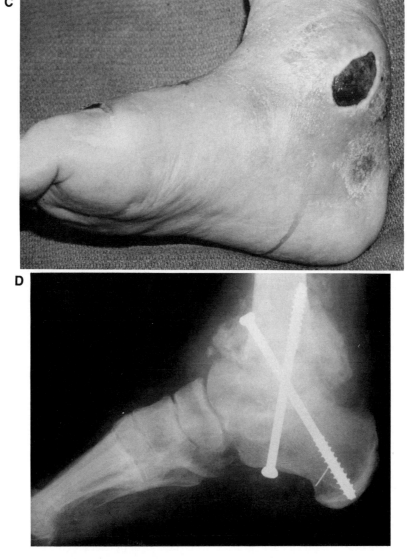

Figure 1, cont'd. *C,* The joint was markedly unstable, and superficial ulceration occurred over the medial malleolus. *D,* This was treated with tibiotalocalcaneal arthrodesis after healing of the ulcer.

of warmth and swelling, and this can be demonstrated clinically and radiographically. Once the neuropathic process has entered a subacute phase, which usually occurs between 2 and 4 months, an alternative to the total-contact cast is a total-contact bivalved cast mold or a Plastizote-lined polypropylene ankle-foot orthosis. Generally deformity in the hindfoot and ankle should be braced permanently with a well-molded AFO. All deformity of the midfoot requires protection with a total-contact molded shoe, or at the least an extra-depth shoe with molded Plastizote inlays.

INDICATIONS FOR ARTHRODESIS

Indications for arthrodesis in the patient with diabetic neuroarthropathy include the following:

1. Acute arthropathy of the hindfoot and ankle that is not amenable to reduction and cast immobilization
2. Acute arthropathy of the midfoot, in which dislocation is present and no bone fragmentation has yet occurred
3. Chronic arthropathy of the hindfoot or ankle associated with recurrent infection, in which bracing has failed or is not feasible
4. Chronic arthropathy of the midfoot associated with recurrent ulceration and infection, in which shoe modifications and brace treatment have repeatedly failed

Despite prompt immobilization and protection, patients may develop significant deformity, some even occurring while immobilized in a cast or brace (Fig. 1). A minority of acute neuropathic dislocations of the hindfoot or ankle are just too unstable for bracing, and reduction of the deformity followed by cast immobilization may not be prudent. This probably is more pertinent to the ankle and hindfoot, where some deformities simply are not amenable to bracing or immobilization (see Fig. 1). Once the hindfoot deviates or drifts into varus or valgus, it becomes increasingly difficult to control. Weight bearing worsens the deformity, and sooner or later ulceration and infection occur. Arthrodesis is indicated in the hindfoot and ankle in both the acute and chronic setting when the deformity is not amenable to bracing.

Enthusiasm for surgery should be tempered by the high incidence of pseudoarthrosis and complications, particularly infection. Surgery for chronic deformity should be performed only during the coalescence or healing phase of neuroarthropathy. We have attempted arthrodesis during various phases of neuroarthropathy, and have learned that surgery should be avoided during the acute stages. During this hyperemic stage, bone fragmentation occurs, and adequate rigid internal fixation usually cannot be achieved. Additionally, the bone tends to be osteopenic and fragments during dissection and attempted realignment.

External fixation is not used routinely because it provides a bacterial pathway and increases the risk of osteomyelitis. External fixation is used, however, when severe focal sepsis is present that cannot be managed adequately by other means (Fig. 2). This is not my preferred method of fixation. There are, however, some patterns of hindfoot and ankle dislocation associated with profound local sepsis and osteomyelitis in which fixation is not easy, but coverage of the wound is impossible without some form of rigid immobilization. I prefer to use rigid internal fixation for the hindfoot and ankle with large cannulated screws, and 3.5 mm cortical, 4.5 mm malleolar, and occasionally 6.5 mm cancellous screws for the midfoot. Occasionally the pattern of dislocation is such that it is not amenable to rigid internal fixation, and under these circumstances, I use large, fully threaded Steinmann pins. These pins may be introduced percutaneously and generally are rigid enough that little motion of the pin-skin interface occurs. They may be left protruding through the skin protected by a povidone-iodine sponge under the cast.

All extremities should be graded according to the Wagner classification for neuropathic ulceration (Table 1). Generally I prefer to restore full epithelialization and to operate only in the presence of healed ulcers. All patients with grade I or II ulcerations therefore are treated with total-contact casting until ulcer healing is obtained. Occasionally severe instability occurs in the presence of ulceration, which precludes the use of casting or bracing before ulcer healing. In these patients a trial of bed rest or strict non–weight bearing may suffice to achieve healing of the ulcer. Alternatively split-thickness skin grafting may be used to obtain coverage, followed by reconstructive surgery as soon as is feasible before breakdown occurs. For the same reason, in rare cases it is necessary to resort to external fixation to achieve stability, and once the wounds have settled down, coverage is obtained and final revision surgery is performed to attempt arthrodesis. Infections in patients with grade III ulcers are treated aggressively with debridement and appropriate antibiotics, and surgery is delayed until the infection is resolved completely and skin coverage obtained.

SURGICAL TECHNIQUE

Prophylactic intravenous antibiotics and a pneumatic tourniquet are used routinely. A standard Kocher-type approach is employed for triple arthrodeses. A transfibular lateral approach is used for all tibiotalar fusions, and extended distally toward the sinus tarsi when tibiocalcaneal, tibiotalocalcaneal, or pantalar arthrodesis is attempted. A limited medial incision frequently is used to allow resection of the medial malleolus and debridement of the talonavicular joint when it is to be included in the fusion. For the midfoot, I use three longitudinal incisions kept 1 inch apart, the first over the dorsal-medial aspect of the first tarsometatarsal joint, the second between the second and third metatarsal, and

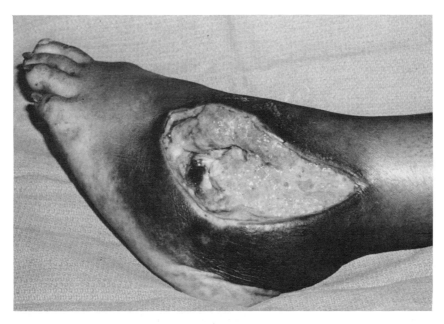

Figure 2 This patient had severe infection associated with osteomyelitis of the talus and acute neuroarthropathy. The primary goal was to attain stability in the absence of infection. The initial treatment consisted of talectomy and external fixation to stabilize the limb, which ultimately healed.

Table 1 The Wagner Classification for Neuropathic Ulceration

Grade	Characteristics of Skin
0	Intact skin
I	Superficial ulceration
II	Ulcers manifested by deep extension to bone, ligament, tendon, joint capsule, or deep fascia without abscess or osteomyelitis
III	Ulcers defined by an abscess, pyarthrosis, or osteomyelitis
IV	Focal gangrene
V	Gangrene of the whole foot

the third between the fourth and fifth metatarsal. I try to preserve full-thickness flaps without protecting local cutaneous sensory nerves. Congruent surfaces are fashioned to allow good bony contact and maximal inherent stability. If the talus is fragmented and avascular, talectomy and tibiocalcaneal fusion are performed. Temporary augmentation with percutaneous threaded Steinmann pins occasionally is performed when the pattern of fracture is not amenable to screw fixation. External fixation is used only when there is an open wound that cannot be controlled or stabilized before the arthrodesis procedure. Final stable rigid internal fixation always is preferable.

I try to position the forefoot plantigrade foot with the ankle in neutral dorsiflexion, 5° to 10° of hindfoot valgus, and external rotation equal to the contralateral side. A copious amount of autogenous bone graft generally is available locally, especially when the malleoli are removed for tibiotalar, tibiotalocalcaneal, tibiocalcaneal, or pantalar fusions. Iliac crest bone graft generally is necessary for midfoot fusions. Meticulous closure in layers is performed over suction drains. A bulky dressing with U and posterior plaster splints is applied. Patients do not bear weight for approximately 3 months and are immobilized in a short-leg cast. This is followed by weight-bearing cast immobilization until radiographic union is present, or in the presence of a pseudoarthrosis, clinical stability has been obtained. Patients then are placed in a polypropylene ankle-foot orthosis indefinitely.

THE HINDFOOT AND ANKLE

As stated earlier, the indications for arthrodesis in the hindfoot and ankle are fairly clear-cut. In chronic neuroarthropathy, surgery is indicated and should be limited to the severely unstable joint that is not amenable to bracing. Included in this group of patients are also those for whom bracing has been attempted, but repeated ulceration occurs. The activity of the neuroarthropathy generally is quiescent by the time severe deformity has occurred, and fragmentation and dislocation of the talus often is present (Fig. 3). Significant thickening of the synovium, multiple fragments, and loose bodies of bone, cartilage, and debris usually are present.

In contrast, surgery also is indicated occasionally during the acute phase of hindfoot neuroarthropathy.

A

B

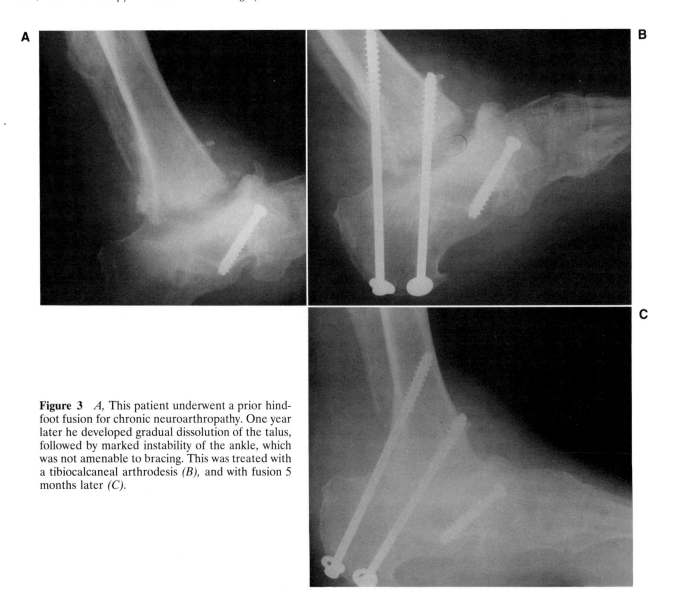

Figure 3 *A,* This patient underwent a prior hind-foot fusion for chronic neuroarthropathy. One year later he developed gradual dissolution of the talus, followed by marked instability of the ankle, which was not amenable to bracing. This was treated with a tibiocalcaneal arthrodesis *(B),* and with fusion 5 months later *(C).*

C

This usually is associated with an acute fracture or dislocation of the ankle, followed by disorderly fragmentation and loss of alignment. In the setting of an acute fracture or dislocation of the hindfoot or ankle that is amenable to open reduction and internal fixation, the standard of care should prevail as it does for patients without neuropathy. I believe that diabetes and neuropathy definitely are not contraindications for internal fixation of acute fractures of the hindfoot, particularly of the ankle. The same judgment and care should be exercised for these patients, recognizing the dire consequences of malreduced fractures, particularly of the ankle. It has been my experience that unless fractures of the ankle are well aligned, deformity and chronic neuroarthropathy predictably ensue. Should one perform an arthrodesis for an acute traumatic ankle fracture? Probably not, since range of motion is far preferable. However, I sacrifice full range of motion in

these patients by immobilizing them for a long period postoperatively until satisfactory healing is evident. Following an acute ankle fracture, patients are kept non–weight bearing for 3 months, followed by protected weight bearing and cast immobilization for a further 3 months or until swelling and all warmth have dissipated. If unprotected weight bearing is resumed prematurely, this may precipitate an acute or chronic arthropathy.

Once the alignment is lost, it has been my experience that continued and perhaps malignant deformity occurs rapidly. In these patients I prefer to perform the arthrodesis early, before inevitable ulceration and infection occur. The same principles apply to any acute dislocation of the hindfoot or tarsal joints, in which the deformity ultimately is going to be difficult to brace (Fig. 4). A good example of this is in the patient with an acute neuroarthropathic dislocation of the navicular. The alternatives to treatment are to follow the course of the

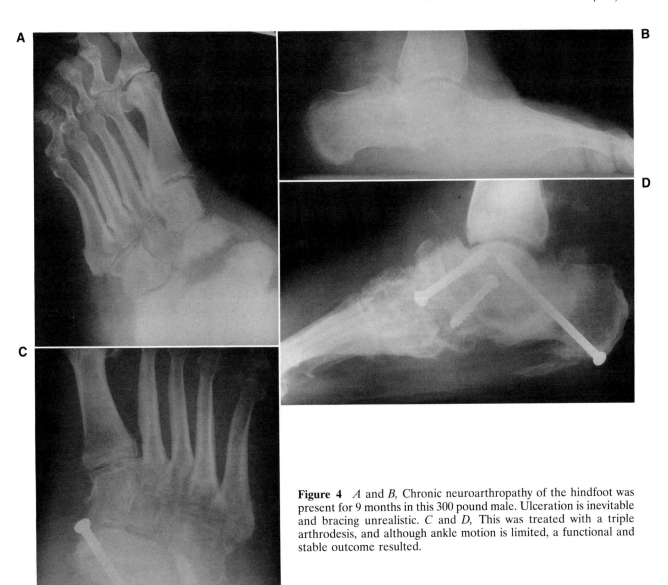

Figure 4 *A* and *B,* Chronic neuroarthropathy of the hindfoot was present for 9 months in this 300 pound male. Ulceration is inevitable and bracing unrealistic. *C* and *D,* This was treated with a triple arthrodesis, and although ankle motion is limited, a functional and stable outcome resulted.

neuroarthropathy with elevation, immobilization, and ultimate bracing in the hope of preventing ulceration. With the deformity, however, it is highly unlikely that the latter can be prevented. Therefore the question arises whether salvage should be performed early or late, once the arthropathy has subsided. Later on either a naviculectomy or an arthrodesis could be performed; the latter is my preference. It is my belief, however, that by waiting, potentially more deformity occurs, and the resulting stresses on the soft tissues may be far more difficult to salvage. Surgery therefore is indicated in acute arthropathy in which the deformity already is severe, or is anticipated to worsen to an extent that would jeopardize the final outcome of surgical salvage.

THE TARSOMETATARSAL JOINT AND MIDFOOT

Unlike the hindfoot and ankle, ostectomy of the midfoot is a reasonable alternative and should be considered when there is recurrent ulceration and deformity refractory to appropriate shoe modifications. However, ostectomy works only where the arthropathy is chronic and the deformity rigid and stable. This is a difficult concept to understand unless one frequently treats this condition. Nevertheless, in many patients, following fragmentation of the tarsometatarsal joints, despite disorderly alignment of the midfoot, the articulation is stable. Bony union often is evident, the midfoot is stiff, and little or no motion occurs across the site of neuroarthropathy. This deformity generally is easy to treat. Bracing usually is not necessary, and we generally use an accommodative shoe with a rocker-bottom sole and the appropriate molded Plastizote orthosis. If recurrent ulceration occurs despite this regimen, ostectomy is indicated, and the offending bone is shaved down whether medial, plantar, or lateral.

This scenario is different from the form of neuroarthropathy in which the articulation is unstable, and motion occurs as a result of an unstable fibrous arthrosis. In these patients ulceration frequently occurs, since the rocker-bottom deformity is extremely difficult to brace: as the forefoot drifts upward and dislocates dorsally, the hindfoot automatically goes into equinus. An Achilles tendon contracture invariably accompanies a rocker-bottom deformity of the midfoot, since the calcaneus is pitched into equinus. Ostectomy is not a good or long-lasting solution in these feet. Although a single bone often can be palpated on the plantar surface of the foot, ostectomy or removal of the bone merely propagates the deformity further.

In these unstable forms of arthropathy of the midfoot, arthrodesis is indicated. This is a most difficult procedure and should not be undertaken unless the surgeon has considerable experience in managing neuroarthropathy. In addition to the surgical principles outlined earlier, the approach must be modified as a result of the chronic dislocation and due care exercised with the bone, which tends to be soft and difficult to secure with any rigid form of fixation. Although I prefer to use rigid internal fixation in the midfoot, I often resort to using large threaded Steinmann pins, which are inserted percutaneously and left protruding through the skin for long periods. Careful bone resection must be performed before the articulation can be reduced. The forefoot gradually is levered down over the midfoot or hindfoot, care being taken not to fragment bone and disrupt the articulation still further. An Achilles tendon lengthening and transfer of the posterior and anterior tibial or peroneal tendons often is required to balance the foot. Iliac crest bone graft generally is necessary for arthrodesis of the midfoot. Unlike salvage of the hindfoot or ankle, a solid arthrodesis of the midfoot is required for success. The articulation is inherently unstable, and despite long-term immobilization, the deformity may recur if a pseudoarthrosis occurs.

Arthrodesis therefore is indicated in chronic neuroarthropathy under the foregoing circumstances. The indications for surgery in the acute setting are less clear. The problem is that of defining the actual onset of arthropathy, since patients rarely are able to give an accurate report of the condition. Arthrodesis is indicated only in documented acute arthropathy before fragmentation of bone has occurred. This indicates that the arthropathy has entered a subacute or chronic phase, in which case it is best to hold off any surgery until the disease is absolutely quiescent. Many neuropathic fractures of the tarsometatarsal joint and midfoot are secondary to the primary pathology, i.e., ligamentous disruption, culminating in the dislocation. During the acute dislocation, before any new bone formation has occurred, the deformity may be treated ideally with arthrodesis. This is extremely controversial but preferable to leaving the foot deformed, which results in inevitable problems at a later date. An arthrodesis, and not open reduction and internal fixation, is the treatment of choice.

My experience with limb salvage by open reduction and arthrodesis in these patients has been satisfying, but extremely challenging. These patients are not compliant, and the perioperative complication rate is high. A Syme or below-knee amputation therefore might be a reasonable alternative in the management of this problem. Ablative surgery eliminates the immediate problem; however, most patients with a Syme or below-knee prosthesis have some limitations in function requiring modifications in life-style. The increased energy requirements of ambulation following amputation are significant, especially in this group of patients who are not infrequently overweight. In addition, the risk that a contralateral amputation will be needed in the future is higher in patients with diabetes than in the general population. Therefore it is my philosophy to attempt limb salvage whenever possible.

SUGGESTED READING

Brower AC, Allman RM. Pathogenesis of the neurotrophic joint: Neurotraumatic vs. neurovascular. Radiology 1981; 139:349–354.

Cleveland M. Surgical fusion of unstable joints due to neuropathic disturbance. Am J Surg 1939; 43:580–584.

Clohisy DR, Thompson RC Jr. Fractures associated with neuropathic arthropathy in adults who have juvenile-onset diabetes. J Bone Joint Surg 1988; 70A:1192–1200.

Harris JR, Brand PW. Patterns of disintegration of the tarsus in the anaesthetic foot. J Bone Joint Surg 1966; 48B:4–16.

Samilson RL, Sankaran B, Bersani FA, Smith AD. Orthopedic management of neuropathic joints. Arch Surg 1959; 78:115–121.

Shibata T, Tada K, Hashizume K, Hashizume C. The results of arthrodesis of the ankle for leprotic neuroarthropathy. J Bone Joint Surg 1990; 72A:749–756.

Stuart MJ, Morrey BF. Arthrodesis of the diabetic neuropathic ankle joint. Clin Orthop 1990; 253:209–211.

TENDONS AND LIGAMENTS

POSTERIOR TIBIAL TENDON INSUFFICIENCY

MARK MYERSON, M.D.

Presentation of posterior tibial tendon (PTT) insufficiency spans a broad range. Early on, patients complain of aching and swelling along the medial foot and ankle. The medial hindfoot, medial ankle, and even distal leg usually are swollen. Tenderness extends along the distal-medial leg, and the PTT is painful to palpation. In the early stage, pain is limited to the medial ankle and medial-plantar midfoot. As the disease progresses, the heel assumes a more valgus position, the midfoot becomes pronated, and the forefoot abducted.

The total excursion of the PTT is 1.5 cm. Any attritional change within the substance of the tendon and any intratendinous tearing or lengthening cause an elongation of the tendon, resulting in tendon insufficiency. As the tendon elongates, it is less able to exert a dynamic pull on the midfoot. As the disease progresses and the hindfoot, midfoot, and forefoot become more deformed, the pain shifts laterally. Typically, no pain is present medially in the late stage, and pain is lateral as a result of a calcaneofibular abutment, periosteal inflammation, peroneal tendinitis, or subtalar synovitis.

The clinical findings in each of these stages are specific. Early on, palpable tenosynovitis is present, and the tendon can be seen and felt to be thickened with underlying edema. The patient is unable to stand on tiptoe, and in doing so, the heel remains in valgus. If the patient is able to stand on tiptoe, a single heel rise test usually is impossible. Toe raises also are painful and difficult to perform and fatigue the tendon. If the patient is able to accomplish these maneuvers, the diagnosis is in doubt. A common diagnostic error is that of a rupture of the spring ligament and talonavicular capsule complex (Fig. 1). The clinical presentation, as well as the

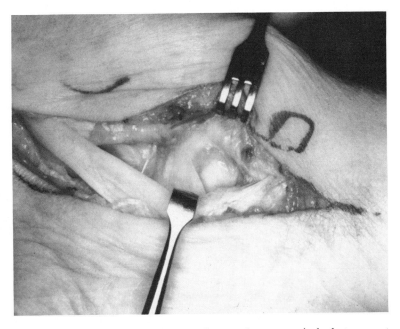

Figure 1 Rupture of the PTT was diagnosed preoperatively, but was not confirmed at surgery, where a tear of the spring ligament and talonavicular complex was found.

⌐s of the foot, are almost identical.
⌐ to try to palpate the PTT
⌐version maneuver.
⌐inversion,
⌐duction,
⌐er of the
⌐ar flexion
⌐o palpate
⌐maneuver,
⌐indicate a
⌐still may be
⌐an intraten-
⌐onally, which

THERAPY

It is important to rule out underlying systemic inflammatory disorders since many younger patients may have a seronegative spondyloarthropathy. The association between psoriasis and posterior tibial tenosynovitis previously has been noted. It is less common for patients with rheumatoid arthritis to have posterior tibial tenosynovitis, although this does occur. In both these patient groups, early tenosynovectomy is important. Patients with psoriatic tenosynovitis develop an aggressive infiltrate in the substance of the tendon, with ultimate erosion and complete attritional tearing of the tendon. Similarly the infiltrative rheumatoid synovitis may cause attritional tearing of the tendon with rapid progression of hindfoot deformity.

A

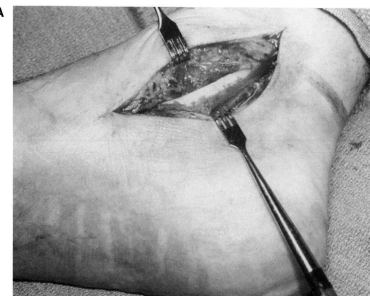

Figure 2 Types of pathology of the PTT are presented. *A,* Tenosynovitis with psoriatic arthropathy. *B,* Infiltrative tenosynovitis.

Continued

B

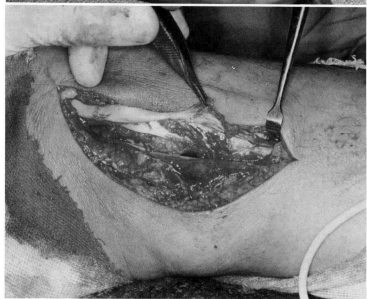

Treatment depends on the age and activity of the patient, the underlying pathologic process, and the extent of deformity. Generally it is useful to initiate conservative treatment in these patients, since many respond to a trial of nonsteroidal anti-inflammatory medication, a ¼ inch medial heel and sole wedge, and a brace or short-leg walking cast for 6 weeks if the symptoms are severe enough.

I believe it is appropriate to be aggressive with surgical treatment with this pathologic condition. The implications of untreated posterior tibial tendinosis are significant. Surgical options are (1) tenosynovectomy, (2) flexor tendon transfer, and (3) arthrodesis.

Although a triple arthrodesis probably is the most reliable of these fusion procedures, an isolated talonavicular fusion, subtalar fusion, or a double ar-

throdesis (talonavicular and calcaneocuboid) also are options that must be considered. Further, a talonavicular arthrodesis or a double arthrodesis can be augmented with a flexor tendon transfer into the cuneiform to add a dynamic component to the procedure. This is helpful particularly when the midfoot collapse is occurring both at the talonavicular and naviculocuneiform joints.

Tenosynovectomy

The indications for tenosynovectomy are tenosynovitis or tendinitis refractory to conservative treatment. Younger patients, particularly those with inflammatory tenosynovitis secondary to a seronegative disorder or those with rheumatoid disease particularly are

C

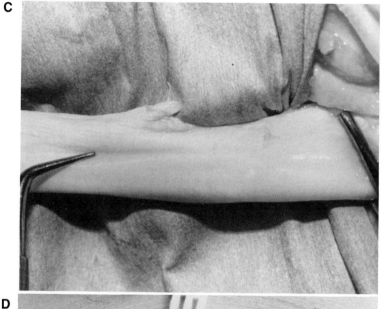

D

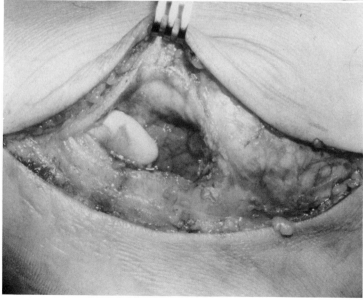

Figure 2, cont'd. *C,* Attritional tearing. *D,* Complete tear.

suited for this operation. Tenosynovectomy seldom is sufficient in older patients with a degenerative rupture. In addition to inflammatory tenosynovitis, intratendinous tearing with tendon elongation already is present.

The procedure is done under a regional anesthetic. The saphenous and deep peroneal nerves, the tibial nerve, and the sheath of the PTT are infiltrated with 0.5 percent bupivacaine with 15 to 20 ml of 1:200,000 epinephrine admixed. An incision is made along the course of the tendon, the flexor retinaculum incised, and the tendon sheath opened. Depending on the underlying pathology, granular or infiltrative synovitis usually is evident (Fig. 2). I find it easiest to use a #15 knife blade to scrape the infiltrative tissue on the surface of the tendon. The undersurface of the tendon sheath also should be cleaned and debrided, which usually is best done with a Metzenbaum scissors. Since this tissue is highly friable, it is prone to bleed; occasionally an ankle tourniquet may be useful temporarily. It is important to rotate the tendon 180° and inspect the posterior surface. This is more of a concern in the older patient who has an attritional tear of the tendon, which usually is on its deeper posterior surface. Superficially, when the tendon lies in the sheath, this tear often is not apparent. Intratendinous tearing also may be visible posteriorly.

Following tenosynovectomy, the wound is irrigated and the tendon sheath and flexor retinaculum closed with absorbable sutures. The tendon sheath is infiltrated with 1 ml of triamcinolone (Kenalog). The adverse sequelae of the injection probably are minimal. The patient remains non–weight bearing for 1 week followed by ambulation in either a brace or a short-leg cast for 5 weeks until swelling and tenderness have resolved. Thereafter, either an Aircast or a shoe with a ¼ inch medial heel and sole wedge is used until the patient is asymptomatic. Patients still benefit from orthotic support of the foot. In the rheumatoid patient we use a softer accommodative-type orthosis. In the younger patient with a seronegative disorder, a biomechanical orthosis made of semirigid materials is used.

Tendon Transfer

I prefer to use the flexor digitorum longus (FDL) tendon, although use of the flexor hallucis longus (FHL) tendon has been described. Tendon transfer is indicated in a patient of normal weight who has a symptomatic flat foot and medial foot and ankle pain only. For tendon transfer to be performed, the foot must be supple with a mobile subtalar and transverse tarsal joint. Any fixed deformity is an indication for an arthrodesis. Once lateral foot pain is present, the tendon transfer cannot be expected to support the foot.

The tendon transfer re-establishes some mechanical support to the foot, which, however, remains in a planovalgus position. It is important to explain this preoperatively to the patient, who may be concerned that the deformity has not been corrected with the transfer.

Obese patients are not suitable for a tendon transfer. In an active female patient who weighs more than 190 pounds, the FDL transfer may not support the foot. To some extent this may not be a function of the tendon transfer itself, but rather the body weight causing further hindfoot drift and lateral impingement.

Radiographs are important to stage the deformity. The PTT has a dominant insertion into the cuneiform, with a major attachment to the navicular and further extension under the first, second, and third metatarsals (Fig. 3). Weight-bearing anteroposterior and lateral radiographs are obtained to determine the pattern of subluxation. Usually the talonavicular joint is subluxed, and the talus collapses plantar and medial with respect to the navicular and first metatarsal. If there is collapse of the naviculocuneiform joint, it may be preferable to transfer the tendon into the cuneiform and not the navicular. Unfortunately the FDL tendon seldom is long enough to transfer through the cuneiform, as is described for the navicular. Other methods, however, are available to attach the tendon to the cuneiform and are discussed subsequently.

The procedure is performed with the patient in the supine position under a regional or general anesthetic. It is important to have adequate relaxation to obtain enough muscle and tendon length for the transfer. A tourniquet is not necessary. An incision is made along the course of the PTT, extending slightly plantarward under the navicular and cuneiform toward the first metatarsal. The flexor retinaculum and tendon sheath are opened and the tendon is inspected (Fig. 4). The FDL tendon lies immediately posterior to the PTT, and it can be approached by incising the sheath of the PTT posteromedially. The PTT now is inspected and its excursion identified. Usually not more than 1 cm of excursion of the tendon is present. If the tendon is stuck down completely with no excursion present, the muscle is not functioning. Under these circumstances, I transect the PTT just proximal to the medial malleolus, and at the completion of the flexor tendon transfer perform a side-to-side tenodesis of the FDL to the PTT. Occasionally, intratendinous tearing with attritional changes are present in the PTT and a Z-step cut shortening of the tendon may be performed if the muscle still is functioning. The step cut is made and the sutures inserted at the completion of the flexor tendon transfer. Although a side-to-side tenodesis of the PTT to the FDL tendon distal to the medial malleolus has been reported. I do not believe that this is a stable construct and invariably fails.

The FDL tendon sheath now is opened and the toes manipulated to ensure that the sheath of the FHL tendon has not been opened inadvertently. The tendon now is exposed on the plantar aspect of the foot under direct vision (Fig. 5). The abductor hallucis muscle is retracted plantarward and the tendon traced to the point at which it overlaps the FHL tendon at the Master knot of Henry. One must be extremely careful not to tear or lacerate the medial-plantar vein, which lies directly under the FDL tendon.

Division of the FDL tendon may be performed slightly more distally by extending the skin incision out

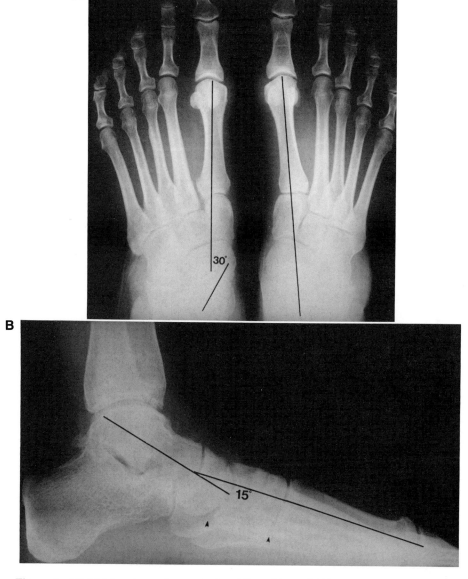

Figure 3 Weight-bearing anteroposterior *(A)* and lateral *(B)* radiographs demonstrate the changes in the talometatarsal angle. Note the subluxation at the naviculocuneiform and tarsometatarsal joints *(arrows).*

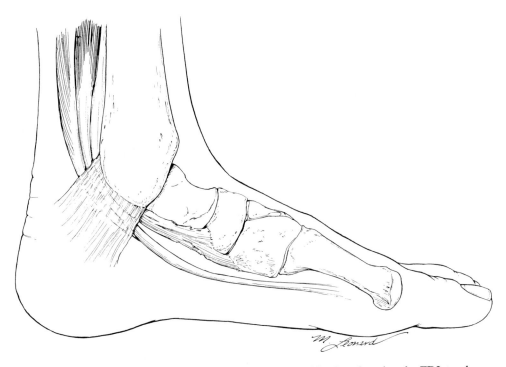

Figure 4 The incision parallels the course of the PTT and lies just dorsal to the FDL tendon.

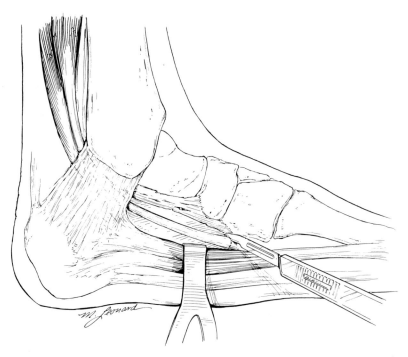

Figure 5 The FDL tendon is retrieved and transected under direct vision in the plantar aspect of the foot.

further along the base of the first metatarsal. Sufficient length, however, always is present provided one cuts the tendon under direct vision just proximal to the division of the tendon into its respective digital branches.

The tendon now is secured with a 2-0 Ethibond whip suture. It is important to insert the suture in such a fashion so as to prevent "bunching up" when the tendon is passed through the bone. A drill hole now is made using a 4.5 mm drill bit in the medial pole of the navicular (Fig. 6). The hole is made from dorsal to plantar approximately 1 cm lateral to the medial tubercle. If the hole is made too medially, the medial wall may subsequently fracture.

A useful technique for passing the tendon from plantar to dorsal is to insert a small suction tip through the drill hole from dorsal to plantar. Clear the soft tissues on the plantar aspect of the foot and insert the suture into the sucker tip. The suture is sucked into it and can be pulled up easily to the dorsum of the foot attached to the tendon. If the tendon begins to bunch on the plantar surface, this can be eased through with a straight hemostat clamp.

The foot now is positioned in maximum inversion with the ankle in approximately 20° of plantar flexion. Before suture of the FDL transfer, a ∪-shaped flap with the base distal is incised into the talonavicular capsule and spring ligament and advanced in a "vest-over-pants" manner. This proximal advancement of the spring ligament complex is an effective and important aspect of the soft tissue procedures (Fig. 7). The tendon then is

sutured back on itself with interrupted 2-0 Ethibond sutures. It also is useful to tack the tendon down to periosteum and other firm soft tissue available in the region (Fig. 8). It is difficult to tighten the flexor tendon transfer too much. Although the FDL muscle initially may not function optimally when stretched maximally, and functions as a tenodesis, the tendon always stretches out and the foot becomes plantigrade shortly after resuming weight bearing. Following the attachment of the tendon transfer, the PTT then is either shortened in a Z-step cut fashion or transected just proximal to the medial malleolus, where it is tenodesed to the FDL tendon with interrupted 2-0 Vicryl sutures.

The foot is immobilized in an equinovarus position in a short-leg cast for 4 weeks. At 4 weeks the foot is positioned in neutral, limited by discomfort on stretching the flexor tendon. By 6 weeks the patient is allowed to commence weight bearing in a short-leg cast, which is changed to either a range-of-motion walker or an Aircast between 8 and 10 weeks. Physical therapy commences with particular emphasis on isokinetic strengthening in plantar flexion and inversion. Semirigid orthoses are used routinely.

A variation of the flexor tendon transfer as described earlier is to insert the tendon into the cuneiform. This is useful when the naviculocuneiform joint is noted to sag considerably on the weight-bearing lateral radiograph. Since the tendon rarely is long enough to be passed through a tunnel in the cuneiform as in the navicular, I attach it to the cuneiform using a screw with

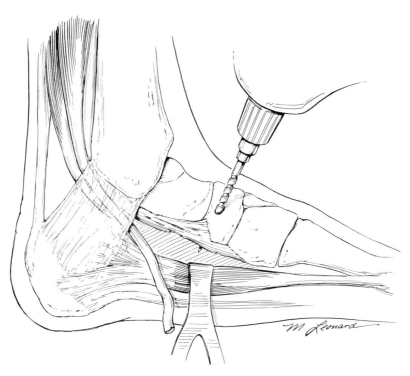

Figure 6 A 4.5 mm drill hole is made from dorsal to plantar in the medial third of the navicular.

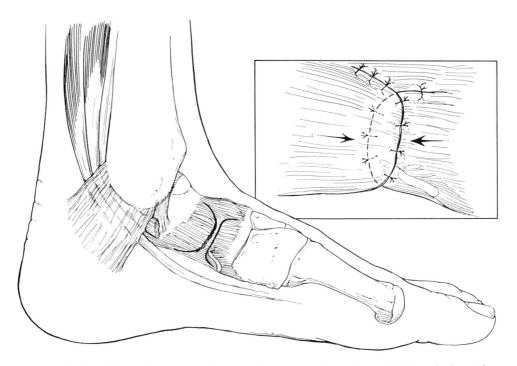

Figure 7 The FDL tendon is passed from plantar to dorsal through the drilled navicular and sutured into adjacent periosteum and, if length permits, back on to itself. The PTT is transected proximal to the medial malleolus and a side-to-side tenodesis to the FDL tendon is performed.

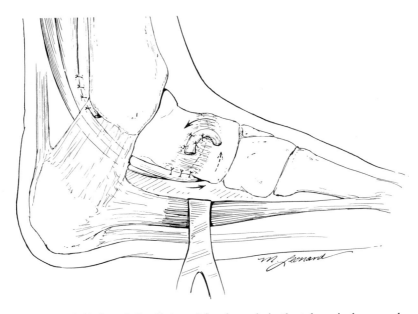

Figure 8 A U-shaped distally based flap is made in the talonavicular capsule and the spring ligament, advanced proximally, and sutured in a vest-over-pants manner.

a spiked ligament washer. The foot is held in an equinovarus position. The bone is predrilled with a 2 mm drill bit. The tendon is pulled distally and is perforated with a #15 blade, and a 20 mm partially threaded 4-0 cancellous screw is inserted through the tendon into the bone. This is highly secure, and the fixation can be augmented with interrupted 0 Ethibond sutures to local periosteal tissue. I use this particular tendon transfer in conjunction with the talonavicular arthrodesis, particularly when naviculocuneiform sag is present.

Talonavicular Arthrodesis

The decision to perform an arthrodesis is determined by the magnitude of the deformity, the presence of lateral foot pain, and obesity. Although re-establishing the medial-longitudinal arch is desirable, this should not be the goal of surgery. Patients who have a hindfoot fusion with the heel left in valgus are asymptomatic. For this reason, one should be cautious when realigning the foot since one easily can overcorrect the hindfoot, causing significant lateral foot pain. Any hindfoot inversion or forefoot supination is poorly tolerated and leads to intractable pain along the plantar-lateral border of the foot. For this reason, it always is preferable to leave the hindfoot in mild valgus.

The indications for a talonavicular fusion are moderate subluxation of the talonavicular joint on the anteroposterior and lateral weight-bearing radiographs (Fig. 9). Although it has been stated that the ideal candidate for this procedure is the elderly patient, I perform this procedure successfully in younger individuals with excellent long-term follow-up. Although the potential for stress transfer to the subtalar and calcaneocuboid joints exists, this should not occur provided the alignment is satisfactory. Therefore it is essential not to overcorrect the talonavicular joint.

An incision is made medial to the anterior tibial tendon, crossing the anteromedial aspect of the foot toward the cuneiform. If the flexor tendon transfer is to be performed simultaneously, the incision is slightly more inferior and extends down toward the cuneiform on the plantar-medial aspect of the foot. It is easy to raise the skin flap on the plantar surface and retrieve the flexor tendon through this incision. The capsule is incised longitudinally and stripped dorsally and medially with sharp dissection.

I find it extremely useful to use a lamina spreader with the teeth shaved off to distract the talonavicular joint. This can be inserted with ease into the irregular contour of the talonavicular joint, and once opened, a regular small lamina spreader with teeth is inserted to hold the joint open while the cartilaginous surface is denuded with sharp fine chisel blades. The joint contour is preserved so that the articulation is repositioned easily.

The foot is adducted and plantar flexed over the head of the talus, and a 2 mm guide pin is inserted slightly inferomedially into the navicular. It is important to insert this off the edge of the naviculocuneiform joint, which otherwise is prone to an erosion from the screw head. Once radiographs confirm adequate alignment, a 7 mm cannulated cancellous screw is inserted over the guide pin. I typically use a 55 mm screw with a short 16 mm thread. Once the arthrodesis is completed, the tendon transfer is performed. It is important at this stage not to overcorrect the forefoot. The flexor tendon is placed at appropriate tension and the forefoot adducted slightly. The tendon is pulled distally on a purse-string suture and then attached to the medial cuneiform by way of a 4-0 cancellous screw and a spiked ligament washer. Patients are kept non–weight bearing for 6 weeks, but commence range-of-motion exercises at approximately 4 weeks, depending on the fixation obtained.

Double Arthrodesis (Talonavicular and Calcaneocuboid)

The indications for a double arthrodesis are lateral foot pain, with or without obesity, a mobile subtalar joint, and moderate deformity. The operation is easy to perform. It is carried out under a regional anesthetic, and although I do not use a tourniquet, the use of an ankle tourniquet is possible. Two incisions are used, one dorsomedial (medial to the anterior tibial tendon) and one over the calcaneocuboid joint just dorsal to the peroneal tendon. If one stays dorsal to the peroneal tendons, the sural nerve is avoided. Each joint is denuded of articular cartilage and a nontoothed lamina spreader is used to distract the joint, facilitating debridement of the articular surface. The contour of the talonavicular joint is preserved.

Once the joints have been debrided, an osteotome should be passed easily from lateral to medial or vice versa across the open joint space. This ensures that adequate rotation of the midfoot occurs. The talonavicular joint is fixed first. It is imperative to position this accurately. The medial border of the talonavicular joint is palpated before inserting the guide pin to ensure that the navicular is not pushed over too far medially, which overcorrects the foot. Intraoperative radiographs are obtained with the guide pins in place to ensure alignment of the talus with the first metatarsal. Cannulated screws are preferred, although power staples are a useful alternative form of fixation (Fig. 10). Postoperatively, the patients commence range-of-motion exercises at approximately 3 weeks and are allowed to start toe touch partial weight bearing at 6 to 8 weeks with full weight bearing usually by 10 weeks.

Triple Arthrodesis

The indications for a triple arthrodesis are moderate-to-severe deformity, particularly associated with a rigid subtalar joint or a fixed valgus heel. In severe cases it is important to assess the mobility of both the ankle and subtalar joint. Even if the subtalar joint is mobile, the range of motion of the ankle should be evaluated with the subtalar joint in the neutral

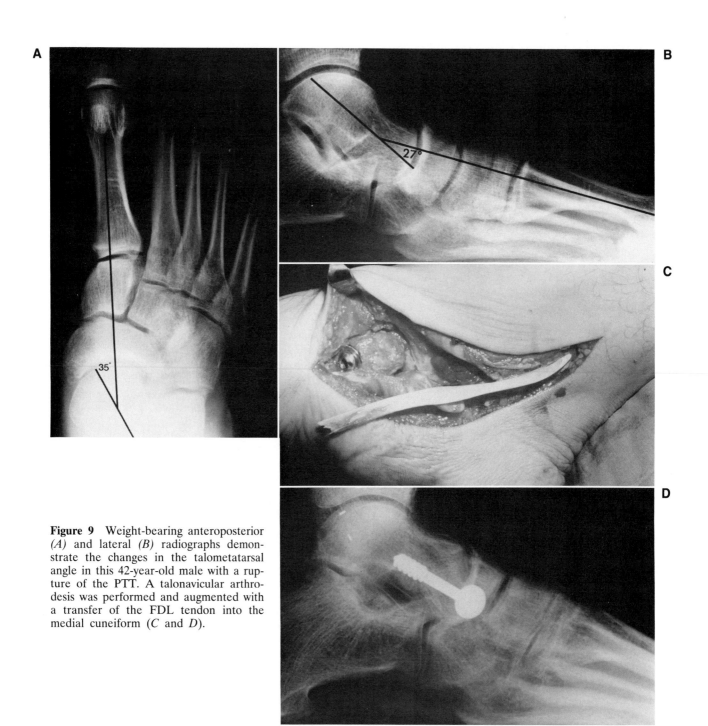

Figure 9 Weight-bearing anteroposterior (A) and lateral (B) radiographs demonstrate the changes in the talometatarsal angle in this 42-year-old male with a rupture of the PTT. A talonavicular arthrodesis was performed and augmented with a transfer of the FDL tendon into the medial cuneiform (C and D).

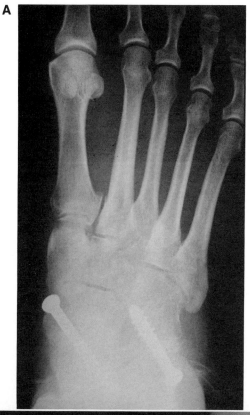

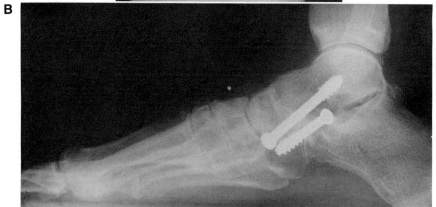

Figure 10 A double arthrodesis performed with cannulated 7.0 mm screws restoring the talometatarsal angle in the AP *(A)* and lateral radiographs *(B)*.

position. If dorsiflexion of the foot is examined with the hindfoot in valgus, a spurious motion occurs through the subtalar and transverse tarsal joints. Once the subtalar joint is locked in the neutral position, an equinus contracture always is evident. Therefore an Achilles tendon lengthening may need to be performed to regain full ankle dorsiflexion. This is performed percutaneously with three stab incisions through the center of the Achilles tendon, and with gentle passive dorsiflexion, the tendon is stretched and elongated. If an Achilles tendon lengthening is not performed, ankle dorsiflexion is limited following correction of the hindfoot valgus. Although this may stretch out, I find that dorsiflexion still is limited, and in the presence of equinus contracture, I gently lengthen the Achilles tendon. In severe cases all the lateral soft tissue structures are contracted, and the peroneal tendons also may require lengthening.

The procedure is performed with the patient supine with a bump under the ipsilateral buttock. Adjunctive bone graft is not necessary. The procedure is performed through two incisions, one dorsomedial, medial to the anterior tibial tendon, and the other lateral paralleling the dorsal surface of the peroneal on the peroneus brevis tendon. If the incision stays dorsal to the peroneal tendons, the sural nerve is protected posteroinferiorly.

It is important to understand that the correction of the hindfoot valgus is attained through translation and rotation of the joints and not through rejection of bone wedges. Only in the most severe cases with fixed valgus deformity and dislocation of the talonavicular joint is bone resection required. I find it useful to transect the calcaneofibular ligament and retract the peroneal tendons inferiorly to visualize the posterior facet. The articular surfaces are denuded of cartilage with fine flexible chisels and the foot gradually brought into correct alignment.

It is important to stabilize the talonavicular joint first. If the subtalar joint is corrected first and brought into neutral, the forefoot automatically supinates and often is locked into this position (Fig. 11). To correct the

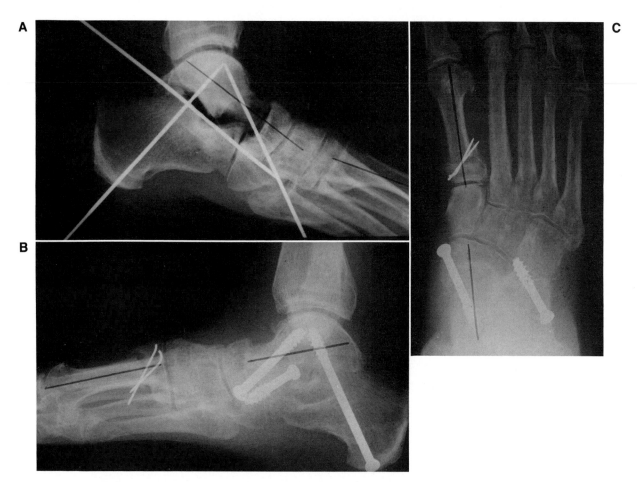

Figure 11 *A,* A severe deformity corrected with a triple arthrodesis. The subtalar joint was fixed first. Intraoperative radiograph demonstrates the position of the guide pins. *B* and *C,* Note the elevated position of the first metatarsal. Correction was obtained with a triple arthrodesis and plantar flexion osteotomy of the first metatarsal.

fixed forefoot supination, the navicular must be forcibly pushed over medially while simultaneously pushing on the talus slightly laterally.

This results in overcorrection of the talonavicular joint. It is therefore preferable to correct the talonavicular joint first followed by the remaining two joints. After stabilizing the talonavicular joint first, the hindfoot may remain in slightly increased valgus, but this is not functionally significant. Stable internal fixation is achieved with 7 mm cannulated screws and the sinus tarsi packed with autogenous bone graft obtained from the talus and calcaneus itself by fish scaling the sinus tarsi.

Following suture removal, the patients are allowed to commence passive range-of-motion exercises followed by toe touch weight bearing at 8 weeks and full weight bearing at 12 weeks.

SUGGESTED READING

Funk DA, Cass JR, Johnson KA: Acquired adult flatfoot secondary to posterior tibial-tendon pathology. J Bone Joint Surg 1986; 68A:95-102.

Jahss MH: Spontaneous rupture of the tibialis posterior tendon: Clinical findings, tenographic studies, and a new technique of repair. Foot Ankle 1982; 3:158-166.

Johnson KA: Tibialis posterior tendon rupture. Clin Orthop 1983; 177:140-147.

Mann RA: Acquired flatfoot in adults. Clin Orthop 1983; 181:46-51.

Mann RA: Rupture of the tibialis posterior tendon. AAOS Course Lectures 1982; 31:302-309.

Mann RA, Thompson FM: Rupture of the posterior tibial tendon causing flat foot. J Bone Joint Surg 1986; 67A:556-561.

Myerson MS, Solomon G, Shereff M: Posterior tibial tendon dysfunction: Its association with seronegative inflammatory disease. Foot Ankle 9(5):219-225.

INJURIES OF PERONEAL TENDONS

G. JAMES SAMMARCO, M.D.

Subtle injuries to the soft tissues of the lateral aspect of the ankle often make diagnosis difficult. In particular, injuries to the peroneal tendons can confuse the signs and symptoms of lateral ankle sprains and lead to misdiagnosis and prolonged disability. The two tendons present on the lateral aspect of the ankle are those of the peroneus longus and the peroneus brevis muscles. The origin of the peroneus brevis muscle is located at the lower two-thirds of the fibula and the anterior and posterior intermuscular septa above the ankle. The muscle belly passes posteriorly in a shallow groove against the surface of the lateral malleolus, where it lies in a common tunnel with the peroneus longus tendon. Beneath and distal to the lateral malleolus, it passes into its own canal above the processus trochlearis on the lateral calcaneus. Below the lateral malleolus it lies superficial to the calcaneofibular ligament and deep to the peroneus longus tendon. It inserts on the styloid process of the fifth metatarsal and functions as an ankle flexor. It also is the strongest evertor of the foot. Variations of the course and insertion of the peroneus brevis occur in 13 percent of cases.

The peroneus longus muscle lies superficial to the peroneus brevis muscle, taking origin from the proximal two-thirds of the fibula, as well as the anterior and posterior intermuscular septa and fasciae. The tendon begins superficial and lateral to the peroneus brevis tendon in the calf, passing posterior to it at the lateral malleolus, where it shares a common peroneal tunnel. Distal to the lateral malleolus, it passes superficial to the calcaneofibular ligament and the peroneus brevis tendon into its own tunnel inferior to the processus trochlearis on the lateral calcaneus. It then turns in a groove beneath the cuboid, where in a third tunnel it passes medially in the third layer of the foot to insert on the first metatarsal and medial cuneiform. It flexes the ankle and flexes the first metatarsal.

Because of the position of the peroneus brevis tendon, it is at risk of injury along with the other lateral ankle structures. This includes acute and chronic tenosynovitis, acute and chronic tears of the tendon, and subluxation and dislocation of the tendon at the lateral malleolus with or without an associated tendon tear. Tendon dislocation can occur because the groove on the posterior surface of the lateral malleolus may be shallow and allows the tendon to be pulled laterally with slight dorsiflexion of the ankle through the tendon insertion on the fifth metatarsal styloid. This may be associated with internal rotation of the leg with respect to the foot. The tendons subluxate anterior to the lateral malleolus and return into their groove when the ankle is plantarflexed.

A shallow groove in the lateral malleolus may predispose the tendons to subluxation.

Inversion of the foot and ankle causes lateral ankle ligament tears and also places the peroneus brevis tendon at risk of injury. Chronic lateral ankle instability places increasing strain on the tendon, usually distal to the lateral malleolus. The tendon acts through muscle contraction as a secondary lateral ankle stabilizer. If instability is present for a considerable period, a tear may occur in this tendon. If pain persists after ankle ligament injury, a peroneus brevis tendon tear should be suspected. The tear occurs distal to the lateral malleolus (Fig. 1). It propagates toward and occasionally proximal to the lateral malleolus. I and others have postulated that compression of the tendon at the lateral malleolus and shearing of the tendon fascicles within the tendon itself distally contribute to tendon degeneration through chronic stress. Chronic lesions of the peroneus brevis tendon also are associated with degenerative arthritis of the subtalar joint and most notably with chronic lesions of other tendons about the ankle joint and tears of the tibialis posterior tendon (Fig. 2). Arthritis of the subtalar joint and posterior tibial tendon dysfunction allow the foot to collapse into valgus, producing stress at the lateral ankle and foot, increasing shear forces within the substance of the tendon, which over a long time create the characteristic longitudinal tear.

Recurrent injury to the lateral ankle ligaments with chronic instability can be associated with tears of the anterior talofibular ligament, fibulocalcaneal ligament, or both. Lateral instability results in recurrent inversion injury and increases the stress on the dynamic evertor muscles of the ankle. These evertors must stabilize the ankle actively in the absence of the passive restraints provided by lateral ligaments. Peroneal muscle strengthening exercises therefore are an essential part of rehabilitation following ankle ligament injury. Instability, which remains for a period of several years, contributes to chronic longitudinal peroneus brevis and occasionally peroneus longus tears. Patients with instability associated with tendon tears were found to have symptoms an average of 8.5 years.

PERONEUS BREVIS TEARS

Symptoms of isolated peroneus brevis tendon tenosynovitis or tears are related specifically to pain at and distal to the lateral malleolus with motion. Pain on inversion of the ankle can occur. Less common is pain over the tendon with rest. Tenderness over the tendon sheath of the inferolateral border of the calcaneus may also be present. Muscle weakness or numbness in the foot usually is not present. Associated conditions also may be present including lateral ankle instability, dislocating peroneal tendons, subtalar joint arthritis and even pain at the medial ankle from posterior-tibial tendon dysfunction. Abduction with plantarflexion of the ankle against resistance may be painful, particularly if acute tenosynovitis is present.

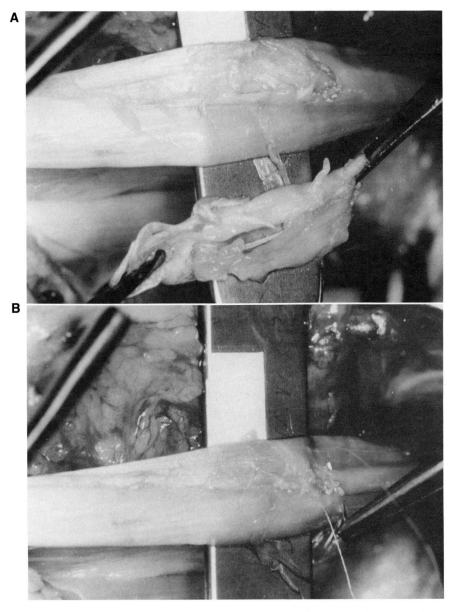

Figure 1 *A*, Operative photograph of the torn peroneus brevis tendon in a 44-year-old man with lateral ankle instability for 15 years. The tear is longitudinal with significant degeneration. The scar tissue has been removed (held with forceps). *B*, Tendon is repaired with a 5-0 Dacron running suture with the knots buried at either end of the tear.

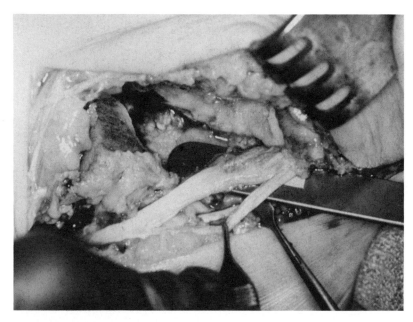

Figure 2 Operative photograph of the lateral ankle in a patient undergoing subtalar arthrodesis for degenerative arthritis. A large tear of the peroneus brevis tendon (forceps) is present. This was repaired with a running suture.

The differential diagnosis includes subluxation of the peroneal tendons, peroneal tendinitis, subtalar arthritis, lateral ankle instability, tear of the peroneus longus tendon at the cuboid, symptomatic anomalous muscle or peroneal muscle, and arthritis of the ankle joint. Stress fracture of the lateral malleolus, talus, or calcaneus also must be ruled out. Radiographic evaluation of the foot and ankle reveals no findings directly attributable to the tendon lesions. No reports of calcification within the torn peroneus brevis tendon have been published, and the sesamoid, which occurs infrequently in the peroneus brevis tendon at the lateral malleolus, would not retract since the tendon rarely ruptures completely. Such migration of an accessory sesamoid has been found in tears of the peroneus longus tendon in diabetics, recreational athletes, and industrial workers if the rupture occurs through or distal to the os peroneum.

Additional diagnostic tests include radiographs of stress testing the ankle in both the coronal and sagittal planes to confirm the existence of ankle laxity. Anterior displacement of the talus from the ankle joint or talar tilt indicates that the underlying problem may be ankle instability rather than an isolated tendon tear. Magnetic resonance imaging (MRI) may be obtained to determine if a significant tear is present or fluid has accumulated within the tendon sheath. A bone scan may be necessary to rule out stress fracture.

Treatment of peroneus brevis tenosynovitis includes immobilization with a brace (ROM walker or Bledsoe foot-ankle orthosis) for 3 weeks and nonsteroidal anti-inflammatory medication. This is followed by rehabilitation therapy including a power-building and flexibility program. A removable ankle orthosis (Aircast) is recommended when resuming increased activity. A shoe may be worn with this brace.

Surgical treatment of a peroneus brevis tendon tear includes repair of the tendon with synovectomy if tenosynovitis is present. This is performed through a 5 cm lateral incision directly over the tendon. Care is taken to avoid injuring the sural nerve. The tendon sheath is opened and debrided. Since most tears are chronic but complete rupture is rare, end-to-end anastomosis, tendon grafting, and tenosynovectomy seldom are necessary. More often findings on surgical specimens reveal degeneration and separation of tendon fibers. Pathologic specimens reveal microscopic findings of chronic infiltration with lymphocytes into the tendon. Treatment is by direct repair of the longitudinal tear using a nonabsorbable braided 4-0 polyester suture with a "swedged-on" tapered needle so as not to cut the remaining fibers of the tendon. A running suture is used, and the knots are buried on either end of the tear.

Underlying problems that may have contributed to the development of the tear should be addressed, e.g., symptomatic osteoarthritis, traumatic subtalar arthritis, or lateral ankle ligament instability. Such procedures as ankle ligament reconstruction, ankle arthroplasty, subtalar arthrodesis and repair of other involved tendons should be performed when indicated. In high-demand ankles, such as observed in high-performance athletes and those who perform contact sports and heavy labor, a modified Elmslie or Christman-Snook procedure may be necessary. The Winfield modification of the Elmslie procedure incorporates the use of half of the peroneus brevis tendon harvested proximally and left attached distally. In patients with lateral ankle instability associated with a tear of the peroneus brevis tendon, the tendon still can be used as a tendon graft. The remaining portion of the tendon then is repaired. The tendon sheath is not closed. If a tear of the peroneus brevis tendon is encountered during reconstruction for recurrent dislocation of the peroneal tendons, repair of the tendon as described earlier is necessary to ensure complete relief of symptoms.

When tendon repair is performed without additional procedures, the patient is immobilized in a cast for a period of 3 weeks followed by range-of-motion exercises in a removable cast boot (ROM walker or Bledsoe). If additional procedures are performed at the same time, such as reconstruction of dislocating peroneal tendons or lateral ankle ligament reconstruction, cast immobilization is maintained for 3 weeks followed by a cast boot for an additional 3 weeks. During this time, gradually increasing the range of motion on the ankle gatch from 10° to 20° is permitted. A rehabilitation program including peroneal strengthening exercises, flexibility, and power building monitored by the Cybex also is prescribed. This is important particularly in high-performance athletes.

Recurrence of the peroneus brevis tears has not been encountered following surgical repair. Observation of the remaining half of the peroneus brevis tendon following removal of half the tendon for graft during a modified Elmslie procedure revealed that no loss of size or additional tears occurred. Rather the repair remained intact, and the tendon hypertrophied over a period of years as described by Snook and others in the few patients in whom the tendon was observed during surgery for other reasons, i.e., reinjury of the ankle.

PERONEUS LONGUS TEARS

Tear of the peroneus longus tendon also occurs and can be confused with peroneus brevis tear caused by the proximity of the two tendons. The peroneus longus tear however, occurs within the tendon sheath inferior and distal to the processus trochlearis of the lateral calcaneus. It may be chronic and longitudinal as are those of the peroneus brevis. Acute avulsion of part or all of the os peroneum also can occur. Chronic symptoms, including pain with walking and running, occur most commonly where the tendon turns beneath the cuboid (Fig. 3). If an acute complete rupture occurs from trauma, a feeling of sudden calf pain and weakness suddenly occur with swelling and tenderness along the lateral calcaneus up to the lateral malleolus. If the os peroneum becomes scarred in its canal beneath the cuboid, pain and disability are compounded by loss of function with failure of the peroneus longus muscle to function as a flexor of the first metatarsal head.

Radiographs reveal no significant findings if the tear is partial and restricted to the tendon. If complete rupture occurs through or distal to an os peroneum (the accessory sesamoid commonly found in the tendon), as

retraction of the tendon occurs, the sesamoid is pulled proximally up the side of the calcaneus toward the lateral malleolus. In cases of mild symptoms, an ankle brace and nonsteroidal anti-inflammatory medication are recommended. Corticosteroid injections are not recommended.

Persistent, debilitating symptoms with or without collapse of the longitudinal arch are indications for surgical repair. Repair of the tendon tear, which is longitudinal, is performed through a lateral incision over the lateral border of the calcaneus and cuboid. Care is taken to prevent injury to the sural nerve. A running 4-0 braided polyester suture with a swedged-on needle is used to repair the tendon. The suture knots are buried at either end of the tear. If complete rupture has occurred with retraction and adhesions of the proximal tendon, excision of the proximal stump and suture of the remaining tendon to the peroneus brevis tendon have been suggested. Partial rupture of the tendon with fibrous ankylosis of the os peroneum within its tunnel beneath the cuboid requires excision of the sesamoid and repair or grafting of the remaining tendon to restore function.

Postoperative care includes immobilization in a cast for 3 weeks followed by a removable cast brace (ROM walker or Bledsoe) with an ankle gatch to allow increasing the range of motion from 0° to 20° in plantar flexion and dorsiflexion. Patients are prescribed a home foot and ankle conditioning program. The long-term outcome in patients with partial tears is good. Those with complete rupture may develop problems of pronation with dorsal bunion if it is allowed to remain uncorrected surgically.

PERONEAL TENDON DISLOCATION

Chronic dislocation of the peroneal tendons at the lateral malleolus with or without tear of the peroneus brevis tendon can be disabling. Acute dislocation may be associated with sports activities and occurs in young individuals. Diagnosis is made by palpating a tender lateral malleolus while moving the ankle. Radiographs of the ankle may reveal a small fleck of bone at the posterolateral border of the peroneal groove, where the retinaculum has been torn from the lateral malleolus. If the tendons cannot be held reduced by cast immobilization, operative repair with reattachment of the peroneal retinaculum to the lateral malleolus is recommended.

Chronic recurrent peroneal tendon dislocation is treated by deepening the peroneal groove at the lateral malleolus with a burr. An incision is made laterally at the malleolus. The groove should be deepened enough so that the tendons do not subluxate when the ankle is put through a range of motion during the operation. Care is taken to avoid removing articular surface of the lateral malleolus. Since the lateral malleolar attachment of the peroneal retinaculum has been lost, the retinaculum is reattached to the bone with a 2-0 Dacron suture.

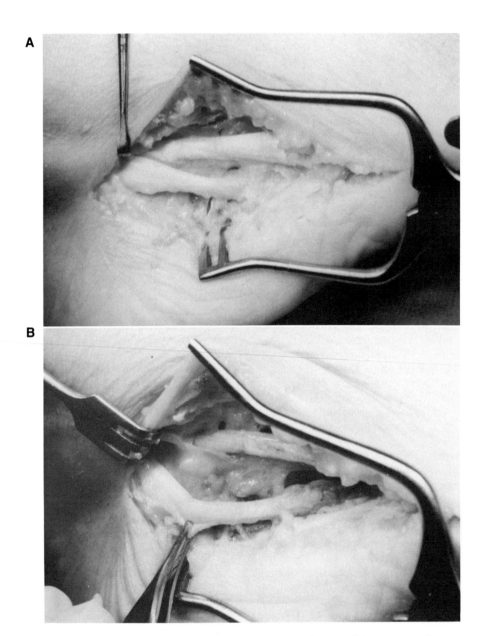

Figure 3 *A,* Operative photograph showing a chronic tear of the peroneus longus tendon. The tendon is partially avulsed from the os peroneum and is somewhat narrowed proximal to its insertion onto the os peroneus. *B,* The tear and associated tendinitis at the os peroneum is visible.

Another option is to reattach the retinaculum with a Mitek suture anchored into the edge of the fibula. Postoperative rehabilitation includes early range of motion in a gatched walker boot (ROM walker or Bledsoe), increasing ankle motion from 0° to 10° dorsiflexion per 10° of plantarflexion 2 weeks postoperatively to 20° of dorsiflexion per 20° of plantarflexion at 3 weeks postoperatively. An ankle splint (Aircast) is used for an additional month along with a foot and ankle rehabilitation program.

SUGGESTED READING

Arrowsmith SR, Fleming LL, Allman FL. Traumatic dislocations of peroneal tendons. Am J Sports Med 1983; 11:142–146.

Elmslie RC. Recurrent subluxation of the ankle joint. Ann Surg 1935; 100:364–367.

Evans JD. Subcutaneous rupture of the tendon of the peroneus longus: Report of a case. J Bone Joint Surg 1966; 48B:507–509.

Munk RL, Davis PH. Longitudinal rupture of the peroneus brevis tendon. J Trauma 1976; 16:803–806.

Parvin RW, Fort LT. Stenosing tenosynovitis of the common peroneal tendon sheath. J Bone Joint Surg 1956; 38A:1352–1357.

Peacock KC, Resnick EJ, Thoder JJ. Rupture of the peroneus longus tendon: Report of three cases. J Bone Joint Surg 1990; 72A:306–307.

Sammarco GJ, Brainard BJ. A symptomatic anomalous peroneus brevis in a high-jumper: A case report. J Bone Joint Surg 1991; 73A:131–133.

Sammarco GJ, DiRaimondo CV. Surgical treatment of lateral ankle instability. Am J Sports Med 1988; 16:501–511.

Sammarco GJ, DiRaimondo CV. Chronic peroneus brevis tendon lesions. Foot Ankle 1989; 9:163–170.

Snook GA, Chrisman OD, Wilson TC. Long-term results of the Chrisman-Snook operation for reconstruction of the lateral ligaments of the ankle. J Bone Joint Surg 1985; 67A:1–7.

Thompson FM, Patterson AH. Rupture of the peroneus longus tendon: Report of three cases. J Bone Joint Surg 1989; 71A:293–295.

Winfield P. Treatment of undue mobility of the ankle joint following severe sprains with avulsion of the anterior and middle bands of the external ligaments. Acta Chir Scand 1953; 105:299–304.

DISORDERS OF THE ACHILLES TENDON

BERT MANDELBAUM, M.D.

The Achilles tendon, as a consequence of its structure and functional demands, is extremely susceptible to acute and chronic injury. Chronic, repetitive, excessive loads may cause tendinitis, and acute rapid loading rates cause rupture of the tendon. These disorders generally have multifactorial etiologies that may be divided in terms of intrinsic and extrinsic factors. This chapter describes the anatomic, structural, and functional aspects of chronic tendinitis and Achilles tendon ruptures and their management.

ANATOMY

The triceps surae include two heads of the gastrocnemius and the soleus muscle. The origin of the muscle is in the distal femur at the femoral condyles and extends into the medial aspect of the calcaneus. This particular tendon is the strongest and largest in the body. It has extreme functional importance in being subjected to the highest of forces and loads. The medial head is clearly the largest and, according to electromyography (EMG) studies, the most active during running. By virtue of its not crossing the knee joint, the soleus muscle is most subject to immediate atrophy with undertraining and/or immobilization. Physiologically, 80 percent of the muscle fibers in the soleus are type I and therefore have a significant potential for atrophic change. There is no synovial sheath around the Achilles tendon, only a peritenon. Microvascular studies indicate a relative area of avascularity just proximal to the insertion into the calcaneus. As a consequence, this area is most susceptible to tendinitis and rupture.

CHRONIC ACHILLES TENDINITIS

Achilles tendinitis is one of the most common injuries in sports. It usually occurs in athletes who spend their time running and jumping. Epidemiologic studies indicate that Achilles tendon injuries constitute 10 to 15 percent of all running injuries. Intrinsic factors leading to Achilles tendinitis include change in duration, intensity, and frequency of running. Extrinsic factors include athletic shoes that may have an inadequate heel wedge or a soft heel counter that does not stabilize the heel. Other structural predisposing factors include tibia vara, tiny hamstrings, and any hindfoot or forefoot deformity. The response to tendon injury is a systemic inflammatory one. As a consequence of Wolff's law of transformation, collagen fiber orientation and response react to the concentration of these forces. It appears the collagen fibers orient and align resisting tensile forces.

Achilles tendinitis occurs with an imbalance of intrinsic and extrinsic factors. Subjectively, athletes complain of pain that localizes to the Achilles tendon. This may be associated with decreased range of motion, swelling, and weakness. Physical examination indicates pain, swelling, decreased range of motion, and in certain cases, a nodular appearance to the distal tendon. It is imperative to define the intrinsic and extrinsic factors that may have a role in causing this process.

Therapy

Initial management includes rest, ice, and nonsteroidal anti-inflammatory drugs. For athletes within the season, it is imperative to have a relative "rest period," including decrease in the duration, intensity, and frequency of training. If there are abnormal structural problems, these may have to be palliated, and clearly the extrinsic factors must be adjusted.

Chronic Achilles tendinitis occurs when this situation is refractory to the usual initial managements. Nodules result, which are mucoid degeneration with fissuring in the tendon. There also is thickening in the peritenon, and it appears as though there is a relative avascularity in the area proximal to the insertion of the calcaneus. The first step in management is a period of relative rest from activity and physical therapy with various modalities.

If all steps are fruitless and the patient continues to have chronic Achilles tendinitis, the next approach is surgical intervention. Surgical intervention is done under a local anesthetic in the outpatient setting. An incision is made over the medial aspect of the Achilles tendon, splitting the peritenon and fish mouthing the tendon. All degenerative mucinous material is excised. Incisions are to be made only in a longitudinal fashion and/or a fish mouth. The patient is kept partial weight bearing for 36 weeks and mobilized gingerly as soon as possible. It is imperative to do this to further activate the gastrocnemius-soleus complex. This particular subsequent physical therapy is required to achieve maximal functional performance results. Preventive measures include strict attention to details of progressive training, as well as specific understanding of the intrinsic and extrinsic factors essential to minimize the probability of recurrence.

ACUTE ACHILLES TENDON RUPTURES

Acute Achilles tendon ruptures usually occur in the mesomorphic male over 30 years of age and also in elderly persons who have been given corticosteroid injections. They occur with rapid loading as the foot and ankle is in dorsiflexion, and the knee is extended with a contracted soleus muscle. At 8 percent strain, the tendon fails and breaks the collagen cross-links. The patient instantaneously feels a pop and feels as though he has been hit from behind. Pain is not the initial response, but the patient describes not being able to run. Individuals should receive immediate orthopedic care. The subject's complaints include pain and an inability to walk on the affected extremity. Physical examination includes palpation of a defect somewhere in the line of the gastrocnemius-soleus complex into the calcaneus. Thompson's test, performed by squeezing the gastrocnemius, indicates discontinuity and lack of a plantar flexor response.

Therapy

The various treatment options are described for the patient. The nonoperative option, which carries a higher risk of rerupture and a lower performance rate, is not recommended for active, athletic individuals. This is reserved for individuals who are not interested in functional performance and high levels of activity.

The surgical option is called the active range-of-motion (AROM) protocol to achieve the highest level of functional performance. The rationale of this procedure is to restore the muscle-tendon-bone complex back to full integrity as soon as possible and achieve rapid stimulation through range-of-motion therapy in the early postoperative period. The risks of any operative inter-

vention include infection and/or skin changes, which can be as high as 5 percent. The AROM protocol does not have any increased risk of infection or any other surgical complication. Using this protocol, there have been no reruptures.

The surgical procedure is done in the outpatient setting. It can be performed with the patient under local, spinal, epidural, or a general anesthetic in the prone position. An incision is made just medial to the gastrocnemius and Achilles tendon. One incision is made down through the peritenon; the peritenon is split and tagged. Most ruptures occur at the muscle-tendon junction. Proximal and distal ends are gathered. Using a #2 Tevdek suture, a Krackow suture technique is used to achieve maximal suture tendon strength without causing tendon necrosis. One suture is placed in the proximal portion and the other on the distal portion. Each of the two legs respectively are tied in plantar flexion. The knots are brought out on the anterior aspect of the tendon. The peritenon is closed with #4 Vicryl, achieving a tubular covering around the repair. At this time the ankle is taken through a full range of motion, and the suture strength is evaluated. If sutures do not break and the load clearly is not a problem, the tourniquet is deflated and the skin is closed with dermal mattress sutures. The patient is placed in a soft bulky

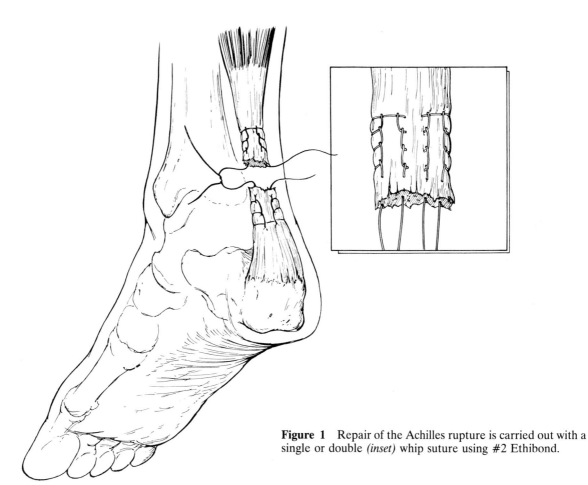

Figure 1 Repair of the Achilles rupture is carried out with a single or double *(inset)* whip suture using #2 Ethibond.

dressing with use of a posterior splint for 2 days.

On the third postoperative day, the splint is removed and the ankle taken through a range of motion. The patient is placed in a posterior shell splint and taken out of the splint on multiple occasions during the day and mobilized through a range of plantar and dorsiflexion. When the wound is acceptable, sutures are removed, and a progressive weight-bearing program is done from week 3 to week 5. The patient is placed in a Walker splint with use of heel pads during this period and converted to using cowboy boots at week 5 to 6. Physical therapy is initiated at week 2, facilitating gentle range of motion and strengthening. The phasic development is depicted in Figure 1.

REPAIR AND REHABILITATION

Tendon repair has long been recognized to follow the three stages of soft tissue healing: inflammation, repair, remodeling and maturation. The inflammation stage ends with the formation of granulation tissue. The repair stage is characterized by a high level of fibroblast activity as the matrix components are produced, leading to a fibrous scar. The remodeling phase overlaps the repair stage as the newly formed matrix begins to undergo organizational and orientational changes. These changes allow for the development of functional healed tissue. In this last stage of maturation, the tendon scar develops cross-linking at the intermolecular and interfibrillar level.

Most researchers today believe that both intrinsic and extrinsic factors contribute to the healing process. It has been shown that rehabilitative care after repair is important in the final outcome of tendon repair. Research under experimental conditions has shown that immobilization of healing wounds compromises wound strength. Conversely, early controlled mobilization of healing canine tendons has led to a significant reduction of adhesion formation and stronger tendons on final healing.

Although the precise mechanisms whereby mobilization assists the healing process of tendons are understood poorly, it is believed that the reduction of adhesions, the stimulation of the intrinsic tendon-healing response, and the promotion of nutrient transport may be operative factors.

The protocol outlined subsequently is adapted from traditional Achilles tendon repair rehabilitation programs and is characterized by a hastened progression of AROM and weight-bearing activities to prevent disuse changes and promote functional strength in healing.

Phase I

Week 1

Weight-bearing Status.   Total non–weight bearing
Instruction in protection of the surgical site

Range-of-Motion Exercise
Out-of-splint AROM
Two sets of five repetitions 3 times daily
Plantar flexion and/or dorsiflexion

Week 2

Weight-bearing Status.   Total non–weight bearing

Range-of-Motion Exercise
Plantar flexion and/or dorsiflexion, 2 sets of 20 repetitions
Inversion and/or eversion, 2 sets of 20 repetitions
Circumduction (both directions), 2 sets of 20 repetitions

Strength Exercise
Isometric inversion and/or eversion, 2 sets of 20 repetitions (in neutral)
Toe curls with towel and weight

Therapy Adjuncts
Gentle manual mobilization of scar tissue
Cryotherapy with caution for any open areas of the wound

Week 3

Weight-bearing Status.   Progressive partial weight-bearing program in Walker splint

Range-of-Motion Exercise
Previous AROM exercise continued
Begin gentle passive stretching into dorsiflexion with strap or towel

Strength Exercise
Isometric inversion and/or eversion, 2 sets of 10 repetitions
Isometric plantar flexion, 2 sets of 10 repetitions, progression to 2 sets of 20 over course of week 3
One rubber band inversion and/or eversion, 2 sets, 10 repetitions
One rubber band plantar flexion and dorsiflexion, 2 sets, 10 repetitions

Conditioning Activities
Stationary cycling begins, 7 to 12 minutes, minimal resistance; water exercise can begin under totally buoyant conditions with use of a flotation device
In the water ankle range-of-motion and running or walking activities can be initiated to preserve fitness in the lower body
No weight-bearing activities can be done in the water

Therapy Adjuncts
Manual mobilization of scar and cryotherapy continues

Phase II

Week 4 to 6

Weight-bearing Status. Progressive partial weight bearing to full load by week 5 to 6

Range-of-Motion Exercise
Previous range-of-motion exercise decreased to one set of 10 repetitions each direction
Passive stretch continues into dorsiflexion with progressively greater efforts, knee at full extension and flexed to 35° to 40°
Begin standing calf stretch with knee fully extended and flexed at week 5

Stretch Exercise
Decrease isometrics to 1 set of 10 inversion and/or eversion and plantar flexion
Progress to 3 rubber band: eversion, inversion, dorsiflexion and plantar flexion, 3 sets of 20 repetitions
Stationary cycling to 20 minutes with minimal resistance

Conditioning Activities
Cycling as previously outlined
Water exercise continues in totally buoyant state

Therapy Adjuncts
Gentle cross-fiber massage to Achilles tendon to release adhesions between the tendon and peritenon
Cryotherapy continues; ultrasound, phonophoresis and electrical stimulation may be added for chronic swelling or excessive scar formation

Phase III

Weeks 6 to 12

Weight-bearing Status. Full weight bearing in cowboy boots

Range-of-Motion Exercise
Further progressed with standing calf stretch

Strength Exercise
Omit isometrics
Continue 3 rubber band ankle strengthening in all directions
Begin double-legged toe raises with body weight as tolerated
Balance-board exercises are begun for proprioceptive training

Conditioning Activities
Stationary cycling
Treadmill walking
StairMaster
Water exercises in chest-deep water

Therapy Adjuncts
As needed

Phase IV

Weeks 12 and Beyond

Strength Exercises
Toe raises should progress to use of additional weight at least as great as body weight, and in the case of athletes, up to 1.5 times body weight
Single-legged toe raises are begun as tolerated

Conditioning Activities
Progress to jogging on a trampoline and then to treadmill running via a walk-run program
Eventually perform steady-state outdoor running up to 20 minutes before adding figure eight and cutting drills
Water exercise performed in shallow water (waist deep)
In the water, begin to include hopping, bounding, and jumping drills
The completely rehabilitated Achilles tendon repair allows 15° to 20° of dorsiflexion at the ankle, and this must be maintained with regular stretching of the gastrocnemius-soleus group. Strength and endurance are developed to preinjury levels, and continued strength and flexibility work is advised.

SUGGESTED READING

Gelberman RH, Botle M, Spiegelman J, et al. Effects of early intermittent passive mobilization on healing canine flexor tendons. J Hand Surg 1982; 7:170–175.
Hitchock TF, Light TR, Bunch W, et al. The effect of immediate controlled mobilization on the strength of flexor tendon repairs. Trans Orthop Res Soc 1986; 11:216.
Hu Han P, Ferris B. Tendons. In: Buckneall TE, Ellis H, eds. Wound healing for surgeons. London: Bailliere-Tindall, 1984:286.
Marske PR, Lester PA. Histological evidence of intrinsic flexor tendon repair in various experimental animals: An in vitro study. Cin Orthop 1984; 192:297–304.

POSTERIOR IMPINGEMENT SYNDROME OF THE ANKLE INCLUDING FLEXOR HALLUCIS LONGUS ENTRAPMENT

RONALD QUIRK, F.R.C.S., F.R.A.C.S.

Posterior impingement syndrome of the ankle is seen when an os trigonum, a large posterior process of the talus, or a fibrocartilaginous bar causes crowding of the structures behind the ankle joint (Fig. 1). The pain comes from crushing of the soft tissues, and it can be relieved by removing the obstructing bone or fibrocartilage. The chief diagnostic clue to this condition is posterior ankle pain on *passive* plantar flexion of the foot.

Another lesion in this area that may coexist and can cause diagnostic uncertainty is flexor hallucis longus (FHL) tendon entrapment within the fibrous flexor sheath behind the medial malleolus. There usually is a nodule on the tendon, and in severe cases this can jam in the fibrous sheath, causing triggering of the big toe. In less severe cases the nodule still can be palpated easily as it moves behind the medial malleolus when the big toe is moved. The surgical solution to this problem is to divide the fibrous sheath.

THERAPEUTIC ALTERNATIVES

In early cases rest, physical therapy, and nonsteroidal anti-inflammatory drugs are worth trying. One or more steroid injections into the back of the ankle joint may help to resolve a posterior impingement syndrome, and the diagnosis may be confirmed by injecting a local anesthetic at the same time. If the pain is abolished by the local anesthetic, the diagnosis almost certainly is correct.

Injections into the FHL tendon should be avoided, because this type of treatment may lead to rupture of the tendon.

PREFERRED APPROACH

Patient Selection

Most patients who come to surgery for either of these conditions are ballet dancers or athletes involved in sports that require jumping. Occasionally the pain results from injury or fracture of the os trigonum. In these patients a bone scan often is helpful to confirm the source of pain, since the trigonal process may not be completely ossified, thereby mimicking fracture.

Timing of Surgery

Surgery should be offered as soon as it is clear that a good trial of conservative treatment has failed to give relief. My experience has been that far too much time usually is spent on unhelpful conservative treatment, and that the patient is referred to a surgeon only after many months of being disabled. It should be possible in 3 months to satisfy all concerned that conservative treatment is not helping, and surgery then should proceed without further delay. This is important particularly in the competitive athlete who may lose an entire season if treatment is delayed.

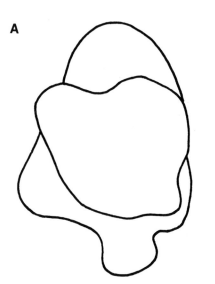 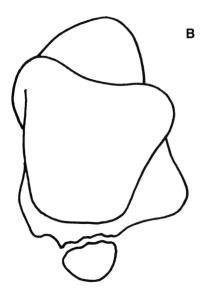

Figure 1 View from above two tali, showing a large posterior tubercle *(A)* and an os trigonum *(B)*.

Preoperative Preparation

It is essential to have a good lateral radiograph of the ankle to show the size of the bony obstruction and whether it is part of the talus or separate from it (Figs. 2 and 3). It is helpful if two lateral views of the ankle are obtained, one in maximum plantar flexion and the other in maximum dorsiflexion.

In cases in which FHL entrapment is suspected, an ultrasound examination often gives useful information about the state of the tendon, including the presence of a partial tear or a nodule.

Choice of Procedure

The back of the ankle can be reached through a posteromedial or a posterolateral approach. I prefer the posteromedial approach for the following reasons: (1) I consider that in all cases of posterior impingement syndrome, the FHL tendon also should be examined, because it is not uncommon to find damage to the tendon even in cases that present as a straightforward posterior impingement. (2) With a medial approach, it is easy to find and protect the neurovascular bundle, whereas in a posterolateral approach there is the risk of damaging the nerve or vessels if an osteotome should slip.

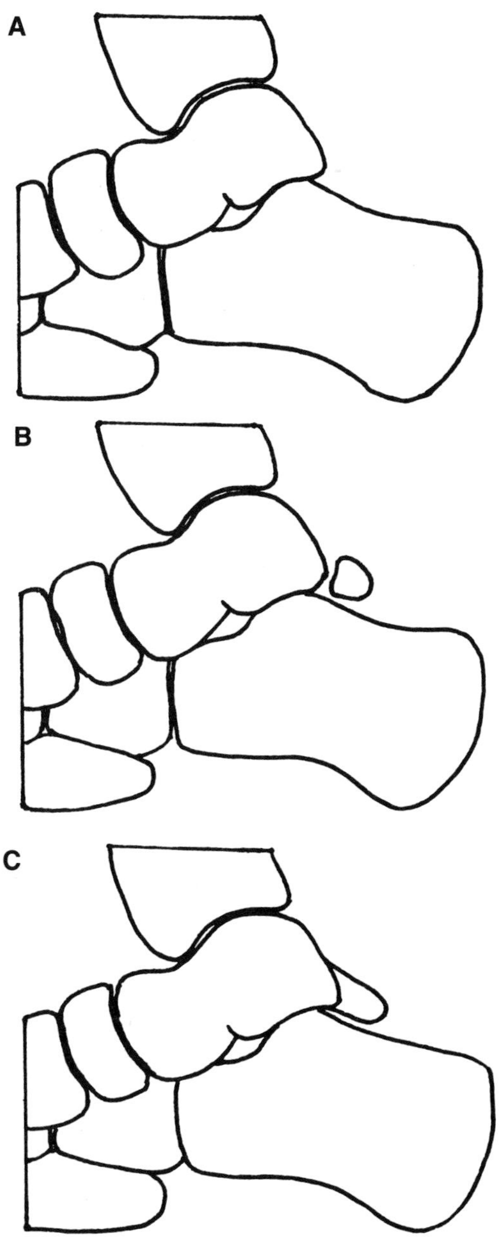

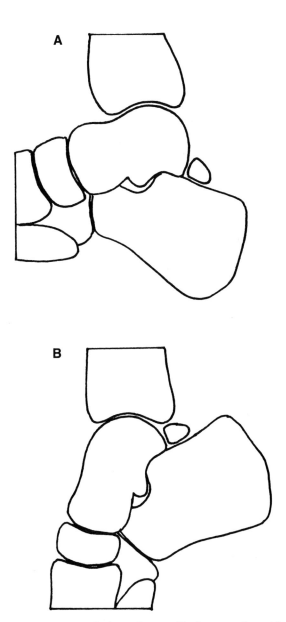

Figure 2 Lateral views of the ankle. *A,* No bony prominence behind the talus. *B,* Os trigonum. *C,* An enlarged posterior tubercle.

Figure 3 *A,* Lateral view of an ankle in neutral position. *B,* Same ankle in forced plantar flexion. Note how the ostrigonum is squeezed between the lower tibia and the upper calcaneum like a nut in a nutcracker.

The steps of the operation are as follows. Make a 4 cm slightly curved incision halfway between the medial malleolus and the Achilles tendon. As soon as the fat is retracted, the neurovascular bundle is observed. Divide the deep fascia and dissect out the nerve, which is posterior to the vessels. Retract the whole bundle forward. The tendon of the FHL in its sheath, is found just deep to the nerve. Divide the sheath vertically and inspect the tendon. If there is a fusiform swelling or a partial tear of the tendon, split the sheath as far as possible in each direction, especially distally. Retract the tendon forward with the neurovascular bundle. It now is a simple matter to open the capsule of the ankle joint and to visualize the back of the talus. An os trigonum or a fibrocartilaginous bar may be removed by sharp dissection, but a large posterior tubercle requires an osteotome and bone nibblers. The wound is closed in layers, with a subcuticular suture to the skin, and a firm pressure dressing is applied.

Postoperative Course

The patient leaves the hospital on the day following surgery and is kept non–weight bearing on crutches until the tenth postoperative day. Dressings then are removed and the wound inspected. If the wound is healed, normal weight bearing is commenced and physical therapy is used to help mobilize and strengthen the ankle. Dancing or athletic activities are commenced about 4 weeks postoperatively and gradually are increased. Normal activity usually is reached within 2 to 3 months of the operation.

Complications

If care is exercised, few complications should occur. Problems that are seen occasionally include (1) wound hematoma as a result of inadequate hemoastasis; (2) damage to the neurovascular bundle; and (3) incorrect diagnosis, which can be avoided if it is remembered that posterior impingement syndrome is the only condition that causes pain on passive plantar flexion of the ankle. In cases of doubt, the injection of a local anesthetic provides confirmation.

PROS AND CONS OF TREATMENT

All cases of posterior impingement syndrome should be treated conservatively at first and many patients will recover. Those patients who do not respond to 3 months of conservative treatment should be dealt with surgically. The operation is a relatively minor one, and in most cases relief is rapid and complete. Operation usually is delayed because the treating doctor cannot make a diagnosis or is unaware of the existence of the condition. In other cases, failure to obtain a surgical opinion early leads to conservative treatment being continued far too long.

SUGGESTED READING

Fricker PA, Williams JGP. Surgical management of os trigonum and talar spur in sportsmen. Br J Sports Med 1979; 13:55–57.
Howse AJG, Hancock S. Dance technique and injury prevention. London: A & C Black, 1988: 114.
Kleiger B. In: Ryan AJ, Stephens RE, eds. Dance medicine. Chicago: Pluribus, 1987: 119.
Quirk R. Talar compression syndrome in dancers. Foot Ankle 1982; 3:65–68.
Sammarco J. In: Jahss M, ed. Disorders of the foot. Philadelphia: WB Saunders, 1982: 1648.
Sarraffian SK. Anatomy of the foot and ankle. Philadelphia: JB Lippincott, 1983: 88.

MODIFIED BROSTROM PROCEDURE FOR ACUTE AND CHRONIC ANKLE INSTABILITY

WILLIAM G. HAMILTON, M.D.

From 1964 to 1966 Lennart Brostrom wrote a series of six articles on ankle sprains, which appeared in the *Acta Chirurgica Scandinavica.* In the last of these, he reported a success rate (good and excellent results) of 58 out of 60 patients, using a new operation for the correction of "chronic" ankle instability. (In one of the earlier articles, he discussed the use of a similar operation for the acute ankle sprain.)

His procedure involved tightening the stretched-out lateral ligaments to restore their normal anatomy without the use of supplemental tissues or "weaving" procedures. It was based on the fact that the anterior talofibular (ATF) ligament lay within the anterolateral ankle capsule (similar to the anterior glenohumeral ligaments of the shoulder), and when the ATF was torn it healed within the capsule in an elongated form. The operation shortened the stretched-out ATF and calcaneofibular (CF) ligaments to their normal lengths and sutured them to their anatomic locations.

In 1980 Nathaniel Gould reported his modification of the Brostrom repair. It consisted of Brostrom's operation followed by mobilizing the lateral portion of the extensor retinaculum, and suturing it to the distal fibula over the ligament repair. This reinforces the

repair, limits inversion and the position of reinjury, and helps to correct the subtalar component of the instability. The last of these factors is important, because the CF ligament is one of the main stabilizers of the subtalar joint. When it is torn, as in third-degree lateral sprains, a combined instability usually is present in both the tibiotalar and subtalar joints. The retinacular reinforcement helps to correct this combined instability, because it runs parallel to the CF ligament and inserts in the lateral calcaneus.

Several advantages to Gould's modification of the Brostrom procedure are as follows:

1. It is a relatively easy procedure.
2. It uses a small cosmetic incision (Fig. 1).
3. The sural nerve should not be in any danger.
4. It does not require the sacrifice of a peroneal tendon.
5. It is anatomic and maintains a full range of motion in the ankle and subtalar joints.
6. Contrary to the various weaving procedures, it is difficult to make the repair so tight that the subtalar joint is locked in eversion.

Because of these factors, it is an ideal procedure for the athlete, ballet dancer, gymnast, or ice skater who needs ankle stability with a full range of motion and no loss of peroneal function. Both Brostrom and Gould described the use of their procedures for acute third-degree sprains in selected high-performance athletes.

INDICATIONS

The modified Brostrom procedure is indicated for chronic symptomatic lateral ankle instability that has not

© Copyright, William G. Hamilton, M.D.

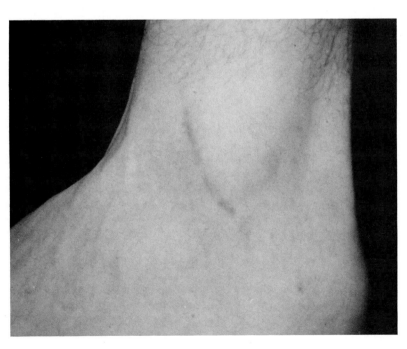

Figure 1 Skin incision (all views left ankle).

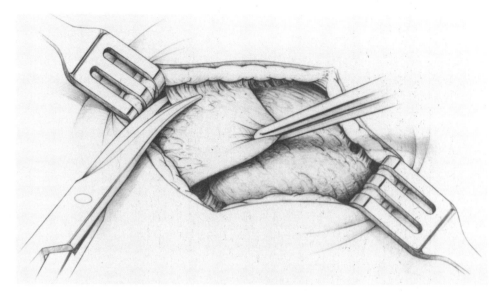

Figure 2 Mobilizing the lateral extensor retinaculum.

responded to physical therapy and rehabilitation (especially proprioceptive training and peroneal strengthening), and for selected cases of acute third-degree ankle sprains (usually in professional-level athletes). The procedure should not be performed on individuals with fixed heel varus. In this instance, a valgus osteotomy of the os calcis should be performed along with the repair. It also is contraindicated in athletes weighing over 225 to 250 pounds. In these individuals I recommend doing the modified Brostrom and then adding an Evans-type repair using half the peroneus brevis. In addition, peroneal weakness, palsy, or dysfunction are relative contraindications.

PROCEDURE

The operation usually is performed on an outpatient basis, with the patient in the lateral decubitus position. A thigh tourniquet is used over cast padding, so a general, spinal, or epidural anesthetic is needed.

After exsanguination of the limb, a curvilinear incision is made along the anterior border of the distal fibula, stopping at the peroneal tendons. (The sural nerve is just below this area, lying directly on the peroneal tendons.) The lesser saphenous vein usually crosses the distal fibula at this level and must be ligated.

The dissection is carried down to the joint capsule along the anterior border of the lateral malleolus. The lateral portion of the extensor retinaculum then is identified. It is dissected off the capsule and mobilized so that it can be pulled over the repair at the end of the procedure (Fig. 2). Care should be taken when working anterior to the malleolus, because the lateral branch of the superficial peroneal nerve often lies in this area and can be damaged by dissection or a sharp retractor. (The mobilization of the extensor retinaculum can be performed either before or after the capsular incision.)

The capsule then is divided along the anterior border of the fibula down to the peroneal tendons, leaving a 2 to 3 mm cuff (Fig. 3). The ATF ligament lies within this capsule, similar to the anterior glenohumeral ligaments of the shoulder. It frequently can be identified as a thickening in the capsule (Fig. 4). It is best to leave a small cuff of tissue on the fibula, rather than taking the capsule off the bone by sharp dissection.

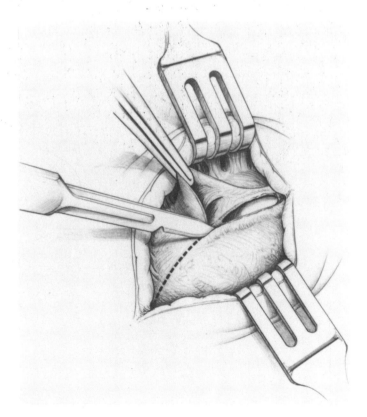

Figure 3 Capsular incision, leaving a small cuff.

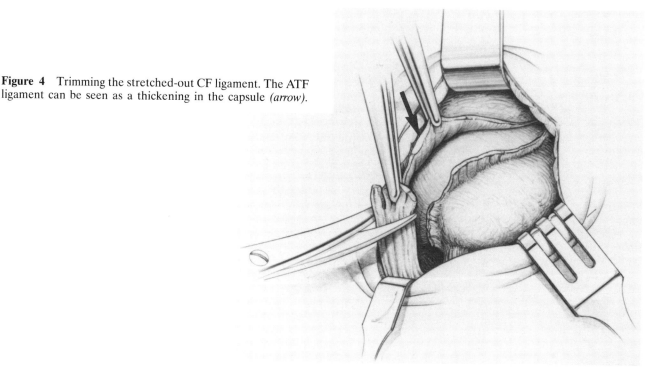

Figure 4 Trimming the stretched-out CF ligament. The ATF ligament can be seen as a thickening in the capsule *(arrow)*.

If the procedure is being done for an acute injury, the tear in the ATF and CF ligaments must be identified and repaired. Obviously, in this case, the insertion of the capsule in the fibula should not be taken down as described earlier.

The CF ligament now must be identified. It lies deep to the peroneal tendons, running obliquely downward and posteriorly to the calcaneus. It often is stretched out and attenuated, or it may be dislodged so that it lies *outside* the peroneals. On rare occasions it can be found avulsed from its calcaneal origin. If it is in continuity, it is divided, leaving a cuff at its insertion on the fibula. By leaving a cuff of tissue at the insertion of the ligaments, the surgeon is able to repair the ligaments in their anatomic locations, thus preserving isometry and an unrestricted range of motion.

The ligaments now must be shortened and repaired. The ankle should be placed in the fully reduced position in neutral dorsiflexion and slight eversion. The stumps of the ligaments are pulled up, and the redundancy is trimmed. The ligaments then are sutured to their anatomic locations with 2-0 nonabsorbable sutures, starting with the CF ligament because it is the most difficult to visualize, and then proceeding to the ATF ligament. This repair can be done by end-to-end suture, pants-over-vest, or into drill holes (Fig. 5).

At this point the ankle should be examined for stability and range of motion. The previously identified lateral extensor mechanism then is pulled over the repair and sutured to the tip of the fibula with 2-0 chromic catgut (Fig. 6). This reinforces the repair, limits inversion (the position of injury), and helps to correct the subtalar component of the instability. (If the CF ligament is attenuated, there must be some degree of subtalar instability—the CF ligament is one of the stabilizing ligaments of the subtalar joint.)

The ankle is checked once again for stability and taken through a full range of motion. A layered closure then is performed with an absorbable subcutaneous suture and steri-strips. The patient is placed in antero-posterior plaster splints and discharged non–weight bearing with crutches.

AFTERCARE

When the swelling has subsided, in 3 to 5 days, a short-leg walking cast is applied for 3 to 4 weeks. The cast then is removed and the ankle is protected with an air splint. Swimming, range-of-motion, and isometric peroneal exercises are begun. Unrestricted activities are allowed at 10 to 12 weeks if full peroneal strength is present.

RESULTS

We began using this procedure for ballet dancers in 1980 and had such good results that we began to use it for all our ligament repairs. All the professional dancers have obtained excellent results and returned to their careers. As of this writing, there has been one failure (as a result of significant reinjury), but no long-term stretch-outs, "redos," or complications.

This operation is thought to be the procedure of choice for the dancer, athlete, and nonathlete who needs a stable ankle with a full range of motion and normal peroneal function.

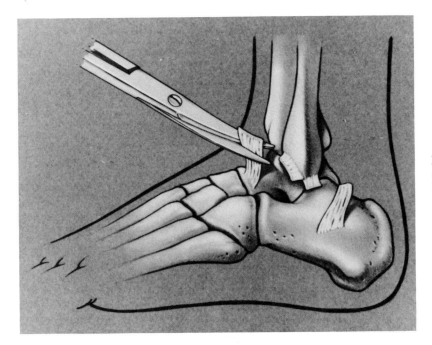

Figure 5 Attenuated ATF and CF ligaments are shortened and reattached in their anatomic locations.

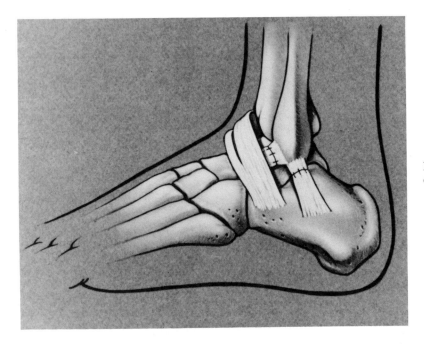

Figure 6 Extensor retinaculum is sutured over the repair.

For a discussion of ankle ligament reconstruction using a split peroneus brevis tendon transfer (Crisman-Snook), see the chapter *Cavovarus Foot*.

SUGGESTED READING

Brostrom L. Sprained ankles. I. Anatomic lesions in recent sprains. Acta Chir Scand 1964; 128:483–495.

Brostrom L. Sprained ankles. III. Clinical observations in recent ligament ruptures. Acta Chir Scand 1965; 130:560–569.

Brostrom L. Sprained ankles. V. Treatment and prognosis in recent ligament ruptures. Acta Chir Scand 1966; 132:537–550.

Brostrom L, Liljedahl S, Lindvall N. Sprained ankles. II. Arthrographic diagnosis of recent ligament ruptures. Acta Chir Scand 1965; 129:485–499.

Gould N, Seligson D, Gassman J. Early and late repair of lateral ligament of the ankle. Foot Ankle 1980; 1:84–89.

Kleiger B. Mechanisms of ankle injury. Orthop Clin North Am. 1974; 5:127.

OSTEOTOMIES

METATARSAL OSTEOTOMY

MARK MYERSON, M.D.

Metatarsal osteotomy typically is performed for metatarsalgia, often as a result of the disparate length of metatarsals caused by prior surgery or trauma. This chapter deals with osteotomies of the lesser metatarsals, focusing particularly on the second metatarsal. Osteotomy of the lesser metatarsals may be performed by a variety of methods, all which purport to offer a modest correction and success. Unfortunately all osteotomies cause a predictable shift of pressure to the adjacent metatarsal. This is less important with the lateral metatarsals, and an osteotomy of the third metatarsal is less likely to be associated with fourth metatarsalgia, and similarly a fourth metatarsal osteotomy is highly unlikely to cause fifth metatarsalgia. Nevertheless, the overall sagittal plane movement of each metatarsal should be assessed preoperatively. The second metatarsal is locked into the mortise and minimal if any dorsal-plantar motion occurs. This is particularly important in hallux valgus correction, since many if not most osteotomies shorten the first metatarsal.

In general, osteotomies either can be fixed or allowed to "float free." I am not a proponent of floating osteotomies. They are imprecise and do not afford one the potential for more precise control when internal fixation is used.

There are a number of different patterns of metatarsalgia: (1) isolated single metatarsal keratosis, (2) second metatarsalgia, (3) third or fourth ray metatarsalgia, (4) second, third, and fourth metatarsalgia, and (5) diffuse forefoot metatarsalgia. Isolated keratosis usually is associated with a prominent single condyle, usually the fibular condyle and is best treated with a condylectomy. Isolated involvement of the second metatarsal is best treated with a shortening osteotomy controlled with internal fixation. The more diffuse patterns of metatarsalgia should be approached carefully. When the second and third or the third and fourth metatarsals are involved alone, some consideration may be given to a floating osteotomy, recognizing that transfer to the adjacent metatarsal is likely to occur. Diffuse forefoot meta-tarsalgia should not be treated operatively. This usually is associated with thinning, atrophy, or forward subluxation of the metatarsal fat pad. If severe and intractable, this diffuse pattern of metatarsalgia is best treated by resection of all the metatarsal heads including the first. This succeeds provided a fixed forefoot equinus is not present.

ISOLATED KERATOSIS

This form of metatarsalgia is easy to discern from a more diffuse pattern of metatarsalgia. It consists of a thin area of keratosis directly under one metatarsal, usually on its fibular side (Fig. 1). It is caused by a prominent fibular condyle and is best treated with condylectomy.

A dorsal approach to the metatarsophalangeal (MP) joint is used for condylectomy. The extensor hood is incised longitudinally and the capsule opened longitudinally. With careful subperiosteal dissection, the capsule and periosteum is freed up off the base of the proximal phalanx to its medial and lateral margins. It is important to preserve the collateral ligament complex with this approach. At this stage the toe usually can be dislocated in a plantarward direction, exposing the entire metatarsal head. If the joint is still tight, more capsular release should be performed dorsal-medially and dorsal-laterally. With the toe plantar flexed, a small osteotome or preferably a chisel is used to remove the condyles as illustrated. No more than ⅛ inch of bone should be removed (Fig. 2). It is important to keep the fragment of bone under direct vision. It is not uncommon

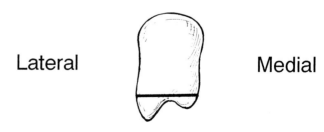

Figure 1 Prominent fibular condyle causing isolated plantar keratosis.

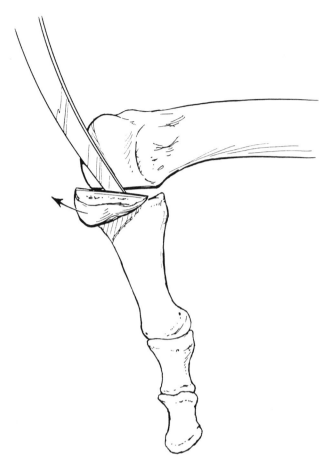

Figure 2 Condylectomy is performed with a chisel or a curved osteotome.

to complete the osteotomy, withdraw the osteotome, and find that the condylar fragment has slipped proximally. A curved spoon-shaped periosteal elevator prevents this proximal migration of the condyle. Following removal of the fragment, the MP joint is reduced and closure made in a routine fashion. If the joint is grossly unstable following this condylectomy, it should be secured with a Kirschner (K-) wire, and removed after 2 to 3 weeks. It is unusual, however, for instability to be present unless complete transection of the collateral ligaments has been performed.

DIFFUSE KERATOSIS

If the keratosis involves all five metatarsal heads, one must be careful in selecting any operative procedure. Diffuse keratosis may result either from a fixed forefoot equinus deformity or from an inherent predisposition to developing callosity. The latter cannot be addressed surgically and should be treated with orthoses. The diffuse form of keratosis as a result of a fixed forefoot equinus (midfoot cavus) may be treated with a dorsal truncated wedge arthrodesis of the tarsometatarsal joint

as described by Jahss, or by dorsal wedge osteotomies of all five metatarsals. This procedure is not precise, and recurrent metatarsalgia under one or more metatarsals may require revision surgery. Diffuse thinning of the metatarsal fat pad in the elderly is a difficult problem, and although modest relief usually is obtained with orthoses, surgery occasionally is warranted. In these patients resection of all the metatarsal heads is highly successful. This is performed through two dorsal longitudinal incisions and a third medial incision over the hallux MP joint.

ISOLATED SECOND METATARSALGIA

Isolated second metatarsalgia is either a result of a short first metatarsal, a long second metatarsal, or both. This is a particularly frustrating problem following hallux valgus surgery, in which the first metatarsal has either shortened or healed with a dorsal malunion. Although shortening of the second metatarsal needs to be performed, the first metatarsal malunion must be addressed simultaneously with a plantar flexion osteotomy. The position and type of osteotomy depend on the original procedure and the position of the malunion. It is difficult to remove a plantar-based wedge from the metatarsal accurately. If this is the method selected, I recommend removing the wedge completely and reversing it by inserting it dorsally to further assist in plantar flexion of the metatarsal (Fig. 3). To some extent this is limited by soft tissue contracture, particularly of the extensor hallucis longus or brevis, which may need simultaneous lengthening. The plantar flexion osteotomy of the first metatarsal requires internal fixation with either K-wires or a low-profile plate. I think it is preferable to use more rigid fixation, and I prefer to use a ¼ tubular plate, which is bent and contoured to the plantar-flexed first metatarsal. Either 3.5 mm cortical or fully threaded cancellous screws are used to affix the plate, depending on the bone quality. This plate cannot be used for dorsal malunion following a distal metatarsal osteotomy. The osteotomy must be performed at the level of the malunion and is best achieved with a dome saw blade oriented with the concavity proximally and directed toward the medial side of the metatarsal as illustrated (Fig. 4). This is an extracapsular osteotomy, and the MP joint does not need to be opened. If the dorsal capsular structures and the extensor brevis tendon are tight, these must be released to plantar flex the metatarsal head. This osteotomy is secured with two or three 0.045 inch K-wires. Regardless of fixation, a plantar flexion osteotomy of either the distal or proximal metatarsal should be protected with restricted weight bearing postoperatively.

In addition to the plantar flexion osteotomy of the first metatarsal, the second metatarsal usually requires shortening simultaneously. This is a difficult decision to make and depends on the position of the first metatarsal that is re-established. This length is relative, since the goal is to create a plantigrade weight-bearing surface of the forefoot. The length itself cannot be re-established

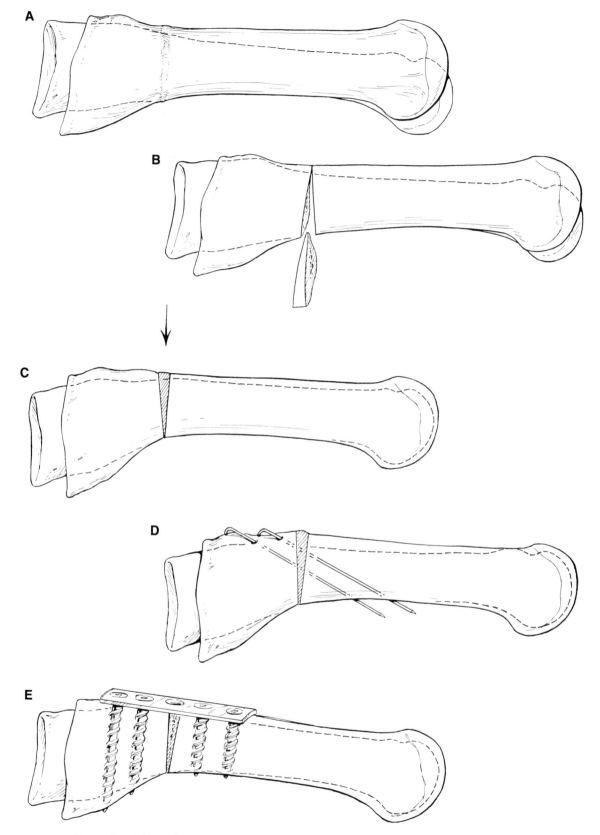

Figure 3 *A,* Dorsal malunion of the first metatarsal following fracture or osteotomy. *B,* A plantar-based wedge removed at the apex of the deformity. *C,* The wedge is reversed and inserted dorsally. The osteotomy is secured with K-wires *(D),* or a five-hole ¼ tubular plate *(E).*

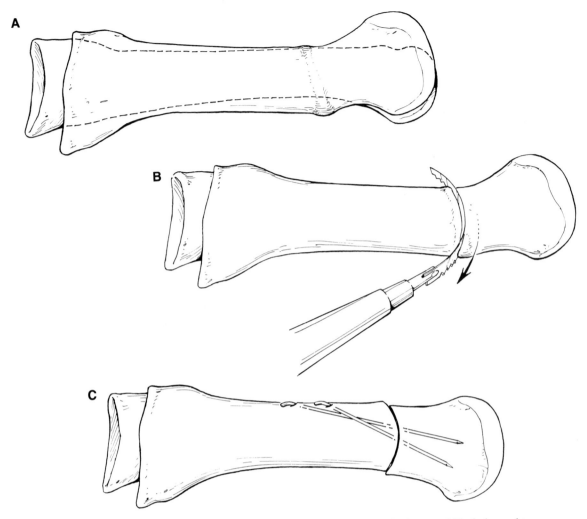

Figure 4 *A,* Dorsal malunion following fracture or osteotomy. *B,* A curved blade is used to correct the osteotomy with the apex facing proximally. *C,* Fixation of the osteotomy is accomplished with two K-wires.

without physical lengthening of the first metatarsal. Because of soft tissue attachments, this is impossible to achieve without causing severe contracture around the MP joint. Instead the plantigrade weight-bearing surface of the foot is achieved by plantar flexion of the first metatarsal. The second metatarsal can be shortened or elevated through a dorsal wedge osteotomy of the metatarsal neck or by resection of a small segment of bone along the shaft of the metatarsal.

An isolated long second metatarsal is best treated by a shortening osteotomy. The problem with any single metatarsal osteotomy is that it is impossible to predict the exact amount of shortening required to unload the metatarsal. Although this makes a floating osteotomy appealing, one cannot assume that the metatarsal "finds" its own level. With controlled fixation, an osteotomy is shortened in a precise manner and then secured with rigid internal fixation. This is best accom-

plished with a long oblique osteotomy made in the proximal metatarsal from proximal and dorsal to distal and plantar (Fig. 5). The metatarsal is predrilled with a 3.5 mm drill bit through one (the dorsal) cortex. The osteotomy is then made at a 45° angle to the plane of the drill hole. It is important not to tear through the plantar periosteum with the saw blade. Once the osteotomy is completed, it is slid proximally by manual pressure under the head of the second metatarsal. Through palpation, one should be able to identify the level of the second and third metatarsal. The fixation is completed while holding the metatarsal in this corrected position. It is important to realize that this osteotomy shortens the metatarsal in two planes. In addition to proximal shift, there is a similar and equal dorsalward shift of the metatarsal (Fig. 5*B*). A 3.5 mm cortical screw is used and should be inserted in a lag mode. It is important to countersink the screw head; ideally this is done with a 4 mm burr, since

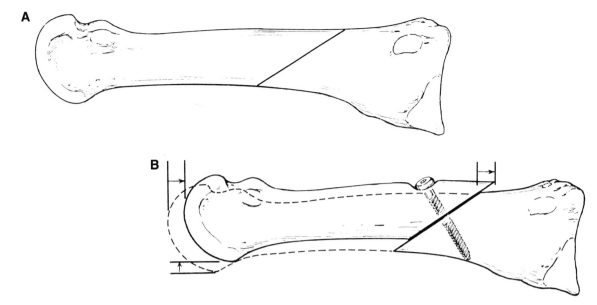

Figure 5 *A,* Proximal-oblique osteotomy for isolated metatarsalgia. *B,* The osteotomy is secured with a 3.5 mm cortical screw inserted in a lag mode.

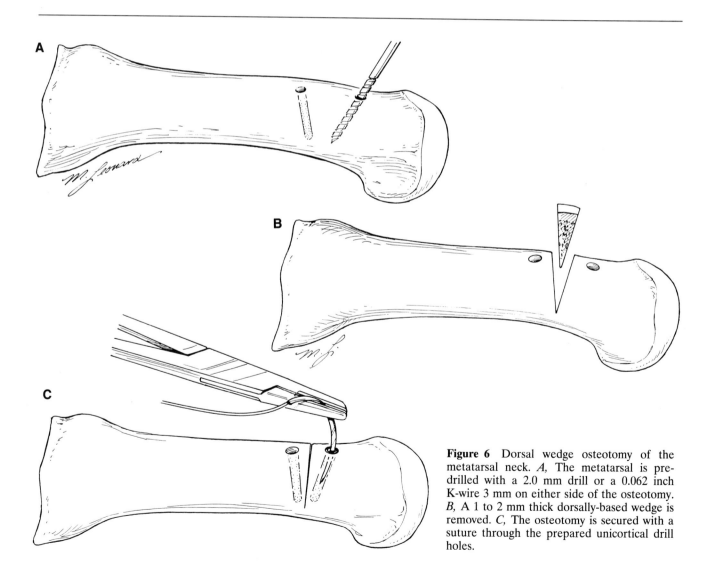

Figure 6 Dorsal wedge osteotomy of the metatarsal neck. *A,* The metatarsal is predrilled with a 2.0 mm drill or a 0.062 inch K-wire 3 mm on either side of the osteotomy. *B,* A 1 to 2 mm thick dorsally-based wedge is removed. *C,* The osteotomy is secured with a suture through the prepared unicortical drill holes.

the counter-sunk head does not prepare the hole adequately for the screw head.

As a rule severe second metatarsalgia associated with a dorsal malunion following bunionectomy and first metatarsal osteotomy is best treated with a revision of the first metatarsal osteotomy, as well as shortening of the second metatarsal. Many methods of performing these osteotomies are available. Some are better than others; those that float the metatarsal clearly are worse.

A dorsal wedge osteotomy of the metatarsal neck is easy to perform. It is indicated in the presence of isolated single metatarsalgia in which one does not need to perform a simultaneous procedure at the level of the MP joint. If the latter is performed, the distal metatarsal head and neck segment becomes unstable, and it is difficult to secure adequately. The metatarsal is approached from the MP joint proximally for approximately 1 inch. The extensor complex is reflected and the periosteum incised dorsally only. It is important not to strip the periosteum excessively. The dorsal metatarsal is predrilled with a unicortical drill hole using a 0.062 inch K-wire and is made at a 45° angle to the metatarsal shaft both distally and proximally (Fig. 6). Each hole should be approximately 4 mm away from the osteotomy site. The osteotomy is made with a small thin blade, and not more than 1/8 inch of bone removed. The osteotomy is not completed, but a greenstick fracture is performed manually, preserving the plantar periosteal sleeve intact. A stout tapered needle then is inserted through the metatarsal from proximal to distal through the osteotomy site. I use a 2-0 nonabsorbable suture, and the knot is tied while the metatarsal is held firmly in the corrected position. Postoperatively patients bear weight on the heel for 4 weeks in a surgical shoe and then are allowed to bear full weight as tolerated.

ISOLATED METATARSALGIA FOLLOWING FRACTURE OR OSTEOTOMY MALUNION

In addition to dorsal wedge osteotomy of the symptomatic metatarsal, one should consider a plantar flexion osteotomy of the dorsiflexed metatarsal. Since the fourth and fifth metatarsals are mobile, this usually applies only to the first or second metatarsal. Severe dorsal malunion of the second metatarsal is difficult to treat with isolated osteotomy of the third metatarsal alone. Even though the fourth metatarsal is mobile, too large an osteotomy of the third metatarsal has to be performed for symptomatic correction. For this reason, I prefer to remove a smaller wedge from the third metatarsal and plantar flex the second metatarsal using a contoured plate and screw technique. A plantar flexion osteotomy of the second metatarsal may be performed simply by a vertical osteotomy through the metatarsal and does not violate the plantar cortex. The metatarsal is cracked, plantar flexed, and then held in that position with the contoured plate. The osteotomy heals by approximately 8 weeks, and weight bearing therefore is avoided during this period. Nonunion may occur, but usually is asymptomatic, since most of the weight is still on the first and third metatarsals.

SUGGESTED READING

Helal B. Metatarsal osteotomy for metatarsalgia. J Bone Joint Surg 1975; 57B:187–191.
Jahss MH. Tarsometatarsal truncated wedge arthrodesis for pes cavus of the fore part of the foot. J Bone Joint Surg 1980; 62A:713–718.
Mann RA. Intractable plantar keratosis. Orthop Clin North Am 1973; 4:647–652.

CALCANEUS OSTEOTOMY

TERENCE SAXBY, M.D., F.R.A.C.S.
MARK MYERSON, M.D.

Osteotomies of the calcaneus are useful for correction of both varus and valgus hindfoot deformity. The calcaneal osteotomy does not of course correct the entire foot deformity, and additional procedures—usually to the midfoot and forefoot—are required, depending on the underlying pathology. The two procedures discussed in this chapter are triplanar osteotomy for correction of hindfoot varus and medial displacement osteotomy for planovalgus deformity.

TRIPLANAR OSTEOTOMY

Although the underlying pathogenesis of the cavovarus foot may be similar, the extent of the deformity often is different; each operation must be planned according to the extent of the deformity.

In addition to hindfoot varus, dorsal angulation of the calcaneus is present, increasing the calcaneal pitch angle. This increased talocalcaneal angle cannot be corrected with a traditional closing-wedge osteotomy of the calcaneus. We also have experienced problems with a standard lateral closing wedge, since a significant amount of bone must be removed to correct the hindfoot valgus. This ostectomy and/or osteotomy therefore significantly shortens the hindfoot. Although a medial opening-wedge osteotomy of the calcaneus may overcome this problem, difficulty with soft tissue closure and wound healing makes this procedure less desirable. A triplanar osteotomy corrects all planes of the cavovarus deformity. The three elements of correction are lateral translation, lateral closing wedge, and dorsal translation.

Procedure

The patient is placed in the lateral decubitus position. The foot should remain internally rotated but preferably perfectly lateral, so that little distortion of the position of the foot is present. For this reason, perfect positioning on the bean bag is helpful. The surface marking for the incision is approximately two finger widths anterior to the insertion of the Achilles tendon and 1 cm inferior to the tip of the fibula (Fig. 1). In this manner both the sural nerve and peroneal tendons are dorsal to the incision. The incision is made obliquely down to the plantar aspect of the foot, so that its inferior edge meets the margin between the normal and plantar skin. At this point the incision should be in line with the fibula.

Dissection is carried on carefully through subcutaneous tissue to identify the sural nerve, which may be running in an aberrant course. Once the nerve is identified, it is retracted superiorly, and the incision is deepened to the periosteum and calcaneus. The periosteum is identified; it is divided with sharp dissection, and the entire calcaneus now should be visualized from its superior to plantar edges (Fig. 2). A small spiked Hohman retractor is inserted into the dorsal and inferior margins of the wound and the soft tissue retracted. A self-retaining retractor often is helpful if placed in line with the skin incision while an assistant maintains the position of the Hohman retractors. A periosteal elevator now is used to strip the periosteum 1 cm on either side to expose the calcaneus further. The entire calcaneus should be well visualized from its superior to inferior extent.

The osteotomy is performed using an oscillating saw in line with the skin incision. The calcaneus is divided commencing dorsally and working toward the inferior margin. Care must be exercised not to overextend the saw cut into the medial soft tissues. Either the saw can be used and careful attention paid to the exact point at which the saw exits medially, or the medial cortex can be perforated with a large blunt osteotome. We find it preferable to remove the triangular wedge of bone laterally before completion of the osteotomy medially. This bone wedge is excised using an oscillating saw (Fig. 3). The size of this wedge varies, but is approximately 6 mm in width from its superior to inferior margin, tapering to its apical surface medially. Once a wedge of bone has been removed, all remaining cancellous bone chips or fragments are removed using either a curette or

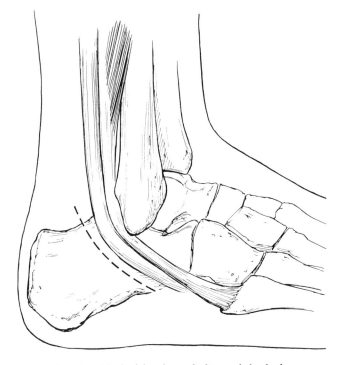

Figure 1 The skin incision is made beneath both the peroneal tendons and the sural nerve and in line with the peroneal tendons.

159

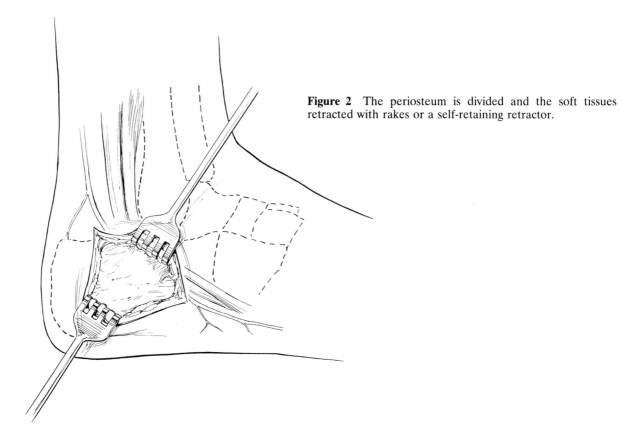

Figure 2 The periosteum is divided and the soft tissues retracted with rakes or a self-retaining retractor.

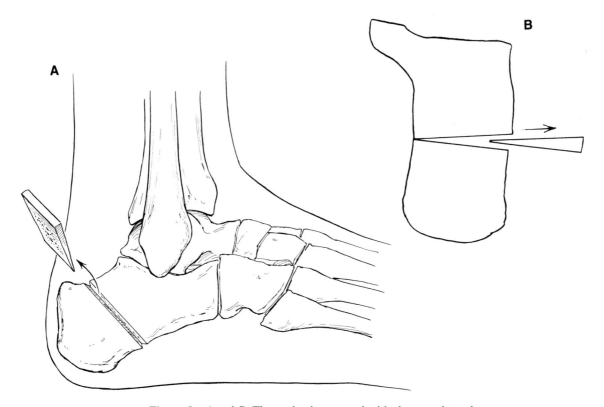

Figure 3 *A* and *B*, The wedge is removed with the apex lateral.

rongeur, and the osteotomy then is completed as described earlier. It is important to divide the medial periosteum to allow translation of the osteotomy. In severe cases the medial soft tissues are extremely taut, and the osteotomy does not close laterally unless this is released completely. The easiest way to release the medial soft tissue from the lateral side is to insert a large lamina spreader into the lateral aspect of the osteotomy site, and then through distraction, the periosteum

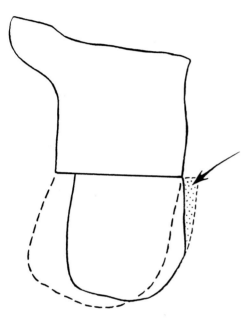

Figure 4 The calcaneal tuberosity is translated laterally, simultaneously closing the wedge.

gradually is stretched and divided. It should be possible to open the medial surfaces approximately 1 cm using this distraction. Only when the periosteum is divided medially does the osteotomy translate as well as close correctly. If the osteotomy still does not close laterally, the contour of the wedge probably is too angulated, and a truncated wedge should be removed. Small bone fragments must be removed, since these prevent correct apposition of the osteotomy.

The posterior portion of the tuberosity now is closed and translated laterally a further 4 mm and then superiorly 4 mm (Fig. 4). The superior translation is important, since it changes the calcaneal pitch angle and decreases the tension on the Achilles tendon. It is easy to palpate this dorsal overhang, and the lateral translation is under direct vision.

While the surgeon holds the osteotomy in the desired position, an assistant inserts one or two guide pins, and the osteotomy then is affixed using a cannulated screw system (Fig. 5). We prefer 7 mm cannulated cancellous screws, using a shorter 16 mm screw thread so that the threads do not traverse the osteotomy site. The screw(s) should cross the osteotomy site at right angles and therefore are started slightly posterior and laterally on the tuberosity segment directed dorsally and slightly medially. It is important to check the position of the osteotomy again after insertion of the guidewires; ideally this is assessed radiographically, using fluoroscopic imaging to ensure that the pin is in the correct position. Once this position has been assessed, the osteotomy is fixed using the cannulated 7 mm screws. The screws typically are 60 mm in length. Excellent compression usually is obtained by one screw. If insufficient compression is achieved, a second parallel screw can be inserted easily. The wound is closed using interrupted 2-0 Vicryl sutures in the subcutaneous tissue and 4-0 nylon sutures for skin. Postoperatively the patient is placed in a posterior plaster splint, with the foot in the neutral position, and does not bear weight for 10 days until the sutures are removed. A short-leg walking cast then is applied for 4 weeks.

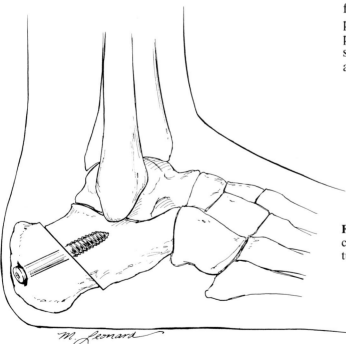

Figure 5 With the tuberosity firmly held, it is secured with a cannulated 7.0 mm screw. Note the dorsal translation of the tuberosity.

Complications

Wound compromise is extremely uncommon with this incision, provided it is made with full-thickness flaps. Injuries to the peroneal tendon or sural nerve are similarly unlikely with careful planning of the incision. We have not encountered nonunion or malunion with this broad cancellous bone surface.

MEDIAL DISPLACEMENT OSTEOTOMY

Indications

A medial displacement osteotomy is used for correction of the valgus foot; typically it is combined with other soft tissue procedures on the medial aspect of the foot for correction of the flexible flatfoot in adolescents and young adults. The rationale of this medial translation of the calcaneus is to improve the tripod effect of the calcaneus, the first and fifth metatarsals. In addition to the osseous translation, the function of the Achilles tendon is improved by translating it medially. In most patients with a flexible flatfoot, the Achilles tendon shifts laterally with the valgus heel and undergoes adaptive shortening or contracture. This is easy to diagnose, since dorsiflexion in the foot with the subtalar joint passively reduced to the neutral position is markedly limited.

Procedure

The patient is positioned laterally with the buttock supported on a bean bag. The incision is identical to the one described earlier, commencing inferior to the peroneal tendon and sural nerve is markedly limited. However, a wedge of bone is not excised, but the osteotomy is performed in the exact same plane as described earlier. It is as important to divide the periosteum medially, since the translation depends on lax medial soft tissues. Once the osteotomy is complete, the inferior portion and posterior aspect of the tuberosity are translated medially. The amount of displacement is judged on the basis of the individual deformity. This usually amounts to 1.5 cm medial translation (approximately one-third the width of the calcaneus). It is important not to let the tuberosity slide proximally, thereby lengthening the Achilles tendon. We prefer to force the tuberosity slightly inferiorly to increase the pitch of the calcaneus.

Once the corrected position is achieved, the surgeon holds the foot while an assistant inserts the guide pin directly from posterior to anterior in the tuberosity. The starting point is immediately under the insertion of the Achilles tendon. A spare guide pin can be placed across the lateral aspect of the foot and used as a guide for

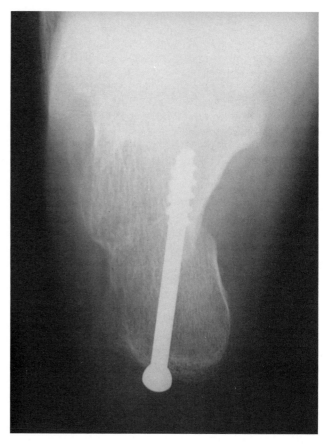

Figure 6 The medial translational osteotomy for a flexible flatfoot deformity is demonstrated with secure rigid fixation.

orientation of the pin to be inserted. One screw usually is sufficient to achieve stable fixation, but if the osteotomy is at all unstable, two screws may be used (Fig. 6). Once the guide pins have been inserted, intraoperative lateral and axial radiographs should be obtained to confirm the position of the osteotomy. The screw typically is 60 mm in length, using a 16 mm thread length.

The wound is closed in layers. The patient is placed in a posterior splint and remains non–weight bearing for 2 weeks. Following removal of sutures, weight bearing is commenced in a short-leg cast for approximately 4 to 6 weeks until union occurs.

SUGGESTED READING

Nayak REK, Cotteril CP. Osteotomy of the calcaneum for symptomatic idiopathic valgus heel. Foot 1992; 2:111–116.
Silver CM, Simond S. Long term observations on calcaneal osteotomy. Clin Orthop 1974; 99:181–187.

SURGICAL MANAGEMENT OF HAGLUND'S DEFORMITY

CAROL FREY, M.D.
GLENN B. PFEFFER, M.D.

Inflammation of the retrocalcaneal bursa often is the result of a prominent or sharply angled posterior-superior margin of the calcaneus. Patrik Haglund described the clinical condition of retrocalcaneal bursitis in 1928, relating it to variations in shape of the os calcis and the wearing of rigid, low-back shoes with flat heels. He described a calcaneus with a prominent posterior-superior border that compressed the Achilles tendon and its surrounding bursa against the posterior shoe counter, causing irritation.

Initial treatment for Haglund's syndrome is nonoperative and includes anti-inflammatory medication, heel lifts, and soft heel counters or backless shoes. If the patient is a running athlete, weekly mileage should be decreased. Achilles tendon stretching is encouraged. The runner should stop training on hills and hard surfaces. Since irritation of the posterior heel by the shoe counter can aggravate the problem, external pressure should be decreased by removing or softening the heel counter or by adding a small felt pad to elevate the heel away from the shoe counter. A heel cup can alternatively be used to protect the area. Tight calf muscles, tight hamstrings, or a cavus foot may be associated with a symptomatic Haglund's deformity. If a biomechanical problem such as a cavus foot is noted on physical examination, proper orthotic devices can be used.

If the above measures do not help to alleviate the discomfort, immobilization in a short-leg walking cast often reduces acute symptoms. Steroid injections are discouraged because fluid leaks out of an inflamed bursa into the paratendinous structures of the Achilles tendon, even if placed into the bursae under image control using radiopaque dye.

PATIENT SELECTION

Although most patients respond to nonoperative treatment, surgical treatment is indicated when adequate conservative or nonoperative treatment has failed to give relief. The objective of the surgery is to eliminate pain by relieving pressure from the underlying bony prominence. Although various angles and lines have been described for evaluating the posterior calcaneus, we have found angles and graphics difficult to measure because of the lack of consistent reference points on the calcaneus. Further, the significance of such measurements has not been proven.

TIMING OF SURGERY

Most patients respond to nonoperative treatment within 6 months. Only after this period of conservative treatment should surgery be considered. One should avoid operating in an area in which there is a blister, open wound, abrasion, or infection.

PREOPERATIVE PREPARATION

Radiographs may assist in the diagnosis by identifying a posterior-superior calcaneal prominence (Fig. 1). Between the tendon and bone on the standing lateral view of the heel, one can observe a thin strip of fat between the tendon and the bone proximal to the insertion of the Achilles tendon. The anterior aspect of the Achilles tendon is outlined sharply throughout its extent by the pre-Achilles fat pad (PAFP). The normal retrocalcaneal bursa is not visible. However, one can identify a radiolucent, wedge-shaped retrocalcaneal recess, which lies between the retrocalcaneal bursa and the Achilles tendon insertion. Retrocalcaneal bursitis is indicated when the sharp definition of the retrocalcaneal recess is lost, and the lucency of the PAFP in this region is replaced by soft tissue density. The distended fluid-filled bursa can project above the calcaneus and into the PAFP. In addition, with retrocalcaneal bursitis, there may be an erosion of the cortex of posterior superior aspect of the calcaneus (Fig. 2). Achilles tendinitis may be noted by a thickening of the tendon and a loss of its sharp anterior interface with the PAFP.

The anatomy of the retrocalcaneal bursa (Fig. 3) can be demonstrated with bursography, but magnetic resonance imaging (MRI) is more helpful not only in demonstrating anatomy but also in differentiating retrocalcaneal bursitis from Achilles tendinitis. Accurate recognition of these entities is necessary for proper management. On the MRI the retrocalcaneal bursa is a potential space that is clearly demarcated only when inflamed. MRI is recommended only in those cases in which a diagnosis is difficult.

CHOICE OF PROCEDURE

Many types of surgical treatment have been described. The objective of each is to relieve pressure from the underlying bony prominence of the calcaneus and thus eliminate the inflammation. A transverse incision over the heel region can be used, splitting the Achilles tendon longitudinally and then resecting the retrocalcaneal bursa and superior prominence of the calcaneus. Although the technique provides excellent exposure, the complications of avulsion of the Achilles tendon and excessive subcutaneous scarring make this method less desirable.

Another approach involves a dorsally based closing-wedge osteotomy of the calcaneus to rotate the superior

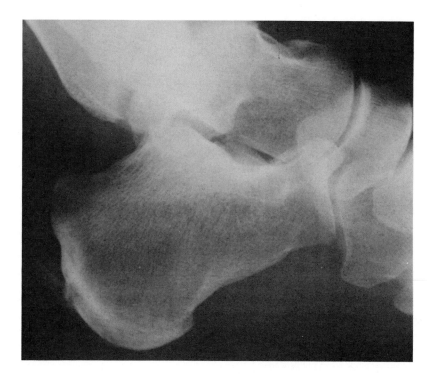

Figure 1 Patient with a prominent posterior-superior tuberosity of the calcaneus in addition to calcification within the Achilles tendon near its insertion on the posterior tubercle.

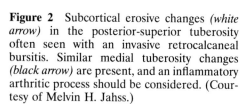

Figure 2 Subcortical erosive changes *(white arrow)* in the posterior-superior tuberosity often seen with an invasive retrocalcaneal bursitis. Similar medial tuberosity changes *(black arrow)* are present, and an inflammatory arthritic process should be considered. (Courtesy of Melvin H. Jahss.)

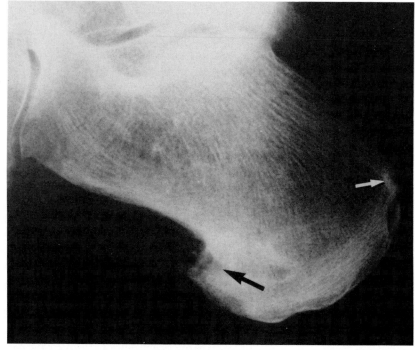

prominence away from the Achilles tendon. Although this technique is somewhat demanding, with rigid screw fixation, patients are able to ambulate almost immediately, and the morbidity is not greater than a simple ostectomy.

We suggest an operative approach that includes resection of the superior prominence of the calcaneus along with associated bursal tissue. A medial and lateral incision along the Achilles tendon can be used for resection of the superior prominence, although we find that complete resection usually can be carried out using just a lateral incision. The addition of a medial incision is useful if the bump is notably medial. In this case the ostectomy through a single lateral incision may leave

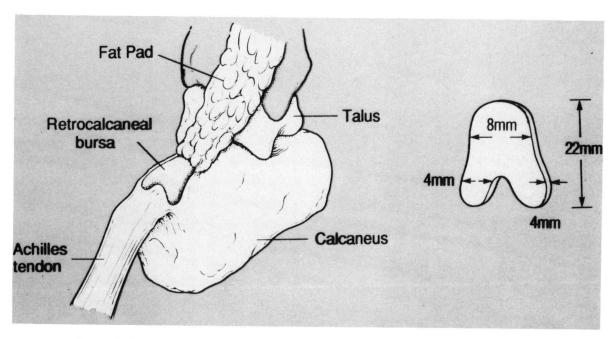

Figure 3 The retrocalcaneal bursa is a disk-shaped structure that overlies the posterior-superior tuberosity of the calcaneus. The average dimensions of the bursa are presented in this graphic depiction.

bone and debris medially. A single incision decreases the incidence of wound problems, as well as the possibility of injury to the superficial medial calcaneal sensory nerve.

PREFERRED PROCEDURE

The patient is placed in the prone position with a bolster under the distal leg. A 5 cm longitudinal incision is made just anterior to the Achilles tendon on the lateral side of the posterior heel, 2 cm proximal to the insertion. The retrocalcaneal area and the superior aspect of the calcaneus are exposed by a combination of blunt and sharp dissection, care being taken to avoid the sural nerve, which lies approximately 1 to 2 cm anterior to the lateral border of the Achilles tendon. The sural nerve should be protected and retracted anteriorly with the subcutaneous tissues. The incision is carried down to the bone, making sure that the insertion site is exposed adequately. If extensive inflammation of the retrocalcaneal bursa is observed, the bursal tissue should be removed. Removal of the bursal tissue is not as important as adequate decompression of the bony prominence. This decompression is carried out using an oblique osteotomy of the superior angle of the calcaneus, starting approximately 1.5 cm anterior to the posterior border of the calcaneus and angling downward to the insertion of the Achilles tendon (approximately 2 cm distal to the superior margin of the calcaneus) (Figs. 4, 5, and 6). The osteotomy is carried out with a power saw, keeping perpendicular to the longitudinal axis of the calcaneus. A ridge of bone always is left at the insertion site of the Achilles tendon and must be removed

carefully with a small curette and power microreciprocating rasp. The microreciprocating rasp also is helpful in rounding off the margins of the calcaneus in all directions, especially on the medial side. The area is palpated often through the overlying skin to make certain that all ridges and prominences are removed. The piece of bone removed must be of adequate size to ensure thorough decompression of the retrocalcaneal area.

It should be kept in mind that the Achilles tendon does not insert at the superior aspect of the calcaneus but significantly more inferior in the apophyseal portion of the calcaneus. The Achilles tendon sweeps backward and away from the tibia to meet the inclined calcaneus obliquely, the bone and the tendon forming an acute angle. We have found that by resecting bone down to the insertion site of the Achilles tendon, adequate decompression of the retrocalcaneal space can be obtained. The Achilles tendon then should be examined for tendinosis. Longitudinal scalpel cuts in the anterior 50 percent of the tendon often reveal necrotic areas of tendon that require debridement. The tendon is repaired with a buried 3-0 nonabsorbable suture such as Ethibond. The wound is closed routinely in layers over a small suction drain.

POSTOPERATIVE COURSE

The patient is placed into a short-leg non–weight-bearing cast with the foot in mild plantar flexion for the first 4 weeks. A short-leg walking cast then is used, with the foot gradually brought up to neutral position for the

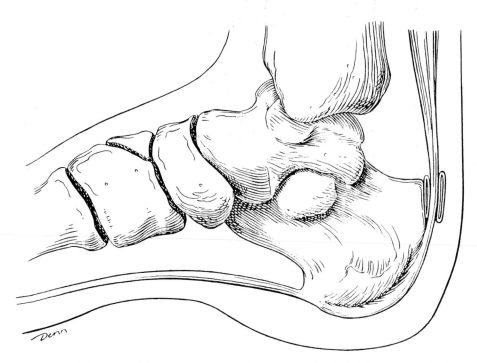

Figure 4 Calcaneus with the retrocalcaneal and superficial Achilles bursae before ostectomy.

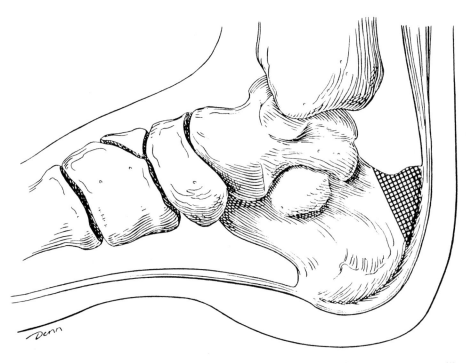

Figure 5 A large portion of the calcaneus needs to be excised surgically or symptoms will recur.

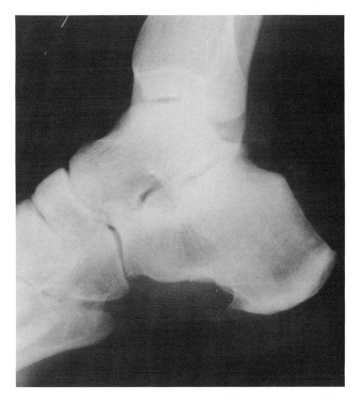

Figure 6 Correctly performed ostectomy of the calcaneus in a patient with Halgund's deformity.

next 4 weeks. When the cast is removed, the patient is placed into a shoe with a ⁷⁄₁₆ inch tapered internal heel lift that gradually is brought down to ³⁄₁₆ of an inch. This is worn for 3 months. General muscle conditioning is begun when the cast is removed.

COMPLICATIONS AND TECHNICAL PITFALLS

Beware of leaving a potentially irritating ridge along the medial calcaneal border, which can become symptomatic. This can be prevented by using a microreciprocating rasp to round off the margins. If the medial ridge still can not be reached adequately with the rasp, a medial incision should be added. We find that this rarely is necessary, however. Make sure that adequate bone has been removed to successfully decompress the retrocalcaneal space. Bone can be removed up to the insertion site of the Achilles tendon. Do not leave a ledge or spike of bone under the Achilles tendon at its insertion site. This potentially is painful and a source of irritation to the Achilles tendon. This bone can be removed with a curette, rongeur, or reciprocating rasp.

It is possible to remove too much distal bone and cut into the insertion of the Achilles tendon. This could allow the tendon to avulse later. Careful exposure of the insertion site of the Achilles tendon at the time of surgery should help the surgeon avoid this pitfall.

Other problems that can be encountered include damage to the sural nerve or the medial neurovascular structures. These problems can be prevented by paying close attention to anatomy and using careful dissection technique. Wound problems are a constant source of worry around the Achilles tendon, and great care should be taken when handling the soft tissues and posterior skin.

SUGGESTED READING

Fiamengo S, et al. Posterior heel pain associated with a calcaneal step and Achilles tendon calcification. Clin Orthop 1982; 167:203.

Fowler A, Philip JF. Abnormality of the calcaneus as a cause of painful heel. Br J Surg 1945; 32:494.

Henneghan M, Pavlov H. The Haglund painful heel syndrome. Clin Orthop 1984; 187:228.

Keck S, Kelley P. Bursitis of the posterior part of the heel. J Bone Joint Surg 1965; 47A:267.

Pfeffer GB, Baxter DE. Surgery of the adult heel. In: Jahss MH, ed. Disorders of the foot and ankle: Medical and surgical management. 2nd ed. Philadelphia: WB Saunders, 1991.

NEUROMUSCULAR PROCEDURES

TENDON TRANSFERS

JOHN D. HSU, M.D., C.M., F.A.C.S.
PETER EDWARDS, M.D.

Transfers about the foot and ankle are not common orthopedic procedures. However, these procedures are useful for the correction of foot and ankle deformities. The purpose of this chapter is to identify the common tendon transfers that are used around the foot and ankle, to discuss their indications, to make the orthopedic surgeon aware of possible pitfalls that could occur when these procedures are performed, and to identify special problems that may be encountered.

GENERAL PRINCIPLES

Tendon transfers around the foot and ankle are used for the correction of a dynamic deformity and as an adjunct for rebalancing the foot after a fixed deformity has been corrected. Knowledge of the underlying disease is of the utmost importance and can guide the orthopedic surgeon in selecting the appropriate procedure, allow for the assessment of the usefulness of the procedure, serve as adjunct measures such as bracing and physical modalities including electrical stimulation, and determine prognosis and success of the procedure for the overall maintenance or restoration of function.

ANATOMIC CONSIDERATIONS

The major muscles that control foot and ankle function consist of the anterior tibial, posterior tibial, the gastrocnemius-soleus, the peroneus longus and peroneus brevis muscles, and the flexors and extensors of the big toe and lesser toes. Dynamically and functionally, balance is maintained so that the foot is plantigrade in the stance phase and the leg advanced through the gait cycle in walking in a smooth, efficient, and coordinated manner. Imbalance of the musculature when one muscle

functions improperly or when it is functioning out of phase can cause gait disorders. Callosities can form with shoe wear. When fixed deformities occur, the position of the major joints of the foot and ankle become distorted, causing pain with weight bearing.

The intrinsic musculature around the foot also is of concern. Many neurologic disorders affect these muscles, and consequently they must be considered in surgical planning.

ANTERIOR TIBIAL TENDON TRANSFER TO THE MIDFOOT

This procedure was described by Garceau and is useful in rebalancing a foot in which the anterior tibial musculature is causing an abnormal pull, causing the foot to turn into varus. This is a common problem following stroke and other neurologic conditions characterized by anterior tibioperoneal imbalance.

Technique

The anterior tibial tendon is exposed at its insertion and detached. The tendon then is brought out proximally and rerouted into the middle of the foot. In most cases it can be anchored to the cuneiform bone (Fig. 1). This position is determined by the magnitude of the deformity, but generally the middle or lateral cuneiform is selected. A bone block is recommended to avoid pull out. This is best achieved by removing a core or dowel of bone from the cuneiform and passing the secured tendon to the plantar foot with a suture attached to a straight or Keith needle. While tension is held on the suture, the foot is brought into the neutral position and the dowel of bone replaced and tamped securely. To enhance stability further, an interference screw (4.0 mm cancellous) can be inserted between the dowel and the edge of the cuneiform, but avoiding the tendon. This greatly increases pull-out strength. Postoperative casting for 6 weeks is necessary to allow the tendon to become incorporated in its new position. If bracing was not needed preoperatively, it generally is not needed postoperatively.

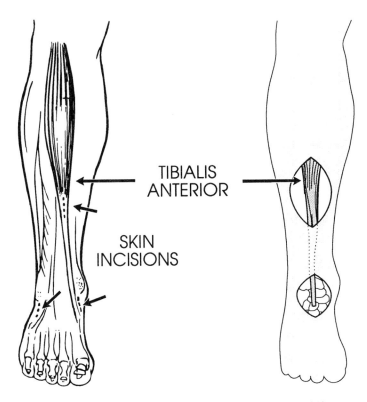

Figure 1   Tibialis anterior tendon transfer to the midfoot.

ANTERIOR TIBIAL TENDON TRANSFER TO THE CALCANEUS

This procedure was described by Peabody and used for the calcaneus foot, frequently observed as a residual of poliomyelitis or in myelomeningocele patients.

Technique

The anterior tibial muscle is exposed distally and detached from its insertion. A second incision is made on the anterior aspect of the midleg, just lateral to the tibial spine. The muscle is retracted laterally with the interosseous membrane exposed. A window is cut out of the interosseus membrane, care being taken not to injure the neurovascular structure. The anterior tibial tendon then is brought posteriorly and anchored to the distal portion of the tendo Achilles or to the os calcis (Fig. 2). As with other tendon transfers, this is best secured using a bone dowel with or without an interference screw. This obviates the need for a button on the plantar foot surface.

A period of casting is necessary for the tendon transfer to incorporate into its new position with the foot in equinus. If there are other weaknesses or imbalances present at the foot, the foot may need to be supported or positioned in a brace.

SPLIT ANTERIOR TIBIAL TENDON TRANSFER

Spastic equinovarus is common in the cerebral palsy, brain-injured, and cerebrovascular accident population. This results in a functional disability. Mild equinovarus deformity can be corrected by the use of an orthosis, but when ambulatory (dynamic) electromyography (EMG) identifies a muscular pattern of premature soleus contraction, spastic midstance anterior tibial action, and decreased peroneal brevis activity, split anterior tibial transfer (SPLATT) is indicated.

Technique

The insertion of the anterior tibial tendon is identified. We prefer to expose the anterior tibial tendon in the midleg region, and after the proximal and distal portions of the anterior tibial tendon are visualized, the lateral one-half to two-thirds of the anterior tibial tendon is released and brought out proximally through the second incision. A third incision is made longitudinally over the dorsum of the cuboid. The lateral portion of the anterior tibial tendon, now split, is passed subcutaneously into this incision. Using the 7/64 inch drill, two converging holes are placed in the cuboid. After the bony channel is smoothed, the transfer tendon is passed through the channel and sutured on itself with the foot slightly everted and dorsiflexed (Fig. 3).

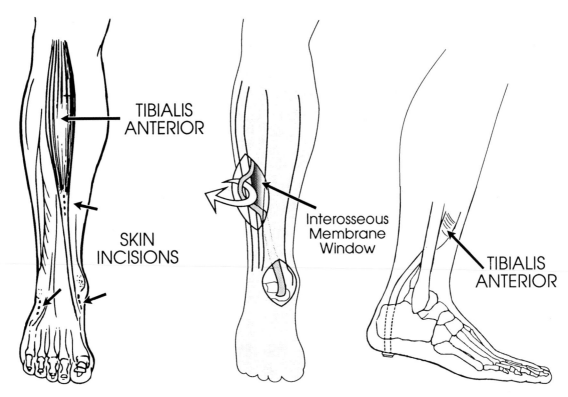

Figure 2 Tibialis anterior tendon transfer posteriorly to the calcaneus.

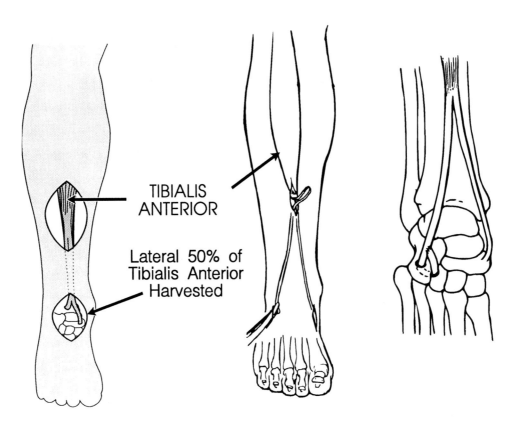

Figure 3 Split tibialis anterior tendon transfer (SPLATT).

Postoperatively, a short-leg walking cast in slight eversion and neutral position of the ankle is applied for 6 weeks. This is followed by an orthosis used for ambulation and splint for nighttime wear over the next 6 months.

The goal of this surgical operation is for a patient to be brace-free, ambulating with improved gait. Paying close attention to patient selection and surgical technique, as well as EMG studies in preoperative planning, aid in this pursuit. The SPLATT operation should be considered only for muscles that have increased tone. For neuromuscular disorders or muscles that have lost strength, transfer of the entire muscle to a new location is a more desirable procedure.

POSTERIOR TIBIAL TENDON TRANSFER ANTERIORLY THROUGH INTEROSSEOUS MEMBRANE

This procedure was initially described by Watkins for the correction of an equinus foot. Footdrop can occur with loss of musculature secondary to poliomyelitis or loss of dorsiflexion because of injury to the peroneal nerve. Additionally, certain neuromuscular disorders, such as Duchenne-type muscular dystrophy or Charcot-Marie-Tooth disease, could allow the posterior tibial musculature to overpower the ankle dorsiflexors.

Technique

The technique of transferring the posterior tibial tendon as described by Watkins is to expose the posterior tibial tendon on the medial aspect of the foot and then bring the tendon out at the medial side of the distal third of the leg. After this is done, an anterior incision is made to dissect the interosseous membrane. Once the interosseous membrane has been exposed, a window is cut out of the interosseous membrane as described in the anterior tibial transfer to the calcaneus. The posterior tibial tendon then is brought to the anterior aspect of the leg. After this is done, the posterior tendon is anchored into the foot, generally in one of the cuneiform bones.

In 1978 Hsu and Hoffer modified this procedure for the neuromuscular patient in whom they felt that prolonged immobilization would result in a rapid loss of musculature and function. They exposed the posterior tibial tendon in a similar fashion, but instead of making a long incision on the anterior aspect of the leg (which would lead to postoperative pain and the need for immobilization), the posterior tibial tendon was brought anteriorly through the interosseous membrane by piercing the interosseous membrane as close to the tibia as possible on the posterior aspect. In this way vessels are not endangered or harmed by the procedure. When excising this window it is useful to stay on bone, gradually lifting up the periosteum and fascia. The vessels lie immediately underneath the membrane and must be avoided. When passing the tendon through, it is useful to widen the window gently with a Kelly clamp. A large-chest Kelly clamp is useful to spread the subcutaneous tissue in the anterior distal leg, since the tendon must not be deep to the exterior fascia. After this is accomplished, the posterior tibial tendon can be brought out to the forward part of the leg. Smaller incisions are used, minimizing postoperative pain and enabling the patient to be mobilized as soon as possible, generally the

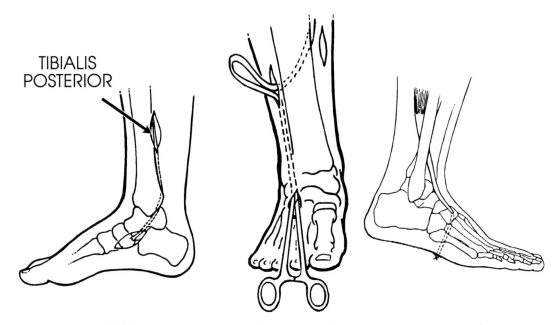

TIBIALIS POSTERIOR

Figure 4 Tibialis posterior tendon transfer anteriorly through the interosseous membrane.

first day after the operative procedure (Fig. 4). Patients are kept non–weight bearing for 2 weeks, after which a walking cast is applied for approximately 4 weeks to allow the tendon to become incorporated into the bone. Once again this is best secured with a bone-dowel technique. When footdrop conditions are being treated, and if there is not sufficient musculature to allow the tendon to function appropriately, an AFO or other brace may be indicated.

SPLIT POSTERIOR TIBIAL TENDON TRANSFER

This procedure is used for the cerebrospastic patient in whom there is an overactivity of the posterior tendon, dynamically allowing the foot to be pulled into equinovarus. The posterior tibial tendon is split in half, and the part that is split laterally is rerouted to the lateral side of the foot or to the peroneal tendon. This allows redistribution of the muscle forces, achieving correction (Fig. 5).

The split posterior tibial tendon transfer (SPLOTT) is useful when the posterior tibial tendon is firing in its proper phase. A walking EMG is recommended and is an integral part of planning this procedure. Also, knowledge of the activity and strength of the anterior tibial muscle is needed, because frequently the correction is insufficient and the anterior tibial muscle continues to pull the foot into varus requiring its release, repositioning, or partial transfer.

PERONEAL TENDON TRANSFER

In a calcaneal valgus or valgus deformity of the foot and ankle, after bony reconstructive procedures such as the Grice in the immature foot or a triple arthrodesis or calcaneal osteotomy in a mature foot, a relatively stronger peroneal muscle may need to be transferred to the heel. This would allow for the correction of the deformity and augmentation of plantar flexion.

LONG TOE FLEXOR AND EXTENSOR RELEASES

Secondary deformity after foot and ankle correction, such as bringing an ankle from a persistent and fixed equinus position to neutral, can cause the big toe and lesser toes to contract. If this presents a problem and causes calluses or pain, fusion at the interphalangeal joint of the toes is indicated. The long toe flexors and extensors then would need to be transferred to a more proximal position to maintain function.

Acknowledgment. The authors gratefully acknowledge the contributions of Lydia Cabico in the preparation of the illustrations.

SUGGESTED READING

Garceau GJ, Manning KR. The anterior tibial tendon transfer. J Bone Joint Surg 1947; 29:1044.

Green NE, Griffin PP, Shiavi R. Split posterior tibial-tendon transfer in spastic cerebral palsy. J Bone Joint Surg 1983; 65A:748.

Hoffer M, Reiswig J, Garrett A, Perry J. Split anterior tibial tendon transfer in cerebral palsy. Orthop Clin North Am 1974; 5:31.

Hsu JD, Hoffer MM. Posterior tibial tendon transfer anteriorly through the interosseous membrane. Clin Orthop 1978; 131:202.

Peabody CW. Tendon transposition: An end-result study. J Bone Joint Surg 1938; 20:193.

Watkins MB, Jones JB. Transplantation of the posterior tibial tendon. J Bone Joint Surg 1954; 36A:1181.

Figure 5 Split tibialis posterior tendon transfer (SPLOTT).

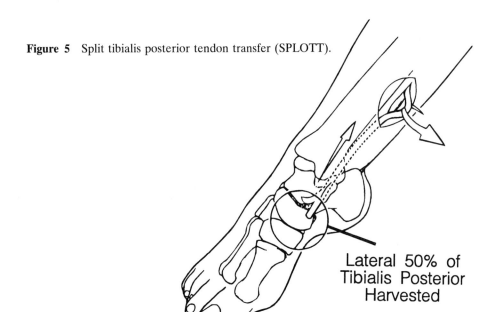

Lateral 50% of Tibialis Posterior Harvested

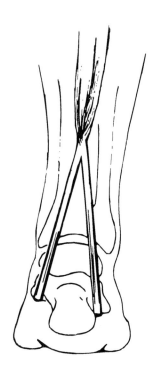

TARSAL TUNNEL RELEASE

LEW C. SCHON, M.D.

Tarsal tunnel syndrome is caused by compression of the tibial nerve in the retromalleolar region. Neuritic symptoms such as burning, shooting, tingling, numbness, or radiating pain may be present from the medial ankle to the toes and/or up the leg. On physical examination, the symptoms are reproduced with percussion of the nerve in the retromalleolar region or along the course of the medial, lateral, or calcaneal nerves. A careful examination must be performed to exclude a more proximal nerve compression in the popliteal fossa, sciatic notch, or spine. A diffuse peripheral neuropathy, tendinitis, or biomechanical malalignment such as progressive pes planovalgus also simulates tarsal tunnel syndrome. Within the tarsal tunnel, the nerve may be compressed by bony residuals following trauma, inflamed tendon sheaths, aberrant muscles, engorged or tortuous vascular structures, or tumors. In over 50 percent of cases, the cause is not identifiable.

Routine examination includes radiographs to evaluate the surrounding bony structures, and electrophysiologic studies. These studies are used to help localize the pathology, to rule out an intrinsic neurologic process, and to help exclude a double-crush or a double-lesion neuropathy. If a space-occupying lesion is suspected, magnetic resonance imaging (MRI) may be of some benefit.

THERAPEUTIC ALTERNATIVES

Conservative modalities must be tried before surgery is considered. Most patients with tarsal tunnel syndrome are placed initially in an ankle stirrup brace (e.g., Aircast) and given vitamin B_6 50 mg PO twice daily for 2 to 4 weeks. Occasionally an anti-inflammatory medication also is started. Injections in the tarsal tunnel have been advocated by some authors with variable results. Orthotic devices and casting, strapping, or bracing to rest the nerve may be of benefit. A trial of tricyclic antidepressant compounds such as amitriptyline (Elavil), nortriptyline (Pamelor), or doxepin (Sinequan) have been effective. Doses begin at 10 or 25 mg and are given about 12 hours before the patient needs to awaken to avoid drowsiness during the day. Patients are instructed that at least 4 weeks often are necessary to determine whether the medication has any effect. Side effects such as drowsiness, irritability, constipation, weight gain, forgetfulness, dry mouth, nightmares, and urinary retention are discussed at great length. If the medications are successful, the patients gradually are tapered off with monitoring for recurrent symptoms. Many patients require 3 to 6 months of treatment and then no longer need medication. Some patients require longer courses of medication. For those patients who do not respond to lower doses after 4 weeks, the dose is doubled, providing the patient has minimal side effects. Other medications can be tried including phenytoin (Dilantin), carbamazepine (Tegretol), and clonazepam (Klonopin). Some of these medications require careful patient monitoring with blood tests and checkups.

INDICATIONS

Patients are selected for surgery based on the localization of their symptoms to the tibial nerve and/or one of its branches underneath the abductor or the flexor retinaculum. Any age group may be affected, but children rarely are symptomatic enough to require surgery. Most cases seen in children resolve with conservative treatment. Older patients with peripheral edema or fatty ankles may be poor candidates for surgery.

Patients with diabetes or other metabolic neuropathies usually do not respond adequately to surgery. Although most patients with the clinical diagnosis of tarsal tunnel syndrome have positive electrodiagnostic studies, the presence of negative or normal studies should not completely deter the surgeon from operating on a symptomatic patient with reproducible and localized findings. It is important to note the specific areas of tenderness with reference to the medial and lateral plantar nerves, first-branch lateral-plantar nerve, calcaneal nerve, and the tibial nerve. Some authors recommend releasing the tibial nerve over the entire course when there is palpable tenderness.

SURGICAL TECHNIQUE

The patient is placed in a supine position on the operating table. If a tourniquet is not used, the patient is placed in a Trendelenburg position to diminish venous back flow. Typically $2.5\times$ loupe magnification is used. An incision is made over the course of the tibial artery, which frequently can be readily palpated. If the artery cannot be palpated, an incision is made approximately 1 cm from the tip of the medial malleolus and about 2 to 3 cm behind the medial edge of the distal tibia (Fig. 1). Distally, once the calcaneal-fibula axis has been passed, the incision should be directed anteriorly in a curved fashion (Fig. 2). Gentle, blunt, sharp dissection is carried out through the subcutaneous tissue with careful attention toward a piercing branch of the calcaneal nerves. Distally the superior edge of the abductor hallucis should be identified. Next the flexor retinaculum is released again with careful attention to any perforating neurovascular structures (Fig. 3). The neurovascular bundles to the medial and lateral side of the foot should be identified in the distal aspect of the incision. Usually it is easiest to follow the course of the veins as they dive deep to the abductor fascia. Partial release of the superficial fascia of the abductor with reflection of the abductor muscle distally permits release of the deep fascia of the abductor overlying the veins that accompany the medial and lateral-plantar nerves (Fig. 4). If a first branch of the lateral-plantar nerve entrapment is suspected, this branch and its vein should be freed.

I do not recommend dissections of the perineural tissue. This destroys its natural protective surroundings, including the fat, artery and veins, and may lead to perineural scarring and adhesions that prohibit nerve gliding and normal nerve function. Often when a more aggressive dissection is done, small branches of the nerve, artery, and vein are inadvertently sacrificed, further adding to the morbidity of the procedure. If, however, there is a specific area in which an entrapment or tumor is suspected, dissection of the nerve in these

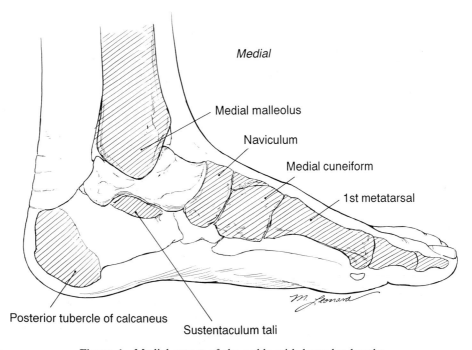

Figure 1 Medial aspect of the ankle with bony landmarks.

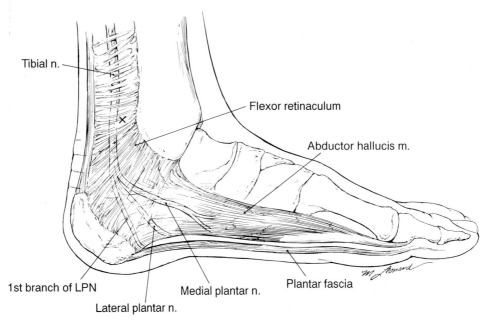

Figure 2 Incision for tarsal tunnel release. LPN, lateral plantar nerve.

locations is warranted. Still, as much as possible, the surrounding veins and arteries should be disturbed minimally.

Once the neurovascular bundle has been freed, the entire course of the bundle and its branches should be palpated gently to identify where further release is necessary. After complete hemostasis is achieved, the wound is irrigated and the skin is closed with nylon everted mattress sutures. A light compression dressing is applied.

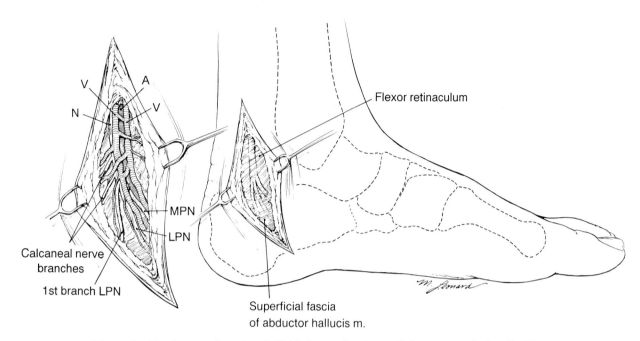

Figure 3 The flexor retinaculum is divided, exposing the medial neurovascular bundle. Note: The veins (V) are superficial to the artery (A), and the nerve (N) is deep and posterior to the vessels. LPN, lateral plantar nerve, MPN, medial plantar nerve.

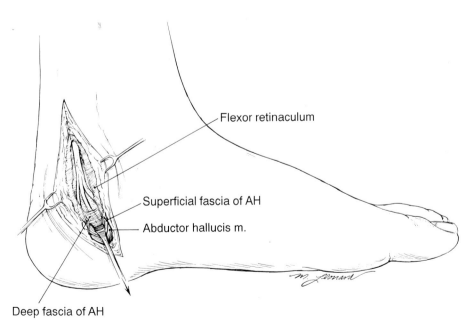

Figure 4 The superficial fascia of the abductor hallucis (AH) is released so that the muscle can be reflected distally, exposing the deep fascia.

POSTOPERATIVE COURSE

The patients are instructed to remain off the foot for 2 weeks following the surgery. During this time, they may use crutches or a walker as they feel comfortable. A wound check is scheduled at 1 week, sutures are removed at 2 weeks, and then the patients may begin gradual weight bearing as tolerated. We encourage resumption of the heel cord stretching and increase in activities as tolerated. Typical recovery should occur within 8 weeks; however, some patients improve within 3 weeks and others take years. Frequently the more extensive the dissection, the longer the recovery.

COMPLICATIONS AND SEQUELAE

Several complications can occur specific to the tarsal tunnel release. The transection of a calcaneal nerve or another branch can lead to a painful calcaneal neuroma. Occasionally this leads to a diffuse tibial neuritis, and in rare instances a reflex sympathetic dystrophy can manifest. A postoperative neuroma or neuritis can be treated with tricyclic antidepressant medications and desensitization physical therapy. In some situations a cast is helpful, but beware of overusing casts and immobilizations because this further increases the likelihood that a nerve may adhere to the scar tissue. Generally it is better to encourage range of motion following the surgery.

It is not uncommon following any nerve release to have a patient initially experience relief of pain only to be disappointed subsequently as the pain partially or completely returns over the next weeks to months. Overall recurrent tarsal tunnel syndrome occurs in about 30 percent of patients. Some of these are a result of inadequate release, inadvertent superficial nerve transection, or repeat trauma, whereas others are idiopathic. It is best to advise patients before surgery that this nerve always will be somewhat more vulnerable to injury, even after a minor insult.

PROS AND CONS OF TREATMENT

This technique of tarsal tunnel release emphasizes a proximal and distal release and avoids extensive dissection of the nerve. As previously noted, the postoperative recovery is much shorter and the likelihood of recurrence is lower. There is much less adhesion of the nerve to the surrounding tissues, and the nerve's natural buffer of the artery and vein is left intact, reducing the incidence of scar pain and persistent Tinel's sign as a result of adherence. One final advantage is that if a wound problem develops with a wound dishiscence, a skin graft can be applied without worrying about the nerves being exposed superficially.

The disadvantage of this technique is that the nerve is not visualized for its entire course. If an area of specific nerve tenderness is not noted and deeper exploration therefore is not adequately performed, both intraneural and extraneural pathology may be overlooked. In many cases in which a tumor is suspected based on clinical findings, an MRI of the tarsal tunnel can prevent this pitfall.

SUGGESTED READING

Cimino WR. Tarsal tunnel syndrome: Review of the literature. Foot Ankle 1990; 11:47–52.
Dellon AL, Mackinnon SE. Tibial nerve branching in the tarsal tunnel. Arch Neurol 1984; 41:645–646.
Havel PE, Ebraheim NA, Clark SE, et al. Tibial nerve branching in the tarsal tunnel. Foot Ankle 1988; 9:117–119.
Heimkes B, Posel P, Stotz A, et al. The proximal and distal tarsal tunnel syndromes: An anatomic study. Int Orthop 1987; 11:193.
Kaplan PE, Kernahan WT. Tarsal tunnel syndrome: An electrodiagnostic and surgical correlation. J Bone Joint Surg 1981; 63A:96–99.
Lam SJS. Tarsal tunnel syndrome. J Bone Joint Surg 1967; 49B:87–92.
Mann RA. Tarsal tunnel syndrome. In: Evarts CM, ed. Surgery of the musculoskeletal system. Vol 4. New York: Churchill Livingstone, 1983:79.

PLANTAR FASCIA AND BAXTER'S NERVE RELEASE

LEW C. SCHON, M.D.

There are many causes of inferior heel pain including plantar fasciitis, stress fractures of the heel, fat pad insufficiency, and local nerve entrapment (first branch of the lateral-plantar nerve). Various systemic disorders may manifest as heel pain including the seronegative arthritides and sarcoidosis. An examination of the patient must therefore include an assessment of the patient's health and appreciation of the stigmata of these conditions. Biomechanical factors such as tight heel cords or a pronated or cavus foot also should be identified. A more detailed discussion of the etiology, pathogenesis, and diagnosis are beyond the scope of this chapter, but should be reviewed to achieve a proper perspective.

For the most part, conservative treatment is successful in approximately 90 percent of patients after 6 months of onset of the heel pain. Patients are encouraged to perform Achilles stretching 3 times a day. Each stretch should be held without bouncing for 10 seconds. Stretching of the symptomatic heel should be alternated with contralateral stretching for the same duration with a total of 10 stretches on each side. It is important to keep the foot perpendicular to the body to prevent overstretching the posterior tibial tendon, especially in patients who may pronate to achieve an effective stretch.

A walking program should be instituted if the patient is relatively sedentary or does not do any recreational ambulatory activity. The patient should start with a 5 to 10 minute walk every day and increase the duration of the walk 10 percent each week until reaching 20 minutes daily. Patients who are avid runners should decrease their daily mileage and gradually build up to their previous level at about 10 percent per week. Low-impact activities such as bicycle riding or swimming should be added to the workout.

Walking or running shoes should have a thick soft sole with a slight heel lift. Occasionally a heel pad or heel cup is useful to decrease the stresses on the heel. Some patients may benefit from either a custom-made or off-the-shelf orthosis. A tapered medial heel wedge or heel lift also can be added to shoes. Some cases of resistant plantar fasciitis respond to temporary casting, splinting, or a strapping of the leg, foot, or ankle.

Occasionally a brief trial of nonsteroidal anti-inflammatory medications may be prescribed for 1 to 2 weeks. Subsequent to this initial dosage, patients may be instructed to take the medication intermittently during an acute flare-up. An injection of cortisone with lidocaine and bupivacaine (Marcaine) may be instilled in the area of the plantar fascia in those patients that are not responding to other modalities. With each injection, the risk of plantar fascia rupture increases. Certainly beyond three injections, the risk becomes significant. Injections may be given every 2 weeks, but typically it is preferable to wait at least 4 weeks between injections. An injection just before surgery should be avoided, since it increases the risk of wound complications and infection.

Only 1 or 2 percent of patients will continue to have pain despite a year of conservative modalities. In these patients who have failed a concerted trial of heel cord stretching, walking program, heel pads or cups, injections, anti-inflammatory medications, a heel lift or medial heel wedge, and occasionally casting or splinting, surgery may be indicated.

PREFERRED SURGICAL APPROACH

Patient Selection

Patients who are to be considered for a plantar fascia release and/or release of Baxter's nerve should be selected carefully. These must be patients who have pain that is reproduced with palpation over the medial tubercle and/or along the course of the first branch of the lateral-plantar nerve (Fig. 1). As mentioned previously, the patient should have undergone a conservative trial of approximately 1 year. In rare cases surgery may be indicated after a shorter period if symptoms are incapacitating and a reasonable trial of therapy has been completely without benefit. Patients with diffuse enthesopathies, seronegative arthropathies, or systemic diseases tend to have a poor prognosis following surgery. No significant differences in outcome have been noted regarding age, sex, activity level, or foot type.

Patients with neuritic symptoms that are reproduced with palpation of the plantar fascia and first branch of the lateral-plantar nerve may be candidates for preoperative nerve conduction velocity tests (motor and mixed) and electromyography. In some cases in which uncertainty exists as to whether there is tarsal tunnel syndrome or a more localized distal nerve entrapment, these tests can be of help. It is important to correlate the clinical examination of the tibial nerve, medial-plantar nerve, lateral-plantar nerve, first branch of the lateral-plantar nerve, and the calcaneal branches with the findings of electrodiagnostic studies. Tenderness along the course of one of the nerves in association with a positive study is an indication for a release of that nerve.

Athletes or those patients with non-neuritic localized tenderness over the medial tubercle of the calcaneus probably are best served with a limited partial medial-plantar fasciectomy. In some of these patients, release of the fascia of the abductor may result in a prolonged recovery.

Routine preoperative use of a technetium bone scan should be discouraged because it does not make a difference regarding prognosis or surgical approach. Nevertheless, in patients with uncharacteristic or diffuse findings, a bone scan may be warranted to rule out a stress fracture of the calcaneus or enthesopathies.

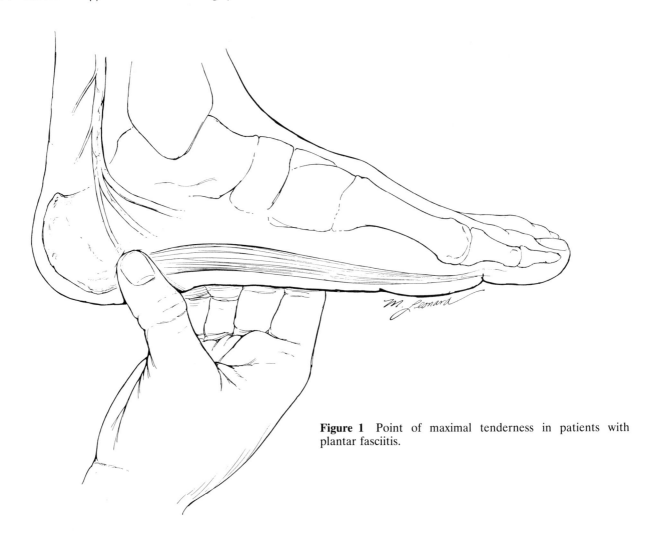

Figure 1 Point of maximal tenderness in patients with plantar fasciitis.

Operative Approach

The surgery may be performed under ankle block anesthesia with or without intravenous sedation or a general anesthetic. A tourniquet is not required, and its use depends on the level of comfort of the surgeon. The patient is positioned supine so that the affected foot can be rotated externally. A 2.5× loupe magnification routinely is used for the surgery. If no tourniquet is used, the patient may be put in a slight Trendelenburg position to decrease venous back flow. Prophylactic intravenous antibiotics may be used at the discretion of the surgeon.

An oblique 3 to 4 cm incision is made along the medial aspect of the heel overlying the course of the first branch of the lateral-plantar nerve and the proximal edge of the belly of the abductor hallucis muscle (Fig. 2). The starting point of the incision may be located by bisecting a longitudinal axial line that runs 1 cm from the posterior edge of the medial malleolus. The incision courses obliquely in a distal and plantar direction and stops at the junction of the plantar and medial skin. Sharp dissection is carried out through the subcutaneous fat, with careful attention directed toward a superficial branch of the calcaneal nerves. Occasionally, before encountering the superficial fascia of the abductor, subcutaneous fascia is identified. This fascia often is confused with the abductor hallucis fascia. Once the superficial fascia of the abductor is identified, a small self-retaining retractor is inserted into the wound. The plantar fascia is identified by passing a Freer elevator from the medial-distal edge of the abductor in a plantar and lateral direction. A small lamina spreader with teeth is inserted at this junction of the abductor fascia and plantar fascia. A Senn retractor is placed distally between the two arms of the lamina spreader to afford better visualization of the plantar fascia.

Once the exposure is complete, the superficial fascia of the abductor is released sharply (Fig. 3). Next, using the Freer elevator, the deep fascia of the abductor is identified. This fascia is concave and is important to visualize before performing the release. Next, using a Senn retractor the abductor muscle is pulled superiorly, and the inferior portion of the deep fascia of the abductor is released with a scalpel (Fig. 4). Beneath this fascia, there is fat, an artery, a vein, and the first branch of the lateral-plantar nerve. Next, the Senn retractor is placed superiorly, pulling the abductor muscle in a distal direction and permitting complete release of the deep

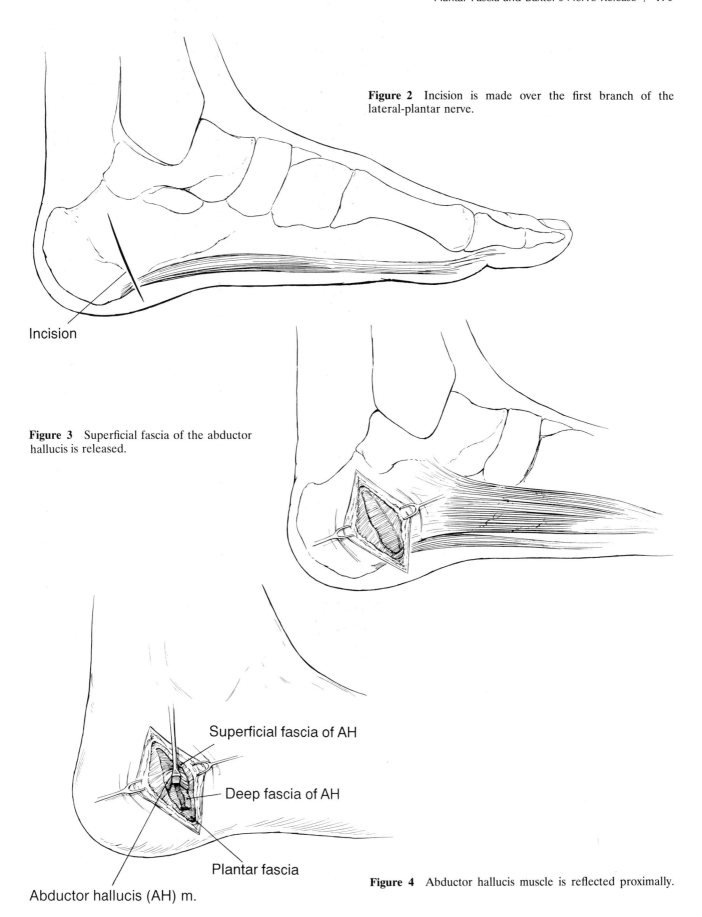

Figure 2 Incision is made over the first branch of the lateral-plantar nerve.

Incision

Figure 3 Superficial fascia of the abductor hallucis is released.

Superficial fascia of AH

Deep fascia of AH

Plantar fascia

Abductor hallucis (AH) m.

Figure 4 Abductor hallucis muscle is reflected proximally.

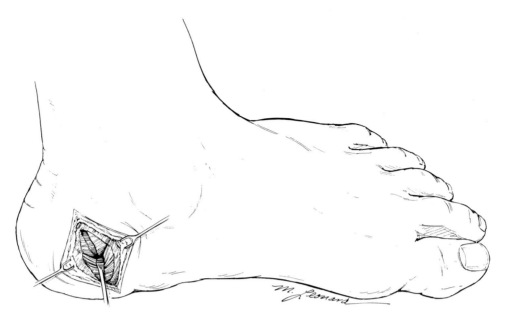

Figure 5 Abductor hallucis muscle is retracted distally.

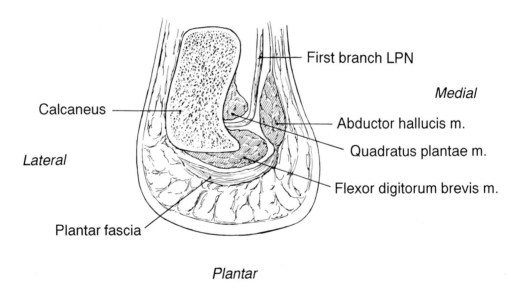

Figure 6 Cross-sectional anatomy of the heel along the course of the first branch of the lateral plantar nerve (LPN).

fascia of the abductor from this direction (Fig. 5). Thus the first branch of the lateral-plantar nerve is released. The nerve may be visualized without dissection in about 20 percent of cases. Routinely, I do not dissect out the nerve because this may cause unnecessary bleeding and trauma to the structures. Occasionally a sharp edge of the medial-caudal border of the quadratus plantae is palpated (Fig. 6). In these patients, a careful release of this fascia is warranted.

Attention now is drawn to the inferior aspect of the wound. The plantar fascia is well visualized medially, and a rectangle measuring approximately 2 to 3 × 4 mm of medial-plantar fascia is resected (Fig. 7). In some patients who have pain throughout the entire insertion of the plantar fascia medially *and laterally,* and who are not athletic, an entire plantar fasciotomy also may be performed. If the entire plantar fascia is to be released, the lamina spreader is inserted in the area of the resected plantar fascia, and the remaining portion of the plantar fascia is visualized and cut.

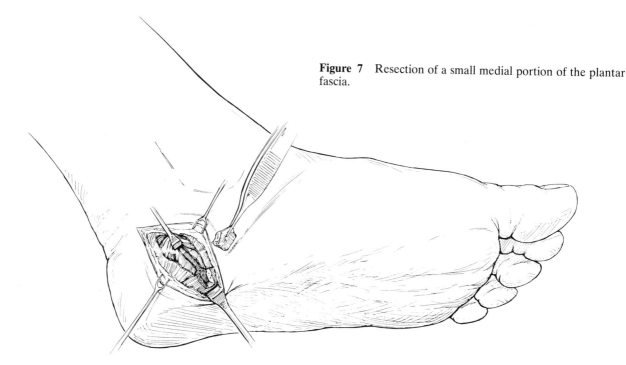

Figure 7 Resection of a small medial portion of the plantar fascia.

If a large spur is present preoperatively and is thought to be contributing to the symptoms, the spur may be resected. This is done by gently reflecting the flexor digitorum brevis off the exostosis. Next, a Freer elevator is placed superior and inferior to the spur. Using a ¼ inch osteotome, the spur is transected. It is important to realize that the first branch of the lateral-plantar nerve lies just superior to the spur, and therefore careful attention must be paid not to damage it during this part of the procedure. After the spur is cut, it is removed using a rongeur. Any edges of bone also are removed with a rongeur or a curette. I do not routinely pack thrombin or bone wax at the cut edge of the bone, but several workers recommend doing this.

Once the deep plantar fascia and spur have been addressed, the release is checked. Typically a small curved hemostat is placed deep to the deep fascia of the abductor and gently spread, palpating for any tight bands. Next the wound is irrigated copiously and final hemostasis is achieved. The skin is closed with 4-0 nylon mattress sutures. A compression dressing consisting of 4 × 4 inch sponge gauzes, a 4 inch Kerlix, 4 inch Kling, and then a 4 inch Ace is then applied.

Postoperative Course

Patients are instructed to remain off the foot for 2 weeks following surgery. During this time, they may use crutches or a walker as they feel comfortable. A wound check is scheduled at 1 week, sutures are removed at 2 weeks, and then the patients may begin gradual weight bearing as tolerated. We encourage resumption of the heel cord stretching and increase in activities as tolerated. The average length of recovery is 3 months with a range from 3 weeks to more than 1 year.

COMPLICATIONS AND SEQUELAE

Routine complications may occur including infections, wound-healing problems, persistent pain, or occasionally some localized paraincisional numbness. Several complications are specific to this operation. If there has been excessive trauma or inadvertent transection of the superficial calcaneal nerve or the first branch of the lateral-plantar nerve, a painful neuroma may continue to generate symptoms. In these cases that do not cool down with time, reoperation with resection of the neuroma may be warranted. Before considering surgery, a trial of tricyclic antidepressant medications (amitriptyline [Elavil], nortriptyline [Pamelor], or doxepin [Sinequan]) may be instituted.

Occasionally, when the entire plantar fascia has been released, the patient subsequently develops strain in the lateral side of the foot with signs of synovitis of the fifth or fourth metatarsal cuboid joints, calcaneocuboid joint synovitis, or stress fracture of the calcaneus, cuboid, or lateral metatarsals. This is hypothesized to result from the loss of the stress-relieving function of the plantar fascia. Typically the arch settles slightly, and the lateral side of the foot begins to absorb more stresses. In these situations a conservative treatment including anti-inflammatory medications, strapping, and shoe modifications have been effective. In patients who do not respond to minor measures or who experience much pain, a short-leg cast is applied until they are asymptomatic for 2 weeks' time.

Other complications can occur. Some patients have a particularly tumultuous postoperative course as a result of their inability to restrict activities. These patients may benefit from casting, strapping, or even an injection. A few patients who have undergone a limited plantar fasciectomy subsequently will have pain in the unreleased portion of the plantar fascia. If these patients do not respond to conservative treatment, reoperation may be warranted with completion of the plantar fasciotomy. The worst complication of this or any operation is reflex sympathetic dystrophy (RSD). This is a rare consequence of the operation. Treatment of RSD requires a concerted effort by the physiatrist, physical therapist, anesthesiologist, and orthopedist.

PROS AND CONS OF TREATMENT

The main advantage of the plantar fascia release as described is that it addresses all components of the heel pain syndrome. The surgery can be tailored readily according to the specifics of the symptoms. If a more proximal release of the tibial nerve is indicated, this is accomplished through proximal extension of the incision. Using this technique, trauma that typically occurs when using a transverse incision paralleling the plantar fascia is prevented for the first branch of the lateral-plantar nerve, medial-plantar nerve, and calcaneal nerves. It is not infrequent after this latter procedure that patients complain of medial heel numbness or dysesthesias along the medial-lateral or calcaneal nerves.

This operation requires detailed knowledge of the anatomy of the region. The surgery requires specific use of the small lamina spreader and Senn retractors to permit adequate visualization. Patients who have been improperly diagnosed with plantar fasciitis but instead have fat pad atrophy or nonspecific heel pain do not benefit from this surgery, since there is no incidental cutting of the calcaneal nerves.

SUGGESTED READING

Baxter DE, Thigpen CM. Chronic heel pain: Treatment rationale. Orthop Clin North Am 1989; 20:563–569.
Baxter DE, Thigpen CM. Heel pain: Operative results. Foot Ankle 1984; 5:16–25.
Henricson AS, Westlin NE. Chronic calcaneal pain in athletes: Entrapment of the calcaneal nerve? Am J Sports Med 1984; 12:152.
Lapidus PW, Guidotti FP. Painful heel: Report of three-hundred twenty-three patients with three hundred sixty-four painful heels. Clin Orthop 1965; 39:178–186.
Leach RE, Seavey MS, Salter DK. Results of surgery in athletes with plantar fasciitis. Foot Ankle 1986; 7:156–161.
Lutter LD. Surgical decisions in athletes' subcalcaneal pain. Am J Sports Med 1986; 14:481–485.
Rondhuis JJ, Huson A. The first branch of the lateral plantar nerve and heel pain. Acta Morphol Neerl Scand 1986; 24:269–280.

PRIMARY AND SALVAGE PROCEDURES FOR MORTON'S INTERDIGITAL NEUROMA

JAMES L. BESKIN, M.D.

Morton's interdigital neuroma is one of the most frequently encountered sources of foot pain. The characteristic symptoms have been well known to surgeons since Thomas Morton's original description in 1876, yet it remains a challenging problem in any foot practice. There have been numerous articles published on the etiology of the disorder. Most authors feel it is a form of entrapment neuropathy related to exogenous and anatomic conditions that compress the common digital nerve at the level of the metatarsal heads. High-heeled fashion shoe wear, which results in an increase in pressure as well as tension of the nerve under the transverse metatarsal ligament, is an often-implicated factor predisposing to neuroma formation. The difficulty in treating patients lies in accurately separating true interdigital neuralgia from adjacent pathology that mimics or provokes nerve pain, simulating a neuroma. Unfortunately, even with an accurate diagnosis, there are significant limitations to both nonoperative and surgical treatments.

PATIENT SELECTION

Morton's neuroma pain often is diffuse and poorly defined. Symptoms of burning, tingling, numbness, or cramping should alert the examiner to nerve pathology. Patients often relate having to remove their shoe or rub their toes to relieve a paroxysmal pain in the forefoot that may radiate proximally into the leg. More often it involves one or two toes of the second or third interspace of the forefoot. Symptoms in the first or fifth toe should raise doubt about Morton's neuroma, since neuroma pathology in these interspaces is rare.

When an examination of the foot is performed for nerve pathology, the entire spectrum of nerve pain needs to be considered. Beyond the local symptoms at the forefoot, one needs to consider proximal lesions such as tarsal tunnel entrapment or lumbar disc disease. In addition, diffuse nerve injury associated with neuropathy or sympathetic dystrophy must be considered in examining a patient with interdigital neuralgia. Careful examination may reveal loss of sensation in the plantar web space of the affected digital nerve; however, a stocking or radicular sensory loss, intrinsic muscle wasting, or reflex changes should raise the question of other neurologic problems. Mulder's sign is elicited by popping a thickened nerve by grasping the forefoot and applying medial and lateral compression of the meta-

tarsal heads. It is a useful but nondiagnostic finding, since a thickened intermetatarsal bursa may create the same response. Pain with compression of the interdigital space also is a consistent but nondiagnostic finding of Morton's neuroma. Comparison with the adjacent interspaces as well as the contralateral foot helps to interpret these findings. Finally, one should be aware of other sources of inflammation of the joints, tendons, or adjacent soft tissues that may mimic Morton's neuralgia.

An injection of local anesthetic is useful to isolate the primary source of the patient's symptoms when more than one interdigital space is involved. Use of corticosteroids also is worthwhile and may provide long-term relief. Although neuromas rarely can occur in both the second and third interspace simultaneously, this diagnosis should be approached cautiously. Excising both the second and third common digital nerves results in significant numbness of the toes, is associated with a higher rate of patient dissatisfaction, and is not recommended at all.

Laboratory studies usually are not helpful in making the diagnosis of Morton's neuroma, but may be important to exclude other sources of foot pathology. Radiographs must be evaluated for signs of erosive synovitis, significant metatarsophalangeal joint subluxation, or active bone disease. When indicated, rheumatologic and neurologic workup should be considered as well. Current techniques of ultrasound or magnetic resonance imaging (MRI) have not been proven useful for routine use in identifying an abnormal interdigital nerve preoperatively, but may identify associated ganglia or other neoplasms compressing the nerve. Recent work with ultrasound, however, has shown it to be an extremely useful modality in aiding differential diagnosis.

TREATMENT OPTIONS

Unfortunately the majority of patients with symptomatic Morton's neuroma do not obtain satisfactory relief with nonoperative measures. However, this treatment phase offers an opportunity to confirm the diagnosis on subsequent visits, as well as provide satisfactory relief for a significant number of patients. I have found injection of corticosteroids into the web space particularly useful. Although recurrence is common after injection, it usually provides significant relief for a period of weeks to months. Pain relief from the injection also increases the surgeon's confidence that the correct interspace has been identified. Other useful measures include mechanical unloading of the pressure on the nerve by use of a wide shoe with a low heel. Metatarsal pads or orthotics also may help alleviate local pressure against the sensitive nerve area. A semirigid or rigid orthosis may help control interdigital compression from excessive pronation during foot flat or roll off.

Despite continued debate on the etiology of Morton's neuroma, the consensus is that the best definitive treatment is neurectomy. Neurectomy as a means of treatment was discovered by Hoadley in 1893, but never was popularized until Betts's report from Australia in 1940. Betts used a longitudinal-plantar approach, which remains popular in many areas of the world including Britain. Some surgeons have modified this to a transverse-plantar incision distal to the weight-bearing area with success as well. In 1943 McElvenny, an American, reported his work that paralleled that of Betts. He used a dorsal web-splitting incision for neurectomy, which remains popular in this country.

Good results from both techniques are well documented. However, the results in larger series confirm that neurectomy is by no means a panacea. Approximately 50 percent of patients have some residual symptoms or restriction in footwear. In addition, there is a 10 to 20 percent reported failure rate, resulting in persistent or recurrent interdigital pain. Therefore it is important for patients to be apprised of this situation preoperatively. Despite this, the vast majority of patients are grateful for the significant improvement that neurectomy affords.

Both plantar and dorsal approaches have their merits and enthusiasts. The advantages of avoiding incisions on the plantar side of the foot, as well as an opportunity to visualize other pathology in the same or adjacent web space, explain the popularity of the dorsal approach. However, the ease of visualizing the nerve, especially proximally, is a clear advantage of the plantar approach. This has proven particularly important when re-exploration is required after a failed primary neurectomy.

SURGICAL TECHNIQUE: DORSAL APPROACH

The dorsal approach typically is performed in an outpatient setting with an ankle block anesthetic. An ankle tourniquet and loupe magnification are preferred; however, many surgeons do not find that a tourniquet is necessary. A dorsal incision is made over the appropriate web space and extended proximally for 3 cm. Care is taken to identify and prevent trauma to the dorsal cutaneous nerves by spreading the tissues with a small hemostat clamp. A small Weitlaner retractor facilitates exposure. The transverse metatarsal ligament serves as a good reference point to find the nerve, which exits immediately below and distal to it (Fig. 1). Plantar pressure in the web space by the assistant may help bring the thickened area of the nerve into view. A hemostat or Freer elevator is a useful probe and helps confirm the location of the ligament, as well as helping separate the nerve from the vessels and adjacent bursa tissue.

Next, the transverse intermetatarsal ligament is divided to allow proximal dissection of the common digital nerve. A small lamina spreader placed between the metatarsal heads greatly improves visibility. Once the nerve is traced proximally as far as reasonably possible, it is transected sharply, allowing the proximal stump to retract proximal to the metatarsal heads and weight-bearing area of the forefoot. This should be transected in between the interossei. The dissection is completed distally, past the thickened neuroma, to the proper digital branches, and the nerve then is removed.

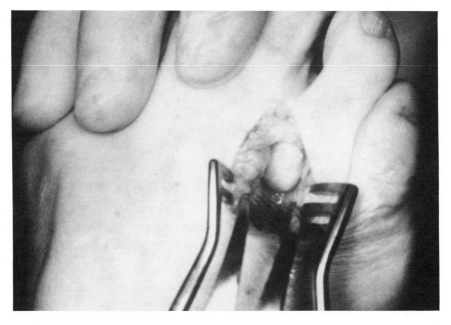

Figure 1 Large neuroma identified at the distal edge of the transverse metatarsal ligament. After dividing the ligament, the lamina spreader aids in proximal dissection of the nerve.

Care is taken to identify and transect small cutaneous branches passing vertically from the common digital nerve plantarward. Occasionally a thickened intermetatarsal bursa is resected as well, but excessive dissection or removal of the plantar fat pad should be avoided. The wound is irrigated and the tourniquet released to obtain hemostasis. Closure is by simple skin sutures. Soft bulky dressings are used along with a stiff postoperative shoe. Patients are allowed necessary ambulation with or without crutches, but are instructed to keep the foot elevated as much as possible for 2 weeks. The wound is checked weekly, and the sutures are removed by 12 to 14 days after surgery. Most patients may resume their usual activities in accommodative footwear by 4 to 6 weeks postoperatively.

RECURRENT NEUROMA PAIN

Recurrent pain following interdigital neurectomy is an especially disquieting problem. Unfortunately the available conservative care measures are no more effective the second time around, and the surgeon is faced with a decision of whether re-exploration will be helpful.

The same process discussed for evaluating a primary neuroma should be repeated. This is necessary to determine whether other concomitant pathology is present, or whether the original diagnosis was a correct foundation for neurectomy. Typically most patients with recurrent neuroma pain have reported little relief from their primary surgery. Although a few patients seemingly are better for awhile after the surgery, the vast majority of failed procedures are evident within a year of the primary surgery. The history and physical findings may not be much different from the primary neuroma. The examiner should check for numbness in the affected web space to determine whether the nerve was resected. Tinel's test may be helpful to localize a potential stump neuroma that may be in the weight-bearing portion of the forefoot. Scrutiny of the adjacent interspace for another neuroma also is important. Use of local anes-

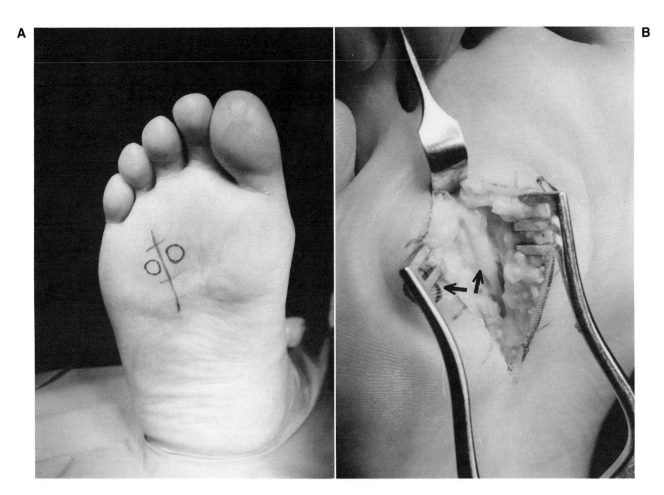

Figure 2 *A,* Placement of the incision between the metatarsal heads for the longitudinal incision approach. *B,* Identification of the remaining nerve. Note the thickened area of neuromatous healing in proximity to the metatarsal heads.

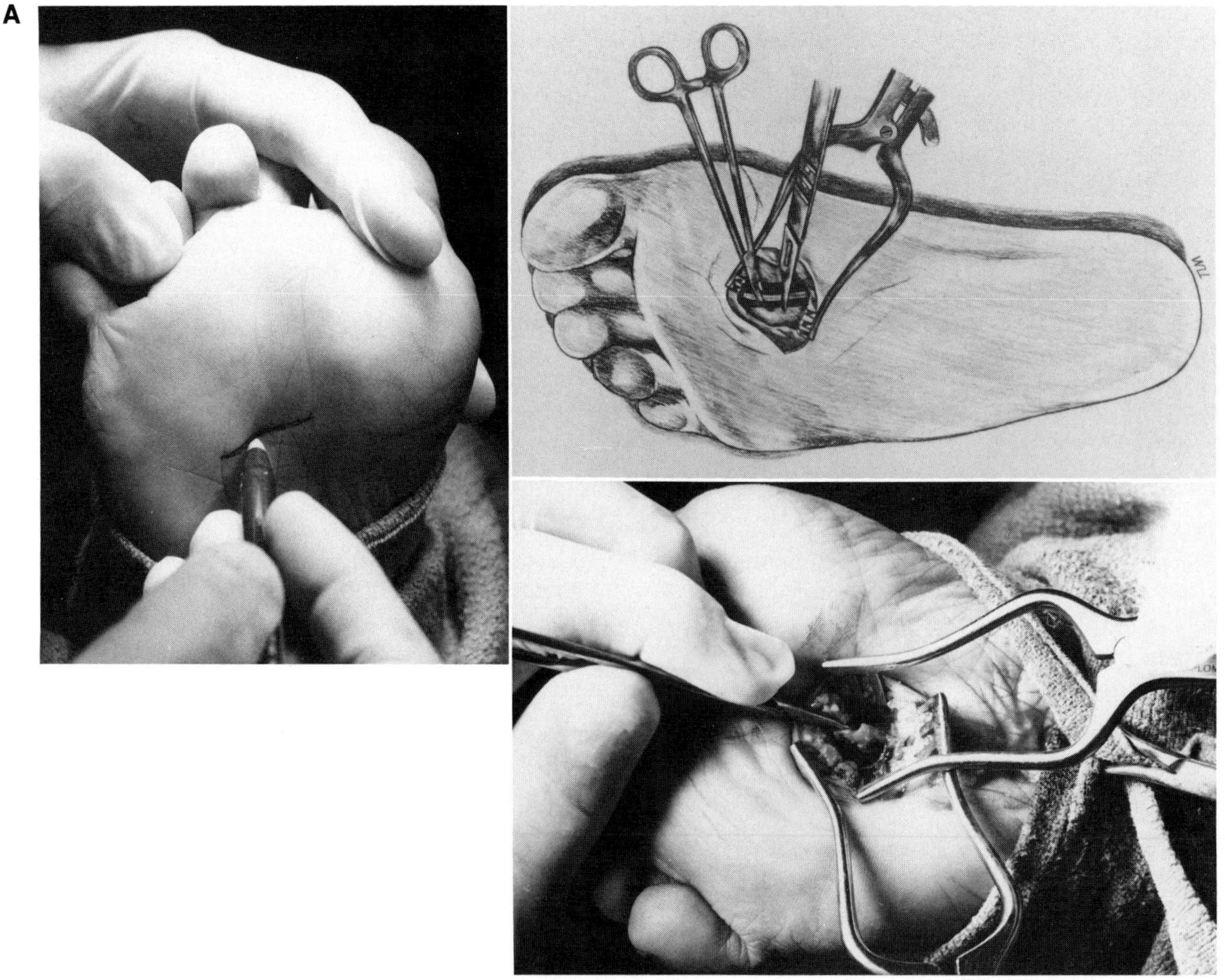

A

B

C

Figure 3 *A,* A transverse incision proximal to the metatarsal heads prevents extension into the weight-bearing area of the forefoot and may be expanded to explore adjacent interspaces. *B* and *C,* The nerve is relatively superficial. It is deep to the plantar fascia septae and superficial to the intrinsic muscles. The ability to explore the distal stump is limited by this method. (*B* from Beskin JL, Baxter DE. Recurrent pain following interdigital neurectomy—A plantar approach. Foot Ankle 1988; 9:32–39; © by American Orthopaedic Foot Society; with permission.)

thetic and steroid injections may help to isolate pathology and provide relief for some patients. Shoe modifications may be worth exploring as well. Finally, one should evaluate the patient's psychological makeup and appreciate their expectations of available treatment options. If symptoms and findings point to a nerve etiology at the same interspace, one of two situations likely exists. Either the nerve or a communicating branch was not excised during the primary procedure, or a true stump neuroma exists in a weight-bearing portion of the foot.

After complete evaluation, the decision of whether to re-explore the nerve should be based on mutual knowledge between the patient and the surgeon that some degree of residual symptoms is likely. Although the literature reports improvement in the majority of pa-

tients (70 to 80 percent), less than 25 percent report complete relief of all symptoms postoperatively after a revision neurectomy.

As with primary neuromas, a dorsal or plantar approach is feasible. However, advantages of a plantar approach under these circumstances is worth emphasizing. Since the anteroposterior diameter of the foot increases from distal to proximal, the ability to identify and explore the nerve proximally becomes increasingly difficult from a dorsal approach. Re-exploration from a plantar approach simplifies the dissection with an acceptably low risk of skin problems postoperatively.

For complete exposure of the web space and evaluation of potential communicating branches at the third interdigital space, a longitudinal incision is preferred (Fig. 2). This requires accurate placement between the metatarsal heads to prevent problems such as fat pad injury, iatrogenic metatarsalgia, or hyperkeratosis. When a stump neuroma is well localized preoperatively by Tinel's testing or an adjacent interspace needs exploration, a transverse-plantar incision proximal to the weight-bearing pad is used. This offers the advantage of preventing extension of the incision over the weight-bearing aspect of the forefoot (Fig. 3).

SURGICAL TECHNIQUE: TRANSVERSE-PLANTAR APPROACH

The preoperative preparation and equipment for a plantar approach are the same as required for a primary procedure previously described. The incision is outlined on the plantar side of the foot over the affected interspace just proximal to the weight-bearing pad and parallel to the natural crease that falls in that area. Palpation of the metatarsal heads helps to provide a reference to the appropriate interspace to be explored. The incision is deepened through the skin to the level of the subcutaneous tissue. Gradual, careful dissection is deepened with a scissors or Freer elevator to expose the septae of the plantar fascia. It is important to remember that these structures, including the nerves, are relatively superficial at this level. Using the small Weitlaner retractor, the incision is opened and the longitudinal septae of the plantar fascia are visualized. Palpation of the metatarsal heads helps to maintain orientation of the interspace being explored. The interval between the plantar fascia septa is opened with the scissors or scalpel. Here, Senn retractors are used to pull the plantar fascia ligament gently aside while the surgeon bluntly explores the interspace with a hemostat or scissors to expose the common digital nerve and vessel. The nerve lies superficial to the flexor brevis muscle and immediately deep to the plantar fascia ligament. Once the nerve is isolated, a 1 to 2 cm segment is resected, allowing the proximal stump to retract into the soft tissues of the arch of the foot. Further distal dissection of the remaining nerve tissue is not necessary, but can be carried out to identify the residual stump of the neuroma. At the third interspace, one should be aware of a possible communicating branch from the lateral plantar nerve. If it is necessary to explore an adjacent interspace, the incision can be extended medially or laterally without crossing the weight-bearing pad of the forefoot. Closure is carried out after obtaining hemostasis by using a simple skin suture. A bulky compression dressing is used, and patients are allowed to perform necessary ambulation for bathroom privileges with or without crutches, using a rigid postoperative shoe. They are instructed to limit activities and keep the foot elevated as much as possible for the first 10 to 14 days. Once the sutures are removed, activity gradually is increased to tolerance, and most patients are in their regular shoes by 4 to 6 weeks.

DISCUSSION

Morton's neuroma is a relatively common source of foot pain and probably related to an entrapment neuropathy of the common digital nerve at the second or third metatarsal interspaces. Most patients eventually elect surgical excision since nonoperative measures offer limited relief for symptomatic neuromas. A 10 to 20 percent failure rate should be discussed with the patient preoperatively when surgery is elected. Dorsal and plantar approaches have been described for both primary and revision exploration procedures. The limited risk for skin complications, as well as facilitated exploration of other potential web space pathology, support the dorsal approach as the recommended procedure for primary neuromas. The comparative ease of exposure after previous surgery, as well as ability to explore the nerve in a more proximal location, make the plantar approach a more desirable procedure for repeat operations. The importance of identifying and resecting the common digital nerve as far proximally as possible at the time of the primary procedure must be emphasized to prevent the potential complication of a symptomatic stump neuroma that may result in persistent pain postoperatively.

SUGGESTED READING

Beskin JL, Baxter DE. Recurrent pain following interdigital neurectomy: A plantar approach. Foot Ankle 1988; 9:34–39.

Friscia DA, et al. Surgical treatment for primary interdigital neuroma. Orthopedics 1991; 14:669–672.

Johnson JE, Johnson KA, Krishnaw Unni K. Persistent pain after excision of an interdigital neuroma. J Bone Joint Surg 70A:651–657.

Mann RA, Reynolds JC. Interdigital neuroma: A critical clinical analysis. Foot Ankle 3:238–243.

PEDIATRIC CONDITIONS

FLATFOOT DEFORMITY

R. LUKE BORDELON, M.D.

FLATFOOT DEFORMITY IN CHILDREN

Flatfoot deformity refers to a deformity in which the foot collapses, or is in a fixed structural position of collapse, so that the foot is not stable to bear the body weight properly during the stance phase of gait. It does not resupinate to form a rigid lever for push off. This produces pain as a result of strain on joints, ligaments, and tendons. Although severe deformity generally results in dysfunction and pain, other stages of deformity do not always correlate with the degree of deformity and pain. Specific patient examination thus is paramount in treatment decision making.

Therapeutic Alternatives

In the young child, some attempts at correction or support with rigid orthotics may be made. In the adult accommodative or biomechanical orthotics are used for symptomatic relief before a surgical procedure is considered.

Preferred Approach

Surgical treatment may be considered for the child with severe flatfoot deformity. Generally there may be some pain with severe flatfoot deformity, but a reduced activity level with fatigue and inability to walk and complete normal activities of daily living may be clinical indications for treatment.

Timing of Surgery

The surgical procedure for severe flatfoot in a child should be done at least 2 or 3 years before the cessation of growth. When the deformity is severe, the procedure may be done at any time down to 3 years of age. The present trend is to do the surgical procedure somewhat younger than in the past, going down to 7 to 10 years of age.

Preoperative Preparation

Before any surgical procedure is done for flatfoot in a child, it is important that the specific foot deformities are evaluated from a biomechanical basis so the surgeon knows precisely which deformities need correction. The family also must be counseled as to what can be expected, and that although the goal is to provide a more normal foot, there is no guarantee that a completely normal foot will result, and that other procedures such as arthrodesis may have to be performed.

Choice of Procedure

The procedure chosen depends on the specific structural deformities. In general, when a severe flatfoot deformity is present, there is an associated forefoot varus, forefoot abduction, heel valgus, and contracture

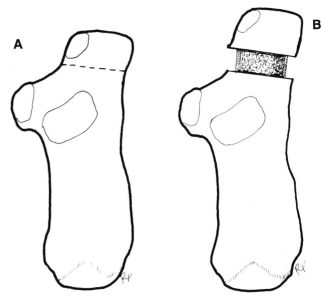

Figure 1 Anterior opening-wedge osteotomy of os calcis to correct foot abduction and heel eversion. *A,* Osteotomy is made completely through the os calcis. *B,* Bone graft is inserted into the osteotomy site. Fixation is with pins and at times a staple. (From Mann RA, Coughlin MJ, eds. Surgery of the foot and ankle, 6th ed. St. Louis: Mosby–Year Book, 1993; with permission.)

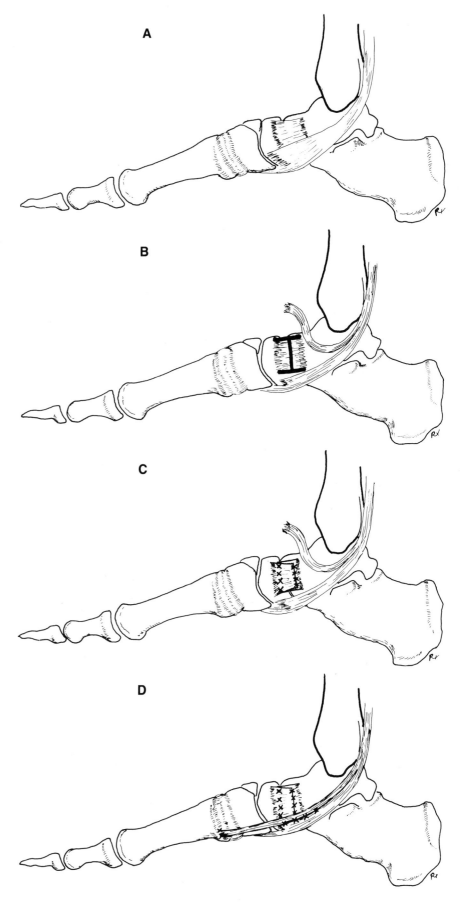

Figure 2 Medial soft tissue correction for flatfoot. This usually is used in conjunction with other procedures. *A,* Illustration of the superior and inferior calcaneonavicular ligaments and posterior tibial tendon. *B,* Release of the dorsal half of the posterior tibial tendon and incision in the superior and inferior calcaneonavicular ligaments. *C,* Vest-over-pants overlapping and shortening of the superior and inferior calcaneonavicular ligaments. *D,* Advancement of the dorsal half of the posterior tibial tendon to metatarsocuneiform joint with proximal side-to-side suturing of the posterior tibial tendon. (From Mann RA, Coughlin MJ, eds. Surgery of the foot and ankle, 6th ed. St. Louis: Mosby–Year Book, 1993; with permission.)

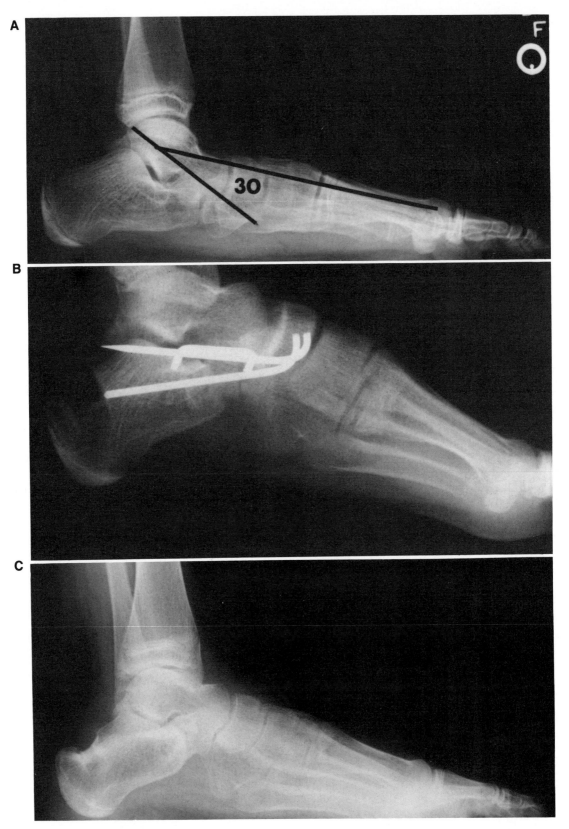

Figure 3 Severe flatfoot deformity in an 11-year-old patient, corrected with tendo Achilles lengthening, Evan's osteotomy, and medial soft tissue plication. *A,* Preoperative standing lateral radiograph with 30° lateral talometatarsal angle. *B,* Postoperative lateral radiograph demonstrating fixation and the area of bone graft of the superior tuberosity of the os calcis. *C,* Postoperative radiograph demonstrating final correction. (From Mann RA, Coughlin MJ, eds. Surgery of the foot and ankle, 6th ed. St. Louis: Mosby–Year Book, 1993; with permission.)

of the gastrosoleus muscle group. All of these deformities should be corrected.

The gastrosoleus group is functionally lengthened by a triple-step cut performed percutaneously or by a modified open procedure. The abduction of the forefoot and valgus of the heel can be corrected by an opening-wedge osteotomy of the anterior part of the os calcis. An incision is made laterally and carried down to the anterior part of the os calcis. The interval between the middle facet and the anterior facet is identified. An osteotomy is made completely through the bone (Fig. 1). The os calcis is spread by an Inge retractor, thus correcting the adduction of the forefoot and the valgus of the heel. Some correction of the forefoot inversion also occurs when this is done. A bone graft bicortical or tricortical is taken from either the posterior portion of the os calcis or the iliac crest and placed into the site. A staple is used to maintain the opening. Smooth pins, ³⁄₃₂ inch in diameter, are inserted from the os calcis to the foot in the region of the cuboid to stabilize the foot and to prevent recurrence of the deformity until healing has occurred. The foot then is approached medially (Fig. 2A). The spring ligament is cut in an H-fashion and shortened (Fig. 2B–D). The dorsal half of the posterior tibial tendon is advanced to the first metatarsocuneiform joint and sutured with nonabsorbable sutures. The

tendon then is resutured to itself proximally (see Fig. 2D). The foot is re-examined, and if the foot is in a biomechanically normal position, no further surgery is performed (Fig. 3). If the patient still has medial instability or forefoot inversion to varus, consideration may be given to a plantar flexion osteotomy of the first metatarsal distal to the epiphysis.

In the event that the deformity is not severe, or one is concerned about limited motion of the subtalar joint and further limitation by changing the subtalar joint axes of motion, one may correct the deformity by procedures around the subtalar joint. The heel may be taken out of the valgus position by an osteotomy through the body of the heel and pinned with two smooth pins (Fig. 4). An incision is made distal but in line with the peroneal tendon and carried down to the body, which is cut through completely, perpendicular to its long axis. The soft tissue on the medial side is spread with a periosteal elevator, and the heel is displaced over approximately half the distance and tilted into the correct position to allow the motion of the subtalar joint from 5° of eversion to 25° of inversion. The osteotomy site is pinned with two smooth ³⁄₃₂ inch pins going from posterior to the anterior part of the os calcis, but without restricting motion of the subtalar joint. The forefoot abduction is corrected by an opening-wedge osteotomy of the cuboid. An incision is

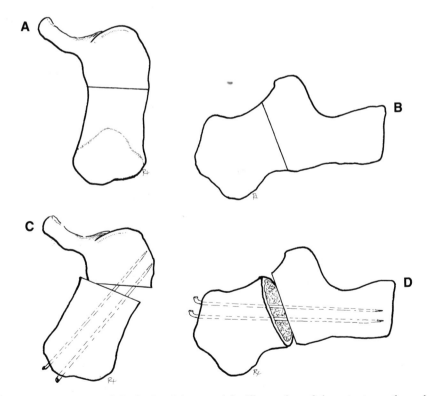

Figure 4 Osteotomy of the body of the os calcis. Illustration of the osteotomy through the body of the os calcis. Cuts are as in *A* and *C*. Displacement and fixation with two pins are as in *B* and *D*. (From Mann RA, Coughlin MJ, eds. Surgery of the foot and ankle, 6th ed. St. Louis: Mosby–Year Book, 1993; with permission.)

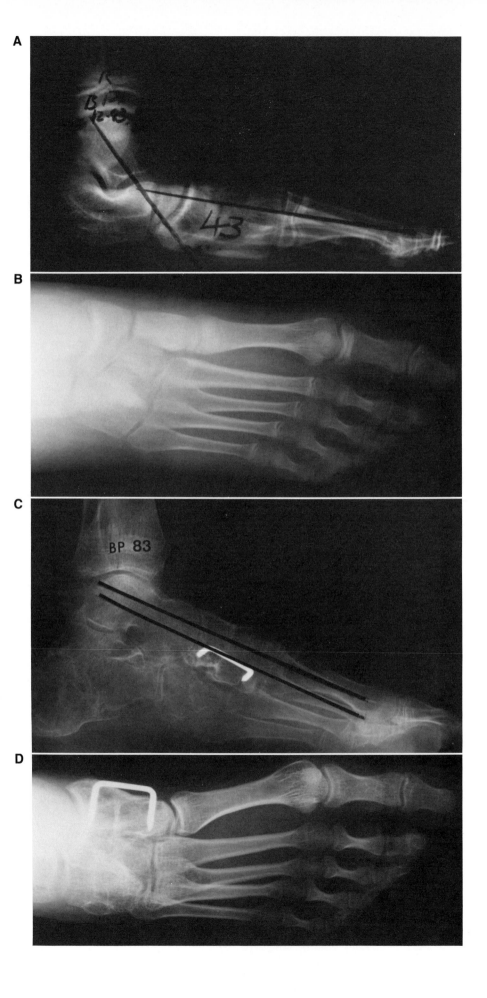

Figure 5 Severe flatfoot deformity in a 13-year-old patient, corrected by a tendo Achilles lengthening, an osteotomy of the body of the os calcis, an opening-wedge osteotomy of the cuboid, and a fusion of the navicular cuneiform joint. *A,* Preoperative standing lateral view. *B,* Preoperative standing anteroposterior view. *C,* Postoperative standing lateral view. *D,* Postoperative standing anteroposterior view. (From Mann RA, Coughlin MJ, eds. Surgery of the foot and ankle, 6th ed. St. Louis: Mosby–Year Book, 1993; with permission.)

made laterally and carried down to the cuboid. The cuboid is split and then wedged apart. A bone graft is taken either from the os calcis or the iliac crest and placed into the area. The osteotomy then is fixed with a staple and pins to prevent recurrence of the deformity. Attention then is directed to the medial side of the foot. The spring ligament is shortened with a vest-over-pants procedure. The dorsal half of the posterior tibial tendon is advanced to the first metatarsol cuneiform joint. The proximal portion is sutured to re-establish the proper tension. If there still is a forefoot varus present or instability of the medial segment, a plantar flexion osteotomy of the first metatarsal or fusion of the navicular cuneiform joint may be performed (Fig. 5).

The patient is placed in a well-padded cast with a section cut out over the front of the cast. Hospitalization usually is for 3 to 5 days. Elevation is maintained until there is no excessive swelling. Partial weight bearing for transfer from the bed to the wheelchair may be allowed. Absorbable sutures are used so suture removal is not necessary. Weight bearing is allowed at 4 weeks according to symptomatic tolerance. At 8 weeks postoperatively, the internal fixation is removed. The patient is placed in another walking cast for 2 to 4 weeks, depending on the status of the healing. The patient then is allowed to ambulate. If the foot is in a good structural position, no support is used. If some deformity still is present, such as residual forefoot inversion to varus, an orthotic may be used. Limited activity without jumping or running may be allowed up to 6 months. At 6 months the patient may begin increased activity depending on the status of the Achilles tendon healing, but generally 12 months is required for recovery to a level of maximal medical improvement.

Complications and Sequelae and Their Treatment

Specific complications following this procedure generally are those of lack of correction of the deformity with continued dysfunction and/or pain associated with joint dysfunction and arthrosis. If the patient has pain as a result of some persistence of structural dysfunction, a biomechanical orthosis may be used to correct this deformity. Because there is a reduced amount of deformity, an orthosis generally is successful in relieving the patient's difficulty. In the event that arthritic changes and/or stiffness of the subtalar joint complex produce severe impairment not responding to an orthotic device and decreased activity, an arthrodesis must be considered. Generally a triple arthrodesis is performed.

The possibility exists for dysfunction of the Achilles tendon, but when the triple-step cut method is used in a young growing child, I have not found it to be a problem.

Pros and Cons of Treatment

Some physicians believe that the hypermobile flatfoot deformity does not cause any trouble. The physician who sees and treats foot deformities, especially those of

adults, is aware that structural deformities of the foot tend to occur as specific deformities with specific problems in older people. All orthopedists agree that some children with a severe deformity who have pain and/or limitation of activities of daily living need surgical treatment of the foot deformity. Deciding who should have surgery is difficult. The general rule is that if a patient has a severe deformity and limitation of activity such that 10 physicians would agree that something should be done, the person should be considered for a surgical procedure, with the other degrees of deformity and dysfunction being evaluated on an individual basis. Certainly a surgical procedure just to improve the appearance of the flatfoot is not for a child who has only a mild deformity or mild limitation of function. It is my opinion that if the specific deformities can be identified and corrected early in those children with a severe deformity, the resultant foot with normal biomechanical position and function will function more normally and with less limitation of activity throughout the patient's life.

ADULT FLATFOOT DEFORMITY

The adult flatfoot refers to the flatfoot in a person who has reached bony maturity with closure of the epiphyses and cessation of growth. Generally this occurs at 13 years in females and 15 years in males.

Therapeutic Alternatives

In the adult with a flatfoot deformity, conservative treatment is recommended with surgical procedures only as a last resort. If a surgical procedure is required, it generally consists of a double or triple arthrodesis. However, limited surgical procedures may be performed to place the foot in a better functional position to try to maintain its mobility without performing a triple arthrodesis. In such an instance, one may consider an opening-wedge osteotomy of the cuboid to correct forefoot abduction or minimal opening-wedge osteotomy of the anterior os calcis. One must be cautious in trying to correct the deformity by doing an opening-wedge osteotomy of the os calcis as is done with a child, because the joint alignment is fixed and the joints may not function properly if excessive correction is performed. One may place the medial segment in a better position to stabilize it and to decrease the forefoot varus deformity by plantar-flexing the first metatarsal or first metatarsocuneiform fusion with the first metatarsal being plantar flexed. Generally, in the adult with a structural deformity, soft tissue procedures medially are not successful. Tendo Achilles lengthening in the adult may be performed in the triple-step cut manner percutaneously or modified open so that only a small cut is made; however, one must be cautious because some patients have persistent Achilles tendon symptoms.

Preferred Approach

Patient Selection

Surgical treatment of an adult with severe flatfoot deformity is limited to those who have not responded to orthotics or supportive devices and who have sufficient pain and limitation of activity level to warrant surgical intervention.

Timing of Surgery

Surgery is performed when the patient can no longer function at an appropriate level. The patient must understand that this surgery is performed to try to decrease the pain and to increase the activity level, but that normal functioning feet are not produced.

Choice of Procedure

The choice of procedure depends on the specific abnormality and what one is attempting to correct. Usually a triple arthrodesis is chosen. However, with certain specific biomechanical abnormalities, a double arthrodesis may be considered.

A double arthrodesis is performed with an incision along the medial side and denuding of the articular cartilage of the talonavicular joint and an incision on the lateral side with denuding of the cartilage of the calcaneocuboid joint. The forefoot then is placed in the proper position using internal fixation). A short-leg non–weight-bearing cast is used for 4 to 6 weeks followed by a short-leg weight-bearing cast for 4 to 6 weeks or until healing occurs.

A triple arthrodesis is performed by an incision on the lateral side of the foot, encompassing the subtalar and calcaneocuboid and lateral talonavicular joints with an incision medially over the talonavicular joint and excision of the articular cartilage. The components of the subtalar joint are placed in such a manner that the foot now is in the normal biomechanical position. It is preferable to fix the talonavicular joint first, correcting the talometatarsal angle. Rigid internal fixation is used. If severe structural deformity is present, appropriate bone removal may be required. However, this rarely is necessary in a mobile adult flatfoot deformity, since correction is achieved by rotation and translation of the joints into the corrected position. A splint with compression dressing is used for 7 to 17 days. Then a short-leg non–weight-bearing cast is used for 4 to 6 weeks. A short-leg weight-bearing cast then is used for another 4

to 6 weeks or until healing occurs. Achilles tendon lengthening may be performed, but generally is not done.

Complications and Sequelae and Their Treatment

Arthrodesis of the foot places the foot in the better position for function, but foot motion is restricted and a loss of shock absorption power occurs. If the patient is not comfortable in ordinary footwear, a soft orthotic to cushion the foot and spread the forces may be used. If a patient has a great deal of difficulty because of some residual deformity, a specific biomechanical type of orthosis may be used to place the foot in a better functional position.

Finally, in the patient who continues to have difficulty because of foot pain as a result of stiffness, a rocker-sole shoe is used.

Pros and Cons of Treatment

Since fusion of the foot does provide a stiff foot, one must be cautious about recommending surgery early in the adult flatfoot. Generally, surgical procedures are recommended only when the person is incapacitated completely.

SUGGESTED READING

Anderson AF, Fowler SB. Anterior calcaneal osteotomy for symptomatic juvenile pes planus. Foot Ankle 1984; 4:274–283.

Bordelon RL. Correction of hypermobile flatfoot in children by molded inserts. Foot Ankle 1980; 1:143.

Bordelon RL. Hypermobile flatfoot in children: Comprehension, evaluation and treatment. Clin Orthop 1983; 181:7–14.

Bordelon RL. Surgical and conservative foot care. Thorofare, NJ: Slack, 1988.

Bordelon RL. Examination of the foot: Foot functions following fusions. Video Orthop Surg 1989; 3.

Bordelon RL. Hypermobile flatfoot in children: Present status of diagnosis and treatment. Semin Orthop 1990; 5:13–22.

Crawford AH, Kucharzyk D, Roy DR, Bilbo, J. Subtalar stabilization of the planovalgus foot by staple arthroerisis in young children who have neuromuscular problems. J Bone Joint Surg 1990; 72-A: 840–845.

Evans D. Calcaneo-valgus deformity. J Bone Joint Surg 1975; 57B:270–278.

Mann RA, Coughlin M, eds. Surgery of the foot and ankle. 6th ed. St. Louis: Mosby–Year Book, 1993.

Phillips GE. A review of elongation of os calcis for flat feet. J Bone Joint Surg 1983; 65B:15–8.

Silver CM, Simon SD, Spindell E, et al. Calcaneal osteotomy for valgus and varus deformities of the foot in cerebral palsy: A preliminary report on twenty-seven operations. J Bone Joint Surg 1967; 49A:232.

INFANTILE CLUBFOOT

RICHARD S. DAVIDSON, M.D.

In spite of the occurrence of clubfoot in more than 1 of every 1,000 live births, its etiology, pathogenesis, pathoanatomy, and treatment remain in dispute.

Treatment, both surgical and nonsurgical, has focused on the correction of deformity by stretching or lengthening the contracted soft tissues. Early correction of the deformity and restoration of the "normal" stresses hope to restore growth and remodeling, as well as to maximize joint motion and strength, while producing a shoeable foot. Proper handling of the soft tissues and cartilagenous anlage of the bones is critical to limit growth disturbances, bone necrosis, and scarring.

A thorough understanding of the deformity requires considerable thought, reading, and experience. Many points remain in dispute. Partial correction may produce a cosmetically acceptable and even flat-appearing foot with underlying bony deformity and stiffness resulting in poor shoe fitting, pressure sores, stiffness, and degenerative joint disease in the second and subsequent decades of life.

CLUBFOOT DEFORMITY

Clubfoot deformity consists of the positional triad of forefoot varus, hindfoot varus, and heel equinus (Fig. 1). Each bone should be palpated in the deformed and maximally corrected positions to gain an understanding of the severity. Often the foot appears corrected while significant underlying deformity persists.

I use two signs to assess the severity of deformity. First, a bony mass can be palpated dorsolaterally on the foot about 1 cm distal to the lateral malleolus in the clubfoot. This represents the head of the talus, which has become uncovered as the forefoot has been displaced medially on the talar head. This positioning can be confirmed at surgery. Complete reduction of the forefoot over the talar head realigns the head of the talus with the first metatarsal and suggests a mild deformity. Partial reduction of the forefoot over this prominence suggests moderate severity, whereas the lack of reduction suggests severe deformity. The traditional sign of medial creasing of the skin parallels talar head prominence dorsolaterally, but is a static test. Moreover, medial creasing often is absent in the most severely (arthrogrypotic) deformed clubfoot where the medial skin is pulled tightly.

The second clinical test is the motion of the ankle or, in practical terms, the movement of the os calcis from equinus to calcaneus. Palpation often reveals that the heel pad has been displaced distally from the os calcis, which remains in equinus. To date, no way has been found to measure this motion reliably and reproducibly for the small varus heel found in the clubfoot. The motion at this joint can be classified simply as coming into calcaneus (found only in postural or extremely mild clubfoot deformities), having some movement, or being fixed rigidly in equinus. The latter implies the most severe deformity.

Both of these tests are useful in determining the success of casting or surgical treatment. Casting is likely to be successful only in feet in which the forefoot can be partially reduced over the talar head *and* the os calcis (hindfoot) is mobile through the ankle. Surgery is likely to be successful in all but the most severely deformed and rigid feet.

RADIOGRAPHS OF THE CLUBFOOT

I do not find that radiographs are helpful in managing clubfoot deformity. They may document the presence of the deformity, but as a static, two-dimensional representation of a dynamic, three-dimensional array of partially ossified tarsal bones, plain radiographs are a poor second to the physical examination. Radiographic measurements are unreliable, not reproducible, and are

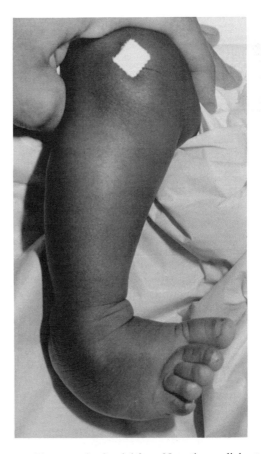

Figure 1 Photograph of a clubfoot. Note the medial rotation of the foot as compared with the knee, hindfoot equinus and varus, midfoot varus, and forefoot supination.

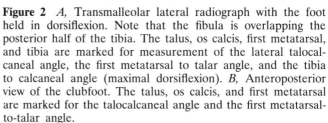

Figure 2 *A,* Transmalleolar lateral radiograph with the foot held in dorsiflexion. Note that the fibula is overlapping the posterior half of the tibia. The talus, os calcis, first metatarsal, and tibia are marked for measurement of the lateral talocalcaneal angle, the first metatarsal to talar angle, and the tibia to calcaneal angle (maximal dorsiflexion). *B,* Anteroposterior view of the clubfoot. The talus, os calcis, and first metatarsal are marked for the talocalcaneal angle and the first metatarsal-to-talar angle.

dependent on positioning. A normal flexible foot can be positioned to produce a clubfoot on a radiograph.

When used, radiographs must be obtained in a consistent manner that demonstrates the maximal correction of the deformed foot. The anteroposterior (AP) view should be taken with the foot rotated laterally toward the line of the tibia and dorsiflexed, and should be eliminated as much of the supination as is practical. The lateral view should focus on the hindfoot, a transmalleolar view should have the foot dorsiflexed to simulate weight bearing. Supination should be eliminated. This technique minimizes spurious "flattop talus" and provides more consistent and reliable measurement of the talocalcaneal angle (Fig. 2).

PREFERRED APPROACH

Patient Selection

Initial treatment of an infant with clubfoot deformity involves stretching in the form of serial casting. Only the mildest of postural deformities that can be fully corrected passively are candidates for stretching alone. Casting should be initiated as soon after birth as is practical. At least 3 months of proper casting by an experienced orthopedist is required before giving up on this treatment and continuing on to surgical modalities. Unless the foot can be derotated on the talus (as evidenced by reduction of the forefoot on the talar head in the resting position) and the heel comes out of equinus, casting has failed and the patient is a candidate for surgical intervention.

Timing of Surgery

I prefer surgical intervention after a child is 3 months of age. This allows for an adequate trial of casting and is an age after which anesthetic is safer. I prefer to operate before the child is 9 months old to maximize the remodeling potential and reduce the deformity produced during growth in the clubfoot position. I have observed an increased incidence of posterior flattening of the talus, synovitis, and flattening of the talar head after a child is 9 months old, particularly when the foot was casted throughout this period.

Choice of Procedure

Understanding the malposition of the talus, os calcis, and navicular is critical to the choice of treatment.

The angular changes measured on the AP, and lateral radiographs define a rotation of the os calcis under the talus. The clubfoot therefore can be viewed as a rotation of the foot on the talus, which is fixed in the ankle mortise.

Stretching the foot to correct the forefoot varus first, then the hindfoot varus, and then the hindfoot equinus is unlikely to correct the clubfoot deformity. Rather such sequential stretching is likely to create secondary deformities by overstretching the relatively normal ligaments and capsules in the midfoot, producing a rocker-bottom deformity. I prefer to derotate the foot on the talus in a single maneuver, which is most simply performed by placing the opposite index finger (e.g., left hand on right foot) from medial to lateral around the back of the os calcis. Next, the radial aspect of the flexed middle finger is placed under the midfoot, and the palmar aspect of the base of the thumb pushes against the medial aspect of the first metatarsal head in a direction of lateral rotation. The tibia is stabilized while the foot is spun laterally on the tibia and dorsiflexed. Once the foot thus is manipulated, a cast is applied. Two hands must hold the foot in the position of manipulation while another two hands apply the cast. Attempting to obtain more correction by forcing the casted foot may result in skin ulceration and cartilage necrosis.

Surgical treatment must aim to correct the deformed foot in a single procedure with minimal damage to the soft tissues. The technique is demanding and requires both a thorough knowledge and familiarity with the infant's clubfoot anatomy. Extreme care must be taken to preserve all major and as many minor vessels as possible in an effort to prevent avascular necrosis of the talar head. Soft tissues must be handled gently to prevent skin slough and scarring. Magnifying loupes are useful, particularly in a child under 6 months of age.

Surgical release of the infant clubfoot must be done under general anesthetic by an experienced anesthesiologist. The patient is positioned prone over bolsters with pneumatic tourniquet(s) set between 200 and 250 mm Hg.

I prefer a Cincinnati incision, which begins over the navicula medially, extends posteriorly to a point 2 mm proximal to the tip of the os calcis (just proximal to the posterior skin crease) and then distally to a point just lateral to the cuboid.

The sural neurovascular bundle and the peroneal tendons are identified and protected. Next, the tendo Achilles is identified and the sheath divided. The tendon must be followed proximally to the musculotendinous junction and then divided for Z-plastic lengthening for maximal length. The posterior neurovascular bundle then is identified under its fascial sheath and protected. The posterior tibialis, flexor digitorum longus, and flexor hallucis longus tendons are identified in the line of the incision and divided in notch fashion for lengthening. Failure to lengthen these tendons impedes adequate correction and interferes with the capsular release. Postoperative scarring from these tendons has not been a problem.

The posterior subtalar joint then is identified and released, care being taken not to damage the posterior talus. The subtalar release then is continued medially to the interosseous ligament, care being taken not to damage the flexor hallucis longus or the posterior tibial neurovascular bundle. The subtalar release then is continued laterally to the lateral interosseous ligament, care being taken not to injure the peroneal tendons or the sural neurovascular bundle. I prefer to leave the interosseous ligament intact as a pivot point on which to spin the foot on the talus.

On the medial aspect of the foot, the talonavicular joint is identified and released medially, superiorly, and plantarly, with care being taken to avoid damaging the vascular supply to the talar neck. Forefoot adduction in the presence of a tight abductor hallucis requires lengthening by making an incision medially over the distal third of the first metatarsal. The musculotendinous junction of the abductor hallucis tendon is identified and divided sharply, leaving the muscle intact.

It may be possible to hold the foot in what appears to be a reduced position. However, careful examination demonstrates that the heel is not reduced, or the talonavicular joint is wedged open, or the forefoot cannot be reduced completely under the talar head, and most importantly, that the ankle joint is not aligned straight with the forefoot. Attention now must be turned to the lateral aspect of the foot. Preserving the vessels overlying the sinus tarsi, the extensor brevis is lifted to identify the subtalar joint distal to the interosseus ligament and the lateral talonavicular capsule. Both structures are released. This then permits derotation of the foot on the talus around a central pivot, the interosseus ligament. The talonavicular joint is reduced and pinned using a smooth Kirschner wire from the posteromedial corner of the talus through the talonavicular joint and out the dorsum of the foot. The pin then is bent and cut with just enough length to pull the pin at a later time. Dorsal displacement of the navicula on the talar head results in cavovarus and limits dorsiflexion. Lateral displacement results in midfoot varus. Plantar flexion leaves the forefoot in equinus, which is problematic particularly in the presence of flattop talus.

The correction then is checked. The heel should be in slight valgus and out of equinus, the pin through the reduced talonavicular joint, and the lateral border of the foot straight. Release of the plantar fascia may be necessary, but I find this only infrequently. The talonavicular and subtalar joints should not be gaping open.

The four tendons then are repaired with the foot held at 90° to the tibia. Overcorrection of the Achilles contracture may result in gastrocnemius soleus weakness. Skin closure should be done with the foot in equinus to remove tension from the incision. A bulky dressing from toes to groin then is applied, keeping the knee extended to improve venous drainage. Careful hemostasis should be employed with electrocautery to reduce the risk of infection, scarring, hematoma, and the need for a drain.

Isolated posterior release or tendon lengthening should be reserved for the foot without fixed rotational deformity. It rarely is indicated.

Postoperative Management

The bulky dressing applied in the operating room is changed after 1 week. The wounds are inspected and a short-leg cast applied after the foot is brought up to 90° to the tibia. If persistent tightness of the posterior skin is observed (the Achilles tendon has been lengthened to allow dorsiflexion), cast the foot in a comfortable position and change the cast in another week. Excessive dorsiflexion may disrupt the tendons.

The cast then is changed monthly for 3 months. If the correction has been successful, the patient then may go into regular shoes or sneakers. Follow-up with radiographs is obtained annually.

COMPLICATIONS AND SEQUELAE

Fewer than 5 percent of patients have required additional surgical intervention, although further follow-up is needed. Loss of position (reduction) may require reoperation. Premature pin removal may occur, either accidentally or through poor placement. The pin should be taped or covered in the postoperative dressings or casts. In my experience, weekly casting instead of monthly casting has prevented reoperation in all but two cases.

Considerable growth remains after this treatment. The feet usually are one to one-and-one-half shoe sizes too small at maturity. The calves typically are narrowed. The tibia may be 2 to 3 cm shorter than in the normal leg. These expectations occur regardless of the treatment chosen.

Flattening of the talar dome or head may result in stiffness and later degenerative arthritis, requiring reconstruction or arthrodesis. Infection may require reoperation for drainage and debridement.

In spite of these complications, early correction is preferable to treatment of the painful stiff foot in a child or early adolescent. Remodeling potential and the ability to realign the now mis-shapen tarsal bones lessens as a child matures.

DISCUSSION

I have described the nonsurgical and surgical treatment of clubfoot deformity that has worked for me. Additional time and study are needed to compare this approach to more traditional ones. I am convinced that, in my hands, the short-term results are better than other methods that I have tried.

The surgical technique is demanding and the potential risks significant. Careful evaluation of the deformity and planning of the release and reconstruction should be done before attempting the reconstruction.

SUGGESTED READING

Crawford AH, Marxen JL, Osterfeld DL. The Cincinnati incision: A comprehensive approach for surgical procedures of the foot and ankle in childhood. J Bone Joint Surg 1982; 64A:1355–1358.

Cummings RJ, Lovell WW. Current concepts review: Operative treatment of congenital idiopathic clubfoot. J Bone Joint Surg 1988; 70A:1108–1112.

McKay DW. New concept of and approach to clubfoot treatment: Section 11–correction of clubfoot. J Pediatr Orthop 1983; 3:10–12.

Simons GW. Complete subtalar release in clubfeet, part 1: A preliminary report. J Bone Joint Surg 1985; 67A:1044–1055.

Turco VJ. Resistant congenital clubfoot-one-stage posteromedial release with internal fixation: A follow-up report on 15 years experience. J Bone Joint Surg 1979; 61A:805–814.

VERTICAL TALUS

RICHARD S. DAVIDSON, M.D.

Vertical talus is a rare congenital deformity of the foot that often is part of a syndrome complex (e.g., nail-patella syndrome, Ehlers-Danlos syndrome) or a neuromuscular disorder (e.g., tethered cord, arthrogryposis). Alternative terms used to describe this deformity include congenital convex pes valgus and congenital rocker-bottom foot. Failure to diagnose the associated or causative disorder before correcting the deformity may result in rapid recurrence. Consultation with a geneticist or neurologist may be indicated.

Clinically the deformity is defined by a forefoot locked in dorsiflexion on the hindfoot (dorsal dislocation of the navicular on the talar head), hindfoot valgus and equinus, and midfoot valgus (Fig. 1). The talar head is prominent palpably in the arch and is weight bearing, often with an overlying callus. This callus may become painful in an older weight-bearing child. These are fixed deformities. Similar weight-bearing posturing (not a fixed deformity) may indicate heel cord contracture and/or marked ligamentous laxity and flexible flatfoot. The dorsiflexed everted foot without heel cord contracture indicates a calcaneovalgus foot, which rarely requires more than stretching. The term *oblique talus* has been used to describe a neuromuscular but similar deformity with subluxation of the forefoot on the talus rather than frank dislocation.

The radiographic and clinical picture must be distinguished carefully from the flexible flatfoot, the flexible flatfoot with tight heel cord, and the calcaneovalgus foot. Although a single radiograph provides a static view, two radiographs, one lateral in plantar flexion and another lateral in dorsiflexion, can document the rigidity of the deformity. Unfortunately no amount of verticality of the talus with respect to the tibia can make the diagnosis and distinguish the rigid deformity from benign ligamentous laxity.

RADIOGRAPHIC TECHNIQUE

Standing anteroposterior (AP) and lateral views are obtained where possible. Additionally, obtain a transmalleolar lateral view in maximal plantar flexion and a transmalleolar lateral view in dorsiflexion. The AP view shows midfoot valgus. The standing lateral view shows the weight-bearing position. The talus, in the congenital vertical talus, is vertical and more parallel to the tibia than normal, although no studies have reliably quantitated the amount of verticality to the severity of the deformity. The angle between the talus and the os calcis on the AP and lateral radiographs is increased, although no measured angle is diagnostic of or distinguishes the flexible foot from the vertical talus (Fig. 2).

The plantar flexed lateral view demonstrates the ability of the forefoot to reduce on the talar head (Fig. 3). In the normal or ligamentous lax foot, the first metatarsal should line up with the axis of the talus (Fig. 4). This is true particularly in the spastic valgus foot of cerebral palsy, in which the forefoot moves into valgus and the hindfoot into eversion in an attempt to dorsiflex in the presence of ankle equinus secondary to the heel cord contracture. Unless bony deformity limits motion, plantar flexion should eliminate the effect of the heel cord contracture, allowing the forefoot to reduce on the talus. Failure of the forefoot to reduce on the talus is diagnostic of vertical talus.

The dorsiflexed lateral view documents the equinus deformity of the hindfoot.

THERAPEUTIC ALTERNATIVES

After the diagnosis has been made and associated anomalies, syndromes, and neuromuscular etiologies

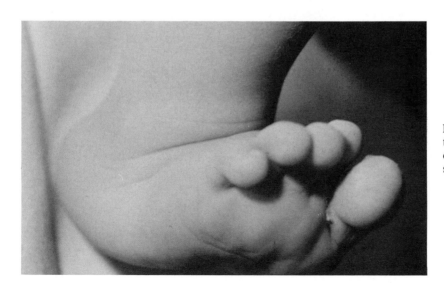

Figure 1 Clinical appearance of the vertical talus foot. Note the heel valgus and equinus, midfoot valgus, and forefoot dorsiflexion.

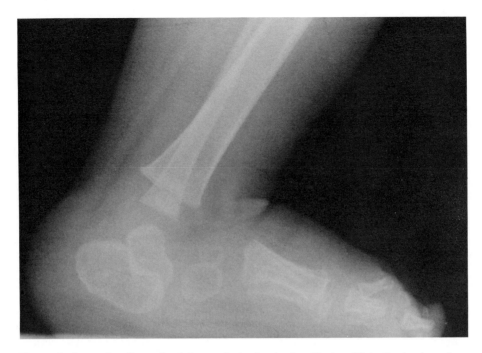

Figure 2 Lateral radiograph of the vertical talus in dorsiflexion. Note the heel equinus, increased angle between the talus and os calcis, and dislocation of the forefoot on the talus.

assessed, treatment can begin. In spite of the dislocation of the talonavicular joint, the foot remains shoeable and often is painless until the second or third decade of life. Weight bearing on the prominent talar head at the medial midfoot may produce a thickened callus and eventually pain. Degenerative changes in the talonavicular joint occur later. It has been suggested by some authors that the late onset of symptoms coupled with failure of early techniques of reduction and the high risk of recurrence should lead the surgeon to postpone treatment until adolescence. At that time bony procedures, such as triple osteotomy and/or arthrodesis should be performed. Unfortunately such delayed treatment may restrict a child's sports activities, and triple arthrodesis may result in a short, wide stiff foot. Soft tissue release at an early age (as young as 3 months) may produce a flexible, "shoeable" foot and lasting results in the absence of a progressive or persistent neuromuscular disorder. Deformities related to such neuromuscular disorders may require repeated releases and later resection arthrodeses.

The deformity is a dislocation of the forefoot dorsally on the talar head with rotation of the subtalar joint (the os calcis rotates laterally under the talus, opposite to the rotation of the clubfoot). Capsular contractures may fix both components of the deformity. Three muscle groups in the ankle demonstrate contractures: the posterior (Achilles tendon), the lateral (peroneals), and the anterolateral (extensor hallucis longus, extensor digitorum longus, anterior tibialis). These structures must be stretched or lengthened to reduce the deformities. It is particularly difficult to stretch the talonavicular capsule

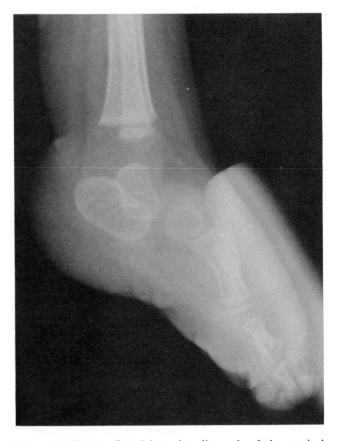

Figure 3 Plantar flexed lateral radiograph of the vertical talus. Note the failure of the forefoot to reduce on the talus.

Figure 4 *A,* Lateral radiograph of the ligamentous lax foot in dorsiflexion. Note the increased angle between the talus and the os calcis and apparent dislocation of the forefoot on the talus. *B,* Lateral plantar flexed radiograph of the same patient. Note the complete reduction of the forefoot on the talus and normal talocalcaneal angle.

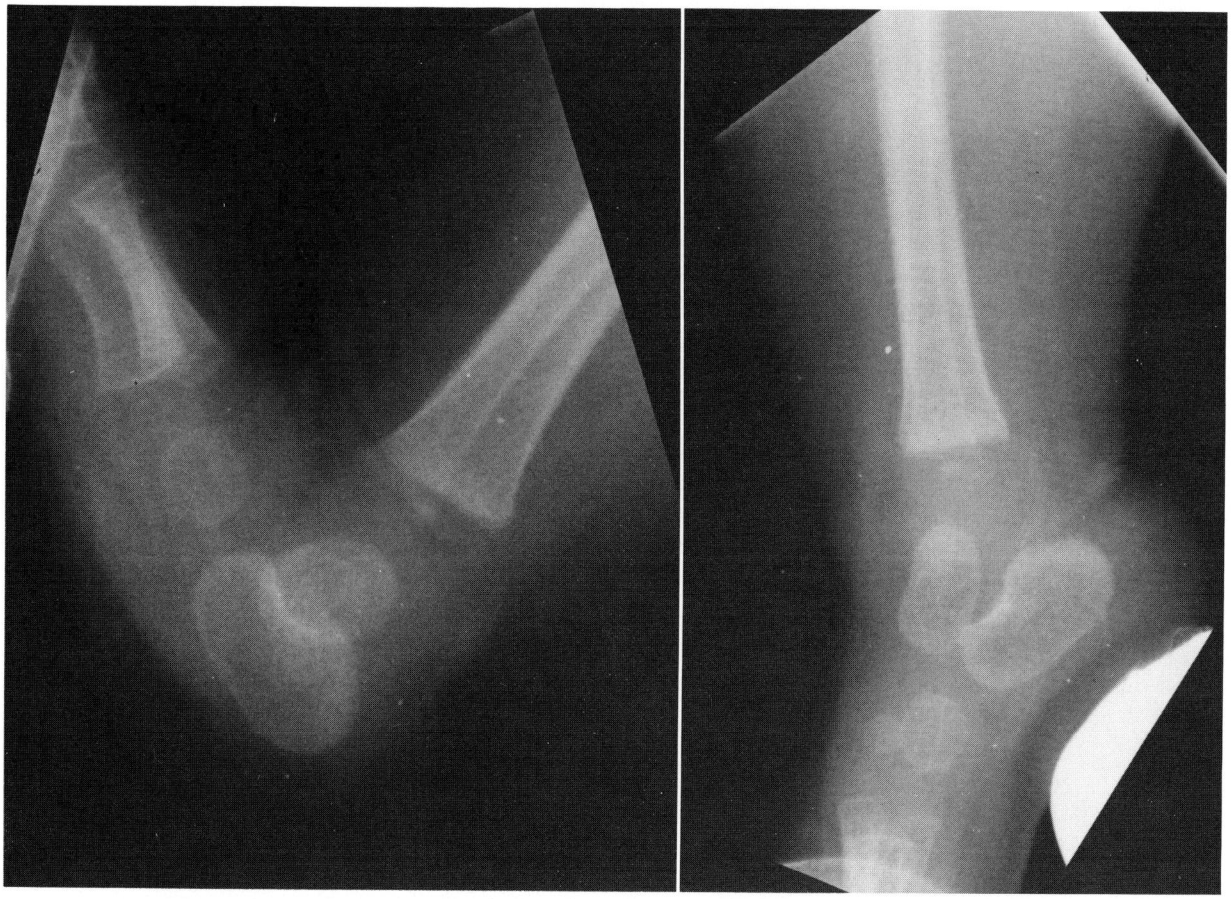

and ankle extensors adequately to allow reduction of the dorsolaterally dislocated talonavicular joint. Application of the cast is difficult, because it must maintain dorsiflexion and inversion of the hindfoot at the same time that it maintains plantar flexion and varus of the forefoot. Failure of casting is the rule, although casting is worthwhile to stretch the soft tissues in preparation for surgical release.

When a child is over 3 months of age and casting has failed to correct the deformity, I believe the patient should undergo surgical release.

SURGICAL TECHNIQUE

The child is positioned supine with a pneumatic tourniquet at the upper thigh. A general anesthetic is necessary because of the young age of the child. The prepared and draped leg then is exsanguinated. An incision approximately 3 cm is made longitudinally, anterior and proximal to the ankle to lengthen the tendons of the anterior compartment. The anterior

tibialis tendon is lengthened in notch fashion, whereas the extensor digitorum longus and the extensor hallucis tendons are lengthened at their musculotendinous junctions by recession.

A Cincinnati incision then is made, extending from the talonavicular joint medially, then posteriorly just proximal to the posterosuperior tip of the os calcis and then laterally to the talonavicular joint. The Achilles tendon is identified and lengthened in notch fashion. The amount of lengthening needed is determined after completion of the release and reduction. The sural neurovascular bundle is identified and protected. The peroneus longus and brevis are identified, released from their tendon sheaths, and lengthened in notch fashion. Infrequently this tendon lengthening alone suffices to reduce the deformity.

The posterior tibial neurovascular bundle then is identified and protected. The medial tendons usually are stretched out and do not require lengthening. The talonavicular joint is identified and divided medially, superiorly, and inferiorly. Attention then is turned to the lateral aspect of the wound. The remaining talonavicular capsule is released. The navicular usually can be reduced onto the head of the talus at this point. However, the talus may remain in plantar flexion and the os calcis in lateral rotation and eversion. Attention then is turned to the posterior aspect of the incision. The posterior ankle joint is released. The posterior, medial, and lateral subtalar joints then are released, leaving the interosseous ligament intact as a pivot when reducing the os calcis under the talus. The talus then should dorsiflex in the ankle. A single pin through the reduced talonavicular joint holds the foot in the corrected position. The tendons are repaired with the foot at 90° to the tibia. The wounds are irrigated thoroughly and closed in layers.

Postoperatively I prefer to use a bulky dressing for the first week. Thereafter I apply short-leg casts at monthly intervals for 3 months. The patients then use regular shoes and sneakers. The pin is removed in the office 5 weeks postoperatively.

I have not found transfer of the posterior tibialis tendon to the talar neck to be useful. Although some patients, particularly those with ligamentous laxity, have continued to pronate, the talonavicular joint has remained stable. Tendon transfer has been shown to stretch out in most cases of pronating flatfoot. If successful, transfer to the talar neck produces ankle stiffness. Skin slough and infection with the Cincinnati incision have been reported in the literature, but I have not encountered these complications as yet.

SUGGESTED READING

Dodge LD, Ashley RK, Gilbert RJ. The treatment of the congenital vertical talus: A retrospective review of 36 feet with a long-term follow-up. Foot and Ankle 1987; 7:326–332.
Lovell WW, Winter RB, eds. Pediatric orthopaedics. 3rd ed. Philadelphia: JB Lippincott, 1990.

CAVOVARUS FOOT

MARK MYERSON, M.D.

Correction of the cavovarus foot depends on the underlying etiology. Although the majority of cavovarus feet are of neuromuscular origin, the idiopathic deformity is not uncommon. These feet are far easier to correct, since tendon transfers are not needed and the deformity usually is less severe. Regardless of the etiology, all components of the deformity should be corrected: (1) hindfoot varus, (2) first metatarsal equinus, (3) forefoot varus, (4) Achilles tendon contracture, and (5) claw toe deformity. The muscle groups that are weak in hereditary sensory-motor neuropathy (Charcot-Marie-Tooth disease) are the anterior tibial, the peroneus brevis, and the intrinsics.

In some patients weakness of all the extrinsic extensors also are present. The planovalgus foot in hereditary sensory-motor neuropathy is less common and is not discussed here. In general, patients with a cavovarus foot present with pain along the plantar-lateral weight-bearing surface of the foot, pain under the first metatarsal head, ankle instability, and painful claw toe deformities including the hallux. Occasionally ankle instability is the presenting problem in an adult patient, and the other deformities, although severe and advanced, are well tolerated. The traditional procedure to correct the cavovarus foot is a triple arthrodesis. I do not favor this operation unless degenerative changes in the subtalar or talonavicular joints are advanced. As a rule, one is able to correct the hindfoot with a triplanar osteotomy of the calcaneus followed by appropriate forefoot correction. Perhaps the worst procedure performed to correct pain in the forefoot associated with hindfoot varus is resection of the fifth metatarsal head. The forefoot pressure associated with hindfoot varus transfers to the distal tip of the remaining portion of the fifth metatarsal and to the adjacent fourth metatarsal.

HINDFOOT VARUS

The hindfoot is corrected with a triplanar osteotomy of the calcaneus, as described in the chapter *Calcaneus Osteotomy*. Osteotomy is my preferred procedure, and a triple arthrodesis is performed only if deformity is associated with severe subluxation of the subtalar joint and/or degenerative changes. It is not possible to correct forefoot rotation with calcaneal osteotomy alone, and if excessive, a triple arthrodesis is required since the forefoot can be partially corrected through the transverse tarsal joint. The arthrodesis is performed through two incisions, one lateral and one medial, as described in the chapter *Posterior Tibial Tendon Insufficiency*. Unlike the triple arthrodesis for the planovalgus foot, wedges

are removed from both the subtalar and transverse tarsal joints to evert the hindfoot and dorsiflex the midfoot. The soft tissues always are tight medially, and even following the wedge resection laterally, the lateral aspect of the subtalar joint does not always appose well. A truncated wedge is removed to prevent undue tension on the medial side of the foot, which would prevent complete closure of the arthrodesis. The size of these wedges is difficult to predict. Nevertheless, minimal bone is resected initially, and once the subtalar and transverse tarsal joints are prepared, it is easy to determine if more bone should be resected (Fig. 1).

ANKLE INSTABILITY

Prolonged hindfoot varus in adulthood leads to varus instability of the ankle. This is associated with attenuation of the anterior talofibular and calcaneofibular ligaments and degenerative changes in the ankle in long-standing cases. It is important to obtain weight-bearing radiographs of both the foot and ankle in these patients. Stress views of the ankle also are helpful and probably required in the presence of lateral ankle pain or instability. If the tibiotalar joint is tilted (into varus) on the weight-bearing radiographs, one assumes that degenerative changes in the ankle have occurred, usually laterally where the joint abuts. I do not regard this as a contraindication to either a calcaneal osteotomy or triple arthrodesis. Debridement of the ankle may be needed, including synovectomy and removal of osteophytes and loose bodies, but an arthrodesis rarely is needed. Realignment of the hindfoot with either an osteotomy or arthrodesis always corrects the tibiotalar tilt by shifting the weight-bearing axis of the leg laterally. If the talus is fixed and rigid, the tilt does not settle, and in the presence of ankle pain, a pantalar arthrodesis should be performed.

The ankle ligament reconstruction is combined with a triple arthrodesis or a calcaneal osteotomy for less severe cases. In patients with hereditary sensory-motor neuropathy, the peroneus brevis does not function and the entire tendon may be used. In cases of hindfoot varus and ankle instability not associated with any neuromuscular imbalance, the peroneus brevis tendon is split and the reconstruction performed after Crisman and Snook (Figs. 2 and 3). The peroneus brevis tendon is transected at the musculotendinous junction, and the muscle fibers are peeled off the tendon sharply. The peroneal tendon sheath is opened proximally, but the pully and sheath of the peroneus longus tendon are not divided distally. Note that the proximal pully contains both the longus and brevis tendons, but distally each tendon is enclosed in a separate sheath and pully. Immediately posterior to the fibula, the peroneus longus lies anterior or superficial to the brevis tendon. This relationship changes distal to the fibula as the tendons rotate, and the brevis tendon then lies more superficially. The brevis tendon can be identified easily since its muscle fibers extend distally on

Text continued on p. 208.

A

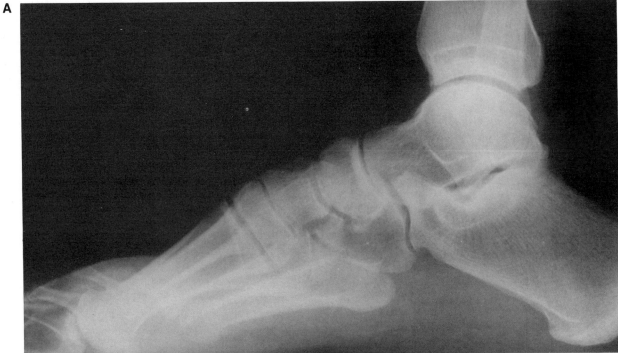

B

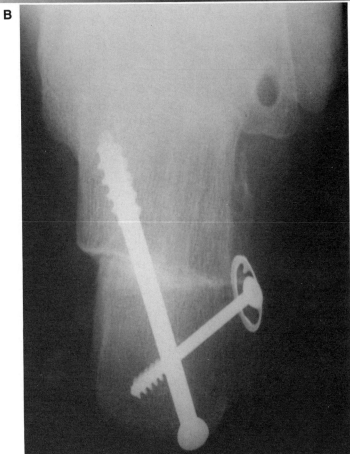

Figure 1 *A,* Weight-bearing lateral radiograph of a 44-year-old male with hereditary sensory motor neuropathy and mild cavovarus deformity with symptomatic ankle instability. *B,* Postoperative axial view demonstrating the valgus and lateral shift of the calcaneus.

Continued.

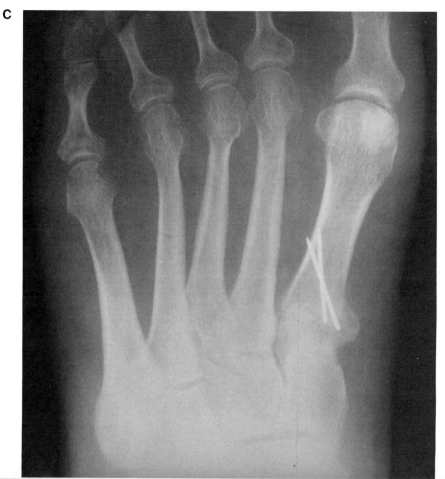

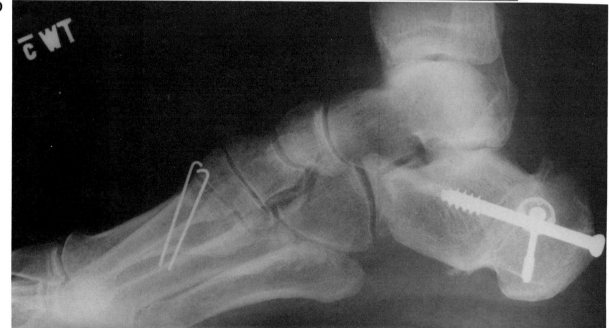

Figure 1, cont'd. *C,* Anteroposterior radiograph demonstrating the dorsal wedge metatarsal osteotomy. *D,* Lateral radiograph demonstrating correction of the hindfoot and forefoot. The 4.0 mm cancellous screw in the calcaneus secures the peroneal tendon used for repair of the unstable ankle.

Figure 2 *A,* The skin incision for the ankle ligament reconstruction is immediately posterior to the peroneal tendon. *B,* The anterior half of the peroneus brevis tendon is split. *C,* A 4.5 mm drill hole is made in the fibula. *D,* The peroneal tendon is passed through the fibula. *E,* The tendon is passed deep to both peroneal tendons and secured to the calcaneus with a 4.0 mm cancellous screw and a spiked 4.0 mm ligament washer. *F,* The tendon is passed superficial to the peroneal tendons and secured to itself and the anterior fibula.

Continued.

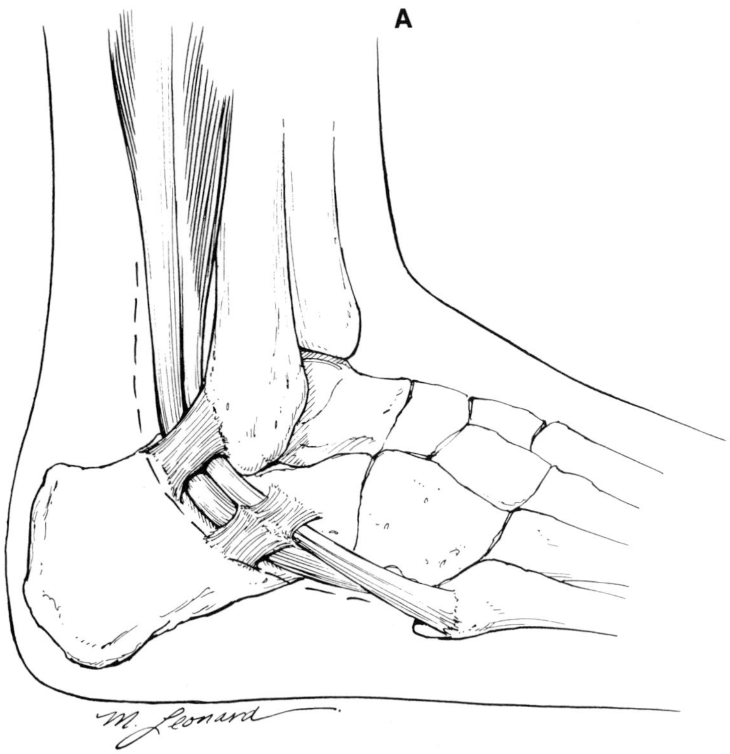

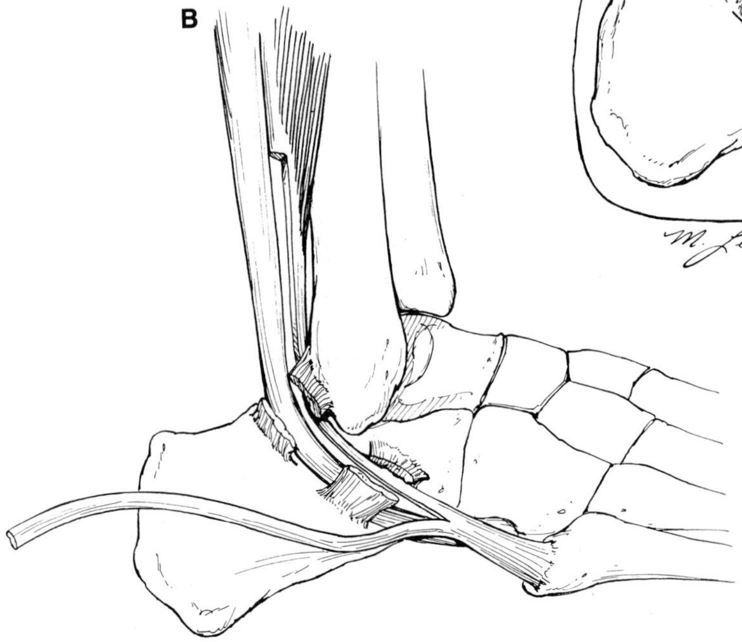

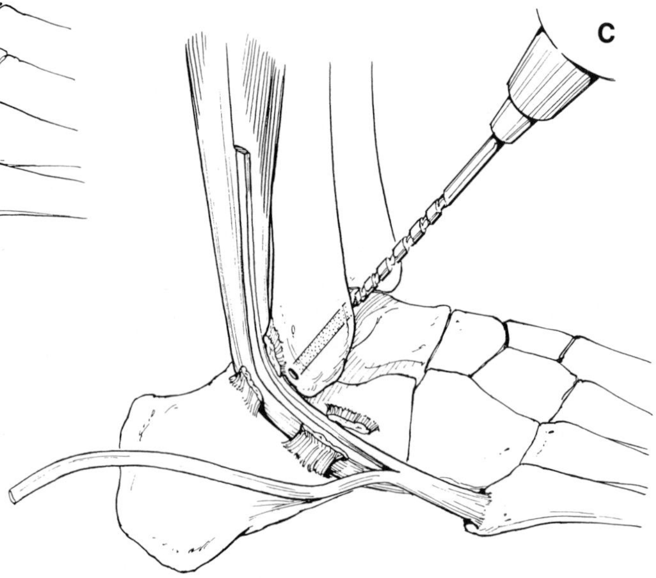

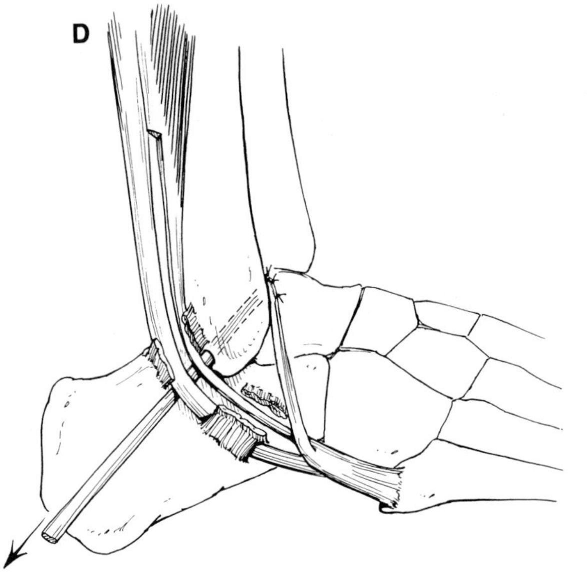

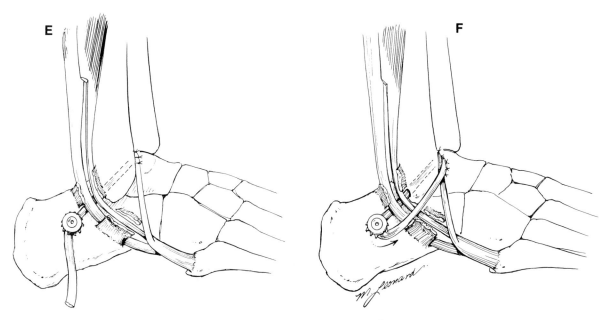

Figure 2, cont'd. For legend see opposite page.

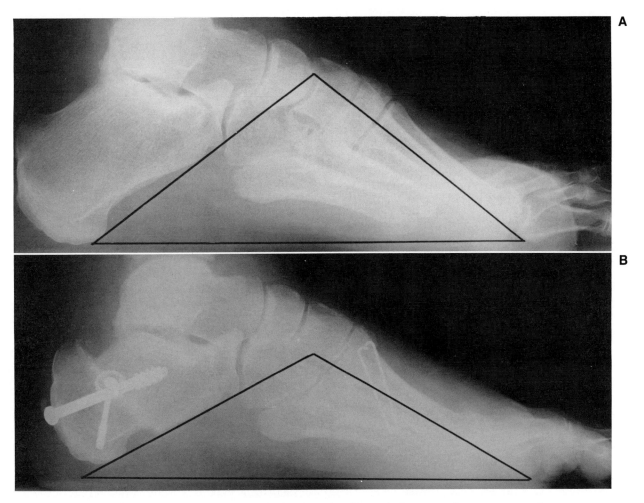

Figure 3 *A,* Preoperative weight-bearing lateral radiograph demonstrating cavovarus and ankle instability. *B,* Correction of the calcaneometatarsal angle and the height of the midfoot following osteotomy of the calcaneus and first metatarsal.

the tendon, unlike the longus tendon, which has no attached muscle at this level. In cases of hereditary sensory-motor neuropathy, in which the entire tendon is used, it is transected 6 cm proximal to the tip of the fibula and the muscle fibers are peeled off the tendon sharply. If half the tendon is used, I split off the anterior half, leaving the posterior half intact, since this segment has a more direct insertion onto the muscle. The separate sheath with the peroneus brevis tendon is divided distally and the tendon delivered into the wound. The distal sheath of the peroneus longus tendon is not opened. The peroneus brevis tendon is split, leaving the distal 1 to 2 inches of the tendon intact. The split tendon is slightly rotated over the more posterior intact portion as it is passed to the anterior edge of the fibula, where it is secured with 2-3 interrupted sutures. A 4.5 mm drill hole is made in the fibula from anterior to posterior approximately 1 cm proximal to the tip of the fibula. The tendon then is passed from anterior to posterior. With the ankle in the neutral position, the tendon is sutured to the periosteum over the anterior aspect of the fibula. The tendon now is passed deep to the peroneus longus tendon and attached to the calcaneus with a 4.0 mm cancellous screw and a spiked ligament washer. I find this modification far easier to perform than creating a bone tunnel in the calcaneus. The tendon is secured rigidly, and I have not noted any screw loosening. A drill hole is made in firm subchondral bone and the medial calcaneal cortex purchased with the screw, which usually measures about 30 mm. An extra 3 to 4 mm should be added to the length of the screw to accommodate the thickness of the washer. The tendon is pulled down inferior to the fibula in the general direction of the calcaneofibular ligament, and a small 2 mm split is made in the tendon with a knife blade. The screw and washer are inserted through the tendon, and while pulling in the axis of the tendon, the screw is advanced. It is not necessary to tap the bone, but if difficulty is experienced with insertion of the screw, the lateral cortex can be tapped. A very firm grasp with the screw should be obtained. If the fixation is even slightly tenuous, I redrill the calcaneus in a different direction. The free end of the tendon, which usually is 2 cm in length, now is passed superficial to the peroneus longus tendon and attached to itself at the tip of the fibula.

Complications

The problem that must be avoided is overtightening of the repair, creating a stiff subtalar joint. When suturing the tendon to the fibula, the ankle joint is positioned in neutral dorsiflexion. The tendon is shortest in this position, and it is easy to check the stability following suture with an anterior drawer test. Stiffness also can be prevented by early postoperative motion. Patients are allowed to ambulate after suture removal in a cast or brace for 2 to 3 weeks, followed by use of an Aircast for 6 weeks. Physical therapy and rehabilitation is commenced at 6 weeks, and return to full sporting activities is possible by 10 weeks.

FOREFOOT VARUS

A plantar fascia release is performed routinely. A 1 inch incision is made along the plantar-medial side of the plantar fascia. The subcutaneous tissue is dissected off the plantar fascia and retracted. A curved clamp is passed deep to the plantar fascia and the fascia transected from deep to superficial. Cutting from superficial to deep risks laceration of the neurovascular structures. It is important to release the lateral band of the plantar fascia. I do not perform a fasciectomy routinely, nor do I find it necessary to strip the fascia off the calcaneus with the exception of the most severe cases. The plantar-flexed first metatarsal is corrected with a dorsal wedge osteotomy performed at the base of the first metatarsal. An incision is made medial to the extensor hallucis longus tendon deep into the subcutaneous tissue, and the periosteum is divided. A 1/8 to 1/4 inch wedge is removed with the base dorsal. It is important not to remove too large a wedge. The size of the wedge can be incrementally increased until the forefoot is plantigrade. The first metatarsal head is pushed dorsally, and the adjacent surface of the second metatarsal head is palpated. The osteotomy is completed and closed dorsally. It is held secure with two 0.045 inch Kirschner wires introduced from proximal-dorsal to distal-plantar.

The hallux and lesser toes are all addressed similarly, with interphalangeal joint arthrodesis and release at the metatarsophalangeal (MP) joint. The dorsal release includes lengthening of the extensor longus tendon, transection of the extensor brevis tendon, transverse dorsal capsulotomy, and collateral ligament release. If the deformity of the hallux is severe, the contracture of the MP joint is fixed. In addition to the soft tissue releases, the entire volar plate is released off the metatarsal neck. This frees up the motion at the MP joint, and the proximal phalanx slides and rotates in an improved arc on the metatarsal head. The interphalangeal joint arthrodesis is performed by extending the incision of the MP joint distally toward the base of the nail fold. A transverse limb is added to the longitudinal incision and extended medially to raise a flap for exposure of the interphalangeal joint. A small sagittal saw is used to make perpendicular cuts to the axis of the hallux, and the arthrodesis is performed with a 4.0 mm cancellous screw reduced through the tip of the pulp of the hallux immediately underneath the nail. It is useful to predrill the distal phalanx, starting with the drill tip at the proximal end of the distal phalanx, so that the drill bit can be perfectly centered on the phalanx. A similar hole can be centered in the proximal phalanx and the position checked with the depth gauge to ensure that the alignment is correct. A 40 or 45 mm 4.0 mm cancellous screw usually is selected, and a compression arthrodesis is performed. In addition to stabilization of the interphalangeal joint, it is useful to pin the hallux MP joint in the neutral position for approximately 4 weeks. This prevents recurrent extension contracture or dorsal migration and translation at the MP joint level.

TENDON IMBALANCE

A posterior tibial tendon transfer should be considered for all patients with hereditary sensory motor neuropathy or for those in whom a dynamic varus deformity is present. If a tendon transfer is not performed, this dynamic contracture of the posterior tibial tendon against a weak or absent peroneus brevis causes the deformity to recur. This occurs even following a triple arthrodesis in which adequate alignment of the hindfoot was thought to have been obtained. The tendon transfer is performed according to the pattern of weakness, although I prefer to transfer the entire posterior tibial tendon through the interosseous membrane and to the dorsum of the foot as described in the chapter *Tendon Transfers*. Not only does this transfer provide dorsiflexion strength, but also balances the hindfoot preventing further varus deformity. If a tendon transfer is to be performed, it is done 6 weeks after the hindfoot osteotomy or arthrodesis. Patients resume weight bearing 2 weeks after the tendon transfer, and the recovery period thereby is shortened.

SUGGESTED READING

Alexander IJ, Johnson KA. Assessment and management of pes cavus. Clin Orthop 1989; 246:273–283.

Coleman SS, Chesnut WJ. A simple test for hindfoot flexibility in the cavovarus foot. Clin Orthop 1977; 123:60–65.

Dwyer FC. The present status of the problem of pes cavus. Clin Orthop 1975; 106:254–262.

Mann RA, Missirian J. Pathophysiology of Charcot Marie Tooth disease. Clin Orthop 1988; 234:221–229.

AMPUTATIONS

AMPUTATIONS OF THE FOREFOOT

JAMES W. BRODSKY, M.D.

Although amputations of the foot hold a measure of repugnance for some surgeons, a well-performed amputation is the key to healing the limb, often after a prolonged attempt at salvage of the nonviable part. A healed amputation represents the first step in rehabilitation of the patient. This chapter highlights the surgical techniques of forefoot amputations; the caveat is that preoperative evaluation of the patient's perfusion is required if the amputation is required for a patient with diabetes, peripheral vascular insufficiency, or distal gangrene. Vascular evaluation can include Doppler ultrasonography pressure measurements, transcutaneous oxygen measurement, arteriogram, and consultation by a vascular surgeon. Once the amputation is healed, the treatment of the patient still is multidisciplinary: the services of qualified orthotists and pedorthists are needed for appropriate fitting of shoe insoles, ankle-foot orthoses, and prescription footwear. For amputations of the forefoot, true prostheses, and hence the services of the prosthetist, are not required.

PRINCIPLES OF AMPUTATION CLOSURES AND HEALING

When a forefoot amputation is done for dysvascularity, diabetes, or infection the healing time can be long. Sutures generally should be left in place at least 1½ to 2 times the usual period, often 4 to 6 weeks or longer.

Amputations of the forefoot have a great advantage over more proximal procedures. Not only are they more cosmetic, but they also allow more normal shoe wear, with enhanced function. It is presumed that a forefoot amputation represents "foot salvage" in itself, so the goal is to choose an amputation level that heals primarily and with a stable scar.

Although the technique of amputation surgery is important, proper decision making is equally important.

A balance must be achieved between the amount of bone resected and the amount of residual soft tissue left to cover. Although defects in skin can be covered by split-thickness skin grafting, exposed bone or joint capsule usually is best covered by local full-thickness tissue, i.e., resection of more bone so that the residual soft tissue flaps can be approximated without tension. As a general rule, at the time the incision is made, the basic flaps should be planned sufficiently so that the surgeon knows to preserve the skin and soft tissue distal to the line of bone resection. In the case of gangrene from peripheral vascular disease or a crush injury, the skin should be incised right at the line of demarcation and then observed for bleeding. Hasty or careless initial flap incisions can force the procedure to the next higher level of amputation for lack of only a small amount of soft tissue coverage. In the case of amputation for infection, multiple debridements often are required before a delayed primary closure is performed. The latter still is preferable to leaving the wound open to granulate in entirely, which in a diabetic often can take several months, require a skin graft, and lead to a less stable scar.

The goal in the insensitive foot (usually that of a diabetic) is to achieve soft tissue healing and a plantigrade foot. In the patient with normal sensation, it also must be painless, which translates into taking precautions not to leave or create otherwise avoidable stump neuromas.

Test the flaps before doing the suturing for a closure. If there is tension, further bone must be resected. Unconventional flaps may be required in some ray or transmetatarsal amputations to save the maximal amount of the foot. Here the surgeon uses what tissue is available, even if it is not, e.g., the typical plantar flap. For example, it might be a medially based, irregularly shaped flap, but if it covers the bone without being put under tension, it is a form of foot salvage. The length of most flaps should not be greater than half the width of the base.

Handle the flaps gently, using the forceps on the subcutaneous layer, rather than on the skin. Palpate through the flaps for any bony prominences or sharp corners on the bone that would be painful or could produce pressure ulceration of the stump. Sharp corners on the bone must be rounded. If the skin is blanched after closure, it usually is too tight. In this case, revise the bone resection more proximally and/or loosen the suture line. Failure of the skin edges to bleed adequately at the time of resection also indicates the need to revise to a higher level.

In the case of an infected foot, an irrigation system is placed at the time of closure, using a #8 pediatric feeding tube brought out through a separate tiny stab to inflow normal saline or Ringer's lactate at a rate of about 40 ml per hour. The irrigation system is applicable to various forefoot amputations that are done for infection, but is especially helpful in ray resections, partial forefoot, and transmetatarsal amputations. They are removed routinely after 12 to 24 hours. A loose closure is necessary, and the fluid escapes through the suture line and saturates the bandage, which is reinforced as needed.

SPECIFIC AMPUTATION TECHNIQUES

Distal Syme Amputation

The distal Syme amputation is indicated for ony-chomycosis, severe nail deformity, and recurrent infection. It is used primarily for the hallux, but can be used for the lesser toes as well. First, the nail is removed with a Freer elevator. Then the entire nail bed and matrix are removed in a single ellipse of tissue. Care is taken to extend the proximal side of the ellipse far enough to include the entire matrix. A single cut is made directly down to the bone. A micro-oscillating saw then is used to resect the underlying bone. The key is sufficient removal of bone from the distal phalanx; at least 1 cm but often more is required. The digit is of course shortened, and to some patients the appearance is less than cosmetic. However, the procedure is effective and definitive (Fig. 1).

Problems

There are two main problems resulting from this procedure. The first is dehiscence caused by overly tight closure, which can be prevented by resecting more bone so that the tension on the soft tissue flaps is relieved. The second problem is a bulbous stump, and this can be corrected by modifying the residual flap sharply.

Amputation of the Great Toe

Although amputation of the hallux can be done most easily as a disarticulation through the metatarsopha-langeal (MP) joint, saving the base of the proximal phalanx produces a better result. A minimum of 1 cm of the bone should be preserved (Fig. 2). The residual base of the proximal phalanx serves to enhance the subsequent weight-bearing function of the first metatarsal by preserving the attachments of the plantar fascia and the tendinous sling of the sesamoids, including the flexor hallucis brevis. This allows at least partial function of the independent plantar flexion of the first ray and reduces

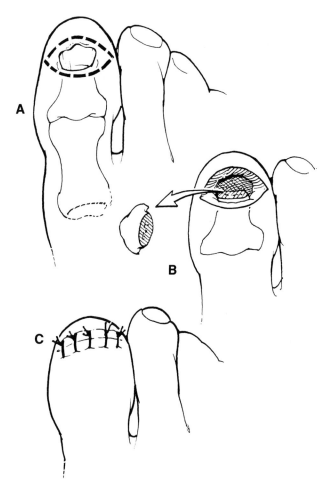

Figure 1 Distal Syme amputation of hallux. *A,* Elliptical incision down to the bone, encompassing the entire nail, nail bed, and proximal matrix. *B,* Amount of distal phalanx to be excised for closure. *C,* Appearance of the closed amputation.

the transfer of pressure to the lesser metatarsal heads, especially the second, which can develop painful plantar keratosis, or in the case of a diabetic produce ulceration.

When disarticulation cannot be prevented, leave the cartilage intact on the metatarsal head; it serves as a barrier against the spread of infection into the bone. Even in an uninfected case, there are no problems by leaving it intact. If possible, make a longer plantar flap and bring the weight-bearing skin up dorsally over the metatarsal head. As in most amputations of the forefoot, closure is done with interrupted sutures of 3-0 or 4-0 nylon monofilament.

Problems

The most common problem in great toe amputations is wound dehiscence. This cannot always be prevented, but can be reduced by thorough preoperative vascular evaluation. If the wound edges show marginal or no bleeding at the time of the amputation, the amputation

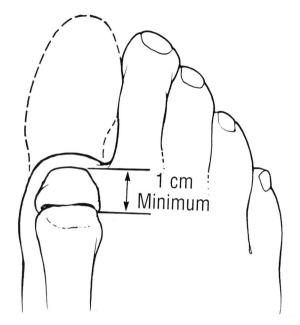

Figure 2 The level of the ideal resection of the proximal phalanx in a great toe amputation that still preserves plantar fascia function.

probably should be revised to a higher level. The other reason for wound breakdown is tension on the suture line, as a result of inadequate bone resection or soft tissue preservation or both.

Postoperatively, once the amputation has healed, a custom-molded shoe insole is manufactured, with additional material in the area of the missing hallux, which serves to block shift of the forefoot in the shoe.

Amputation of the Lesser Toes

Amputation of the lesser toes can be done either as a disarticulation at the MP or interphalangeal joints or by transecting through the bones of the phalanges. Although preservation of the weight-bearing function of the lesser metatarsal head is not as important as in the hallux, there is another reason for preservation of as much bone as feasible, i.e., partial toe amputation. The base of the toe that is saved serves to block the two toes on either side, which tend to migrate gradually, one in varus the other in valgus at the MP joints, as they drift into the defect created by the absent digit. This is not just a cosmetic advantage, but serves to reduce the subsequent secondary ulcerations and painful lesions in insensitive and sensate patients, respectively.

Skin flaps can be either side-to-side or dorsal-plantar "fish mouth" in shape, which work best in a partial toe amputation. A racquet-shaped incision is used at the MP joint (Fig. 3).

Problems

Problems and complications in the lesser toes are similar to those in the hallux, e.g., dehiscence as a result of dysvascularity or incorrect balance of bone and soft tissue resection levels. The drift of the adjacent toes has been mentioned earlier. Late dorsal migration sometimes occurs after partial toe amputation and can produce symptoms if the remnant is sufficiently large. This is treated by MP joint capsulotomy and extensor release, procedures that should be performed at the time of the original amputation if such deformity is present.

Ray Amputations and Partial Forefoot Amputations

Amputation of a toe with part or all of its corresponding metatarsal is a commonly employed procedure for ischemia, trauma, and infection. When two or three contiguous or noncontiguous rays are amputated, the procedure is termed a partial forefoot amputation. Ray amputations are durable, and many patients are able to fit into many shoes with only minor modifications. The complete or partial amputation of one or two rays usually produces a functional foot. Once a third or even a fourth ray is resected, the rate of success of the procedure diminishes. A foot with only one or two residual metatarsals is more likely to be painful as a result of the concentration of pressure on such a diminished area; in the insensitive foot, the result can be ulceration beneath the remaining few weight-bearing points of the forefoot.

The border rays (first and fifth) are the easiest to resect and close. Straight medial and lateral incisions are used, respectively. The distal portion of the incision encircles the corresponding toe ("the racquet"), leaving an ample cuff of soft tissue to allow closure without tension on the suture line. Once the incision has been made, full-thickness flaps should be created down to the bone that is to be excised. Once the metatarsal has been removed, debride the remaining soft tissue to remove infection or necrosis, and save as much viable skin and soft tissue as possible.

Amputation of a single central ray is more difficult in terms of soft tissue coverage, because the flaps cannot be mobilized easily. It is essential to resect the necrotic or injured tissue right up to the edge of viable skin for maximal salvage. If possible, it is best to preserve the base of the resected metatarsal to diminish subsequent instability of the Lisfranc or tarsometatarsal joint. The toes adjacent to the resected toe may drift reciprocally into the defect created by the absent digit, just as they would with a simple toe excision. A filleted flap can be harvested from the amputated toe in some instances by doing a full-thickness subperiosteal dissection of all or part of the toe and turning it proximally to close the defect. The incision usually is dorsal, and the filleted flap is turned on to the dorsal surface, exposing the plantar side of the skin of the toe.

During the healing period, weight bearing is modified and the patient wears a surgical shoe. Once single ray or partial forefoot amputations are completely

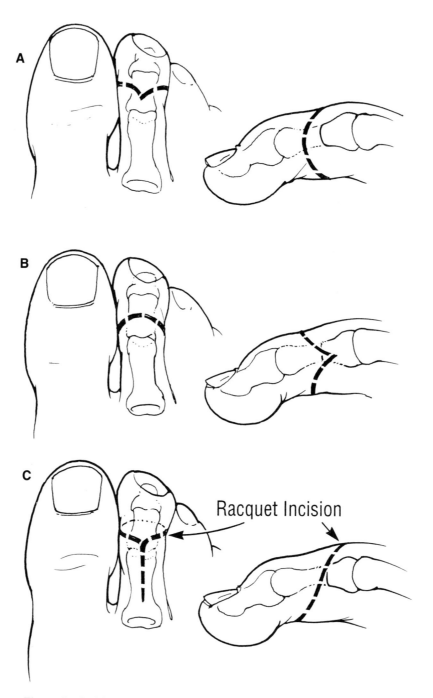

Figure 3 Incisions for an amputation of a lesser toe. *A,* Side-to-side flaps. *B,* Dorsal-plantar flaps. *C,* Racquet-type incision.

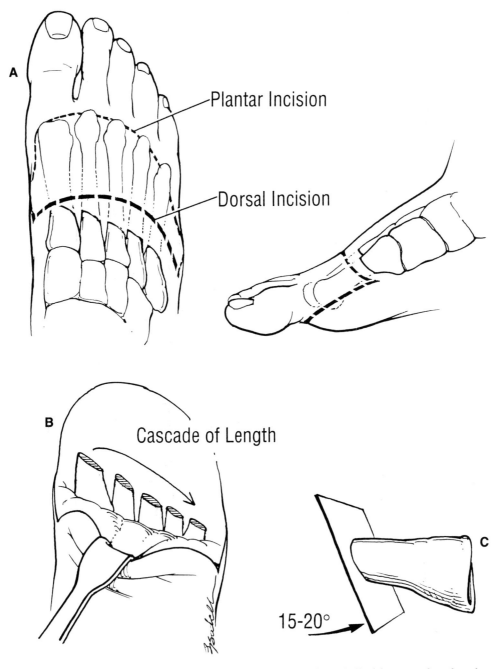

Figure 4 The technique for the transmetatarsal amputation. *A,* Incisions on dorsal and plantar surfaces of the foot. *B,* Level of resection of the metatarsal shafts ("the cascade of length"). *C,* Angle of resection to bevel the distal metatarsals.

healed, patients should be fitted in shoe wear with additional depth and a custom-molded, accommodative insole containing a block for side-to-side sliding of the narrowed forefoot.

Amputations of the lateral forefoot rays generally fare somewhat better than medial partial forefoot amputations because of the destabilizing effect of amputation of the first metatarsal. Once three or more metatarsals need to be resected, the patient usually, although not always, is better off with a transmetatarsal amputation.

Problems

The main problems and complications center on inadequate soft tissue for local wound closure and recurrent pain or ulceration caused by the shift of weight-bearing pressure to a diminished surface area of the forefoot. In most cases local tissue suffices for closure, but occasionally a split-thickness skin graft is necessary to cover a wound. The skin grafts generally function better on the dorsum of the foot and conversely have more recurrent breakdown on the plantar surface. The molded insole helps to distribute and diminish the concentration of pressure under the residual forefoot; recurrent breakdown is an indication for conversion to a transmetatarsal amputation.

Transmetatarsal Amputations

Transmetatarsal amputations are among the most durable and functional of all foot amputations. One of the major characteristics of most transmetatarsal amputations is the preservation of the insertion of the anterior tibialis tendon. This allows active dorsiflexion despite loss of the toe extensors and diminishes the postoperative equinus deformity. However, tendo Achilles lengthening still may be required because of the imbalance in strength between the two muscle groups.

A longer plantar flap usually is developed, and this is brought up over the end of the transected metatarsals (Fig. 4A). Dorsal skin still is highly superior to skin grafts and should be used if plantar skin is not available. Irregular or partial medially or laterally based flaps can and should be used as well to gain coverage and keep the amputation at the forefoot level. The dorsal incision is curved gently in a proximal direction from medial to lateral to correspond to the cascade of length of the metatarsals beneath (Fig. 4B). A full-thickness skin flap is developed sharply down to the bone and then lifted as a single layer by pushing proximally on the dorsum of the metatarsals with a wide elevator. The metatarsals are resected with a power saw to prevent the splintering that osteotomes produce, and the saw cuts are beveled at approximately 15° from dorsal distal to plantar proximal (Fig. 4C). The extensor tendons to the toes are pulled down, cut, and allowed to retract. The anterior tibialis is preserved, or if necessary, reattached through drill holes in the bone.

Each metatarsal is cut at least 2 to 3 mm shorter than the one just medial to it, producing the "cascade" referred to earlier (Fig. 4B). The fifth metatarsal usually is cut 5 mm shorter than the fourth, because it tends to be more mobile and can produce later pain or pressure as it droops plantarward. In the diabetic with significant neuropathy, every attempt is made to preserve the base of all five metatarsals to diminish the risk of developing a subsequent Charcot midfoot collapse.

The plantar flap usually must be thinned to obtain closure. This should be done evenly, avoiding excessive focal thinning that would endanger the viability of the flap. Puckering or bulging at the medial or lateral corner is particularly common, and appropriate trimming is done to obtain skin contact. Closure, especially in a foot with infection, is done with interrupted, nonabsorbable, monofilament sutures that are placed through the full thickness of the entire flap. Sutures usually are left for a minimum of 4 weeks and usually longer. The patient is kept non–weight bearing initially.

The Lisfranc amputations, or disarticulations through the tarsometatarsal joints, are easier technically since transection and shaping of the metatarsal stumps are unnecessary. Disadvantages over a transmetatarsal amputation include the frequent need to reattach the anterior tibialis tendon and the fact that a shorter foot is the result.

Shoe fitting for the patient with a transmetatarsal amputation is not difficult, but usually is not as cosmetic as for the ray amputee, since a lace-up is needed to hold the shoe on the foot, and often a high-top shoe is required. A filler must be placed in the shoe for the missing forefoot, and the sole sometimes must be stiffened. Variations in shoe fitting depend on the length of the stump.

Problems

The most common and difficult problem after this amputation, especially in a diabetic, is the formation of a recalcitrant or recurrent ulceration of the plantar-distal edge of the stump. Almost always, this is the result of apparent or subtle equinus deformity. The equinus can occur as a result of contracture of the Achilles tendon and/or a plantar flexion contracture of the midfoot at the talonavicular and calcaneocuboid joints. Treatment can require proximal reconstruction such as Achilles tendon lengthening, ankle and subtalar joint capsulotomies, and others.

DISCUSSION

Forefoot amputations, although commonly required, still do best with a significant measure of attention to technical detail. Realistic preoperative discussion with the patient and appropriate planning help the surgeon make correct preoperative and intra-operative decisions on the correct level of amputation.

Generally, patients are better served by a more proximal but definitive, stable, healed amputation than multiple unsuccessful attempts to save a nonviable or poorly functioning portion of the foot.

SUGGESTED READING

Brodsky JW, Chambers RB. Effect of tourniquet use on amputation healing in diabetic and dysvascular patients. Perspect Orthop Surg 1991; 2:71–76.

Due TM, Jacobs RL. Molded foot orthosis after great toe medial ray amputation in diabetic feet. Foot Ankle 1985; 3:150–152.

Harris WR, Silversten EA. Partial amputations of the foot: A follow-up study. Can J Surg 1964; 7:6.

Hodge MJ, Peters TG, Efird WG. Amputation of the distal portion of the foot. South Med J 1989; 82:1138–1142.

Jacobs RL. The diabetic foot. In: Jahss MH, ed. Disorders of the foot and ankle. Philadelphia: WB Saunders, 1991.

Larrson U, Andersson GBJ. Partial amputation of the foot for diabetic or arteriosclerotic gangrene. J Bone Joint Surg 1978; 60B:126–130.

Wagner FW. The dysvascular foot: A system for diagnosis and treatment. Foot Ankle 1981; 2:64–122.

AMPUTATIONS OF THE MIDFOOT AND HINDFOOT

MARK MYERSON, M.D.

INDICATIONS FOR AMPUTATION SURGERY

Although amputation of the foot is performed in the context of trauma and congenital deformity, in this chapter I focus on the insensate and ischemic foot. The indications for surgery in these patients are (1) uncontrolled infection, (2) uncorrectable deformity, and (3) protecting the foot at risk.

PREOPERATIVE EVALUATION

Clinical Examination

The foot should be examined systematically, with attention to the extent of infection, the neurovascular status, and an analysis of the plantar weight-bearing surfaces. The essential points on examination other than obvious infection, ulcers, fissures, and gangrene are the color, temperature, and nutritional state of the skin.

It is essential to select a level of amputation likely to result in recovery with a functional plantigrade foot. In amputations resulting from trauma, tumor, or congenital anomalies, length is preserved at the most appropriate level consistent with prosthetic rehabilitation. In diabetic and dysvascular amputations, no well-defined criteria exist and the level is determined by functional considerations, the presence of infection, the status of the circulation, and the age and activity level of the patient.

Vascular Evaluation

If arterial insufficiency is present, salvage may be possible following bypass surgery, permitting an amputation at a more distal level than would otherwise have been possible without revascularization. The status of the arterial circulation is the major determinant of wound healing and should be relied on to assist in determining the level of amputation.

Arteriography reflects the status of the larger arteries only and not the arterioles and skin capillaries, which also are important in healing. Further, involvement of the major vessels usually is patchy, and if these vessels are occluded gradually, a collateral blood supply develops, which may support an adequate peripheral circulation. Therefore the absence of pulses in major extremity vessels does not necessarily indicate severe ischemia. This has the same implications for arteriography, since conservative amputations still may heal despite arteriographic occlusion.

Of the various modalities available to assess the circulatory status, the most economic, efficient, and reliable is Doppler ultrasonography. Transcutaneous Doppler ultrasonography can be used to measure arterial flow patterns and to assess quantitative blockage of the arterial tree. Brachial systolic pressures are obtained simultaneously with various points along the leg, foot, and distally to the toes; each lower extremity pressure is divided by the brachial artery pressure to calculate the ischemic index. An ischemic index of 0.45 or greater indicates sufficient local perfusion for healing following amputation. Doppler ultrasonography measures the status of the larger arteries and not the skin capillaries, which also are important in healing and therefore may be unreliable in the presence of obstructed or calcified vessels. Cutaneous temperature has been well correlated with skin blood flow, using venous occlusion plethysmography. Many commercially available skin thermistors and thermocouples are accurate enough for determining the level of amputation.

On a practical level, I have been satisfied with the accuracy provided by the Doppler ischemic index. In some patients with extensive peripheral vascular disease or sclerosis of the vessels, measurement of the Doppler index is impossible, because the vessel walls cannot be compressed. If pulsatile flow is audible, the amputation level is determined based on the overall skin condition, the temperature, and the presence or absence of infection.

Management of Infection

Definitive amputation with wound closure never should be performed in an attempt to gain control of advancing sepsis; the infection first should be brought under control. The success of amputation surgery depends on adequate control of the local ischemic and infective processes. Unless tissue is debrided aggressively, viable tissue is harmed further, probably as a result of septic thrombosis extending through normal tissue.

Any necrotizing process and active infection should be stabilized by surgical drainage, bed rest, elevation, warm compresses, and antibiotics. Surgery should be delayed until the infection and patient's general nutritional status have improved. Following debridement, ulcers and gangrenous lesions are cultured and broad-spectrum antibiotics commenced until the results of the culture and sensitivities are obtained. The nature of the infection does not have any prognostic value provided the patient is receiving appropriate antibiotics. Patients then are placed on strict bed rest, the extremity elevated, and warm compresses applied. Once the cellulitis and wet gangrenous process can be brought under control, minimal mechanical debridement needs to be performed.

Nutritional Evaluation

The patient's general metabolic and nutritional status always should be considered impaired. It has been shown that the preoperative white blood cell count, temperature, and fasting blood sugar level are significantly correlated with operative success or failure. The basal energy expenditure of a 70 kg male is approximately 1,800 kilocalories, but this energy requirement is increased by about 40 percent during severe infection. Catabolic losses are worse during hospitalization. Severe nutritional depletion is indicated by an albumin concentration less than 3.0 and a total lymphocyte count (the percentage of lymphocytes multiplied by the white blood cell count) less than 1,000. These patients benefit from nutritional supplementation during hospitalization for infection.

SURGICAL TECHNIQUE

General Surgical Principles

A general anesthetic is not necessary for surgery in patients with diabetes. Even with a Syme amputation, a regional anesthetic is sufficient. These patients have significant cardiorespiratory and renal problems, which may be contraindications to a general anesthetic, and since most of these patients have a profound neuropathy, a local or regional anesthetic works well. Occasionally infection may cause a well-localized tissue acidosis, and the anesthetic cannot be injected locally since it is inactivated by the acidosis. Even in this setting, however, a regional anesthetic succeeds and is preferred.

I attempt to preserve as much of the foot as possible. In each case, however, the operative procedure must be tailored to the limitations imposed by infection and deformity. Preservation of length is applicable particularly in the patient with intact circulation. In this group of patients, the infective process is associated with abscess formation and a wet type of gangrene. Although ischemia may be present, metabolic disturbance is the principal problem.

In the second group of diabetic patients, gangrene is caused principally by ischemia, and instead of a florid infection, the affected part usually is dry and associated with a necrotic process that has been present for some time. Revascularization is of particular help in these patients.

The soft tissues always are tenuous; incisions are made carefully, and minimal subcutaneous dissection is performed. Although all surgery is carried out meticulously, this may be accomplished without any concern for precise anatomic landmarks. At no time is the skin or soft tissues firmly grasped with forceps. Skin hooks and rakes are used wherever possible, and overzealous skin retraction always is avoided. Soft tissues and muscle always are retracted gently and protected. Bone cuts are made with sharp instruments, preferably using power equipment. All bone edges are beveled carefully and smoothed with a rongeur and a rasp. All infected gangrenous tissue needs to be debrided radically.

I do not use a tourniquet during diabetic amputation surgery. This more clearly indicates the general perfusion of the foot and also minimizes post-tourniquet ischemic swelling. Post-tourniquet metabolic changes occur and can compromise an already tenuous extremity. If for any reason a tourniquet must be used, it should be inflated after elevating the limb, and not by exsanguination.

Wound Closure

All incisions are closed loosely with absolutely no tension, using 2-0 or 3-0 nylon sutures for skin only, and subcutaneous sutures are not used. This loose approximation of the wound prevents necrosis of the wound edges, which are marginally ischemic. If the incision cannot be completely closed without tension, it is preferable to leave the wound open and allow healing by granulation or to cover it with split-thickness skin grafts. These grafts can be obtained as pinch grafts at a later stage, or split-thickness grafts can be obtained with a dermatome and meshed for immediate application from the amputated part. I have found that the application of these pinch grafts may stimulate the formation of further adjacent granulations, which in turn can be covered with additional grafts and speed closure. If there is insufficient skin for definitive and complete coverage, the foot should not be shortened further by bone resection. I prefer to leave the dorsal wound open and obtain coverage with split-thickness skin grafts—which does not, however, work on the plantar foot surface. Unless a guillotine amputation has been performed for severe sepsis, all incisions are closed loosely, using only nylon sutures for skin.

Drains

Drains always should be used and are placed subcutaneously through the dorsum of the foot into the operative site. During closure of the wound, suction is placed on the catheters to maintain their patency. Once the wound is closed completely, the catheter is irrigated with a continuous infusion. I use Ringer's lactate and not antibiotic solutions. The irrigating fluid exiting between the sutures functions to dilute the bacteria and hematoma, simultaneously washing out debris. There is some question as to the exact role of topical surface antibiotics, and given the potential for systemic toxicity with topical neomycin, either Ringer's lactate or other physiologic solutions are preferable.

The Lisfranc- and Chopart-Level Amputations

Amputation at this level often is not successful as a result of equinus or equinovarus deformity postoperatively, which usually is followed by plantar ulceration. However, if performed correctly, this complication almost never arises. The advantage of amputation at this level is that patients are not dependent on a prosthesis and are able to wear a regular shoe with an ankle-foot orthosis and a shoe filler. Therefore whenever possible, I attempt a Chopart rather than a Syme amputation.

The Chopart amputation is indicated when more

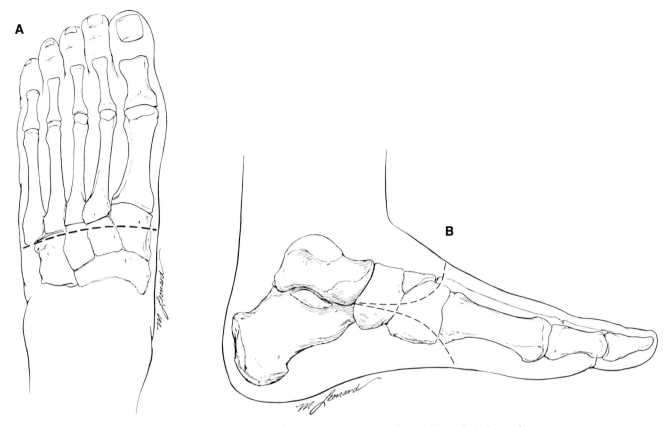

Figure 1 Skin markings for a Chopart amputation. *A,* Dorsal. *B,* Lateral.

extensive necrosis and gangrene of the forefoot preclude performing a transmetatarsal amputation.

The problems of equinus contracture and deformity can be lessened or eradicated by carefully planned surgery. An Achilles tendon lengthening, easiest performed percutaneously, is essential in Chopart's amputations and, I believe, even in transmetatarsal amputations. Additionally, transfer of the extensor tendons and the anterior tibial tendon to the dorsum of the foot must be performed to prevent equinus deformity.

Unlike the skin flap in a transmetatarsal amputation, a long plantar flap is not as important, and I prefer a closure in which the plantar skin is just slightly longer than the dorsal, performed through a large fish mouth incision (Figs. 1, 2, and 3). The plantar flap should join the dorsal skin at the weight-bearing margins of the forefoot. Occasionally the plantar flap is compromised because of necrosis, and the design for closure is modified so that even more of a fish mouth–type flap closure is present.

For the Lisfranc level, the foot is disarticulated at the tarsometatarsal joints. However, a low transmetatarsal amputation is a better functional level since the attachments of the anterior tibial and peroneal tendons are not disrupted completely. I attempt to preserve as much of the soft tissues around the amputation site as possible, including the intrinsic muscles through subperiosteal dissection of the metatarsals. These local muscle

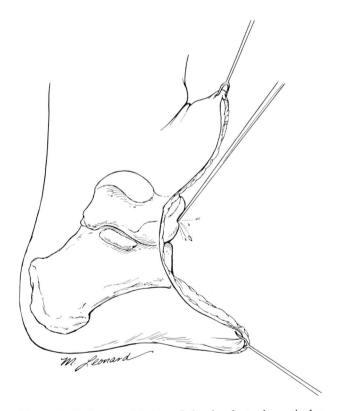

Figure 2 Following ablation of the forefoot, the articular surfaces of the talus and calcaneus are denuded.

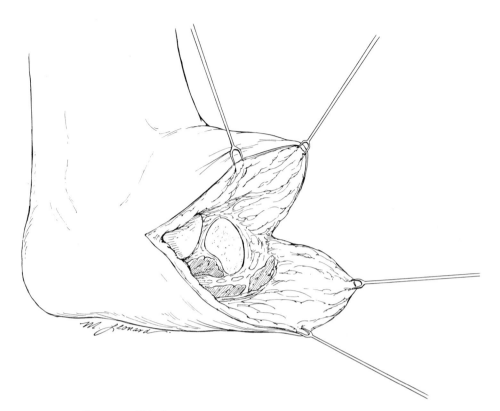

Figure 3 Skin flaps are checked to ensure closure without tension.

pedicles can be of immense importance in the presence of inadequate flaps distally, and provide extra bulk to the flap. When resecting the first and second metatarsals, the first dorsal and plantar interosseous muscles are carefully dissected out to preserve the dorsalis pedis and its perforating branch. These muscles then can be sutured loosely to the adjacent periosteum.

For Lisfranc's amputations, the balance of the extrinsic flexor and extensor tendons must be preserved. The posterior tibial tendon insertion is preserved at this level, and with the loss of the peroneal attachments, the foot tends to drift into varus with time. The anterior tibial tendon insertion can be preserved carefully, although part of this usually is compromised by the resection of the first metatarsal. With the loss of the function of the extrinsic toe extensors, the foot also develops an equinus contracture, although not as severe as with the Chopart amputation. Both the varus and equinus deformity can be prevented by careful reattachment of the extensor and anterior tibial tendons to the dorsal-lateral aspect of the foot. Insertion into the lateral cuneiform usually is adequate.

At the Chopart level, an Achilles tendon lengthening is part of the procedure, since a postoperative equinus contracture otherwise is impossible to prevent. Varus deformity usually is not a problem at this level, since the posterior tibial tendon insertion is sacrificed distally, and the anterior tibial tendon should be attached to the neck of the talus. This can be sutured to the periosteal remnant at this site or passed through a

drill hole in the neck of the talus. I find, however, that the easiest method of attachment of the tendon is by way of a power staple device (Fig. 4).

Closure of the skin, placement of drains, and irrigation postoperatively are as described earlier. The foot requires careful postoperative immobilization in dorsiflexion in a cast or with a carefully molded splint.

Calcanectomy

The surgical approach to acute and chronic infections of the calcaneus presents considerable difficulty in the diabetic patient. Calcaneal osteomyelitis in the diabetic patient is best treated with a total calcanectomy, rather than repeated debridements, which usually fail. A plantar-longitudinal incision is used, through which the ulcer is excised as an ellipse, and any infected tissue or pus is evacuated from the deep fascial space. The insertion of the Achilles tendon, the talocalcaneal interosseous ligaments, and the capsules of the subtalar and calcaneocuboid joints are sectioned. It is important to remove all debris and potentially infective tissue, followed by loose closure of the subcutaneous tissue and skin. These wounds tend to continue draining for a long period, but I have applied a total-contact cast as soon as the acute inflammatory phase has settled, even in the presence of continued drainage, changing the cast more frequently under these circumstances. Patients finally ambulate with a polypropylene splint with a Plastizote and foam filler in the region of the heel defect.

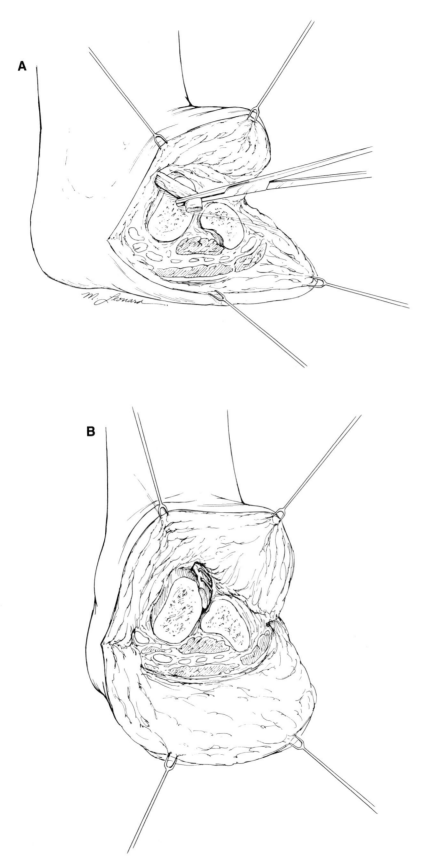

Figure 4 The anterior tibial tendon is pulled into the wound *(A)*, and secured with staples to the lateral surface of the talus *(B)*.

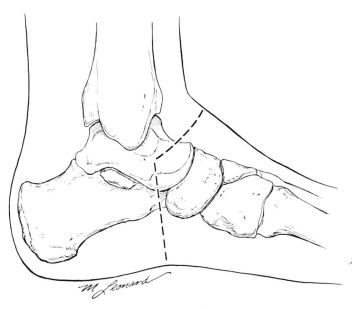

Figure 5 Surface markings for a Syme amputation.

Syme Amputation

The Syme amputation is recommended because the longer length of the leg makes rehabilitation and prosthetic wear far easier. With final maturation of the stump, patients are able to walk short distances without a prosthesis, which may be all that is required in some elderly diabetic patients.

Patients who are candidates for this procedure must be able to weight bear in a prosthesis, and the heel pad ideally should be free of wounds. In addition, the Doppler systolic pressure at the ankle must be 70 mm Hg or more and the Doppler index greater than 0.45. There also should be no acute infection in the ankle or more proximally, and intraoperative bleeding should occur in the skin of the flaps within 3 minutes after release of the tourniquet.

A two-stage amputation is indicated particularly in cases in which extensive infection in the forefoot is present, whereas the single-stage amputation is indicated more in cases of dry gangrene or chronic ulceration. In the first stage of the amputation, an incision is made directly anterior to the ankle, approximately 1.5 cm distal to the malleoli (Fig. 5). This incision is deepened without any dissection of subcutaneous tissue planes. The tendons are incised and allowed to retract. The neurovascular bundle, which lies immediately posteromedially, needs to be preserved carefully, because the posterior tibial artery supplies the entire flap. The Achilles tendon attachment is divided carefully from the calcaneus without perforating the skin. It is important to dissect out the calcaneus in a plane beneath the periosteum so that the fascial septae and the heel pad are preserved (Figs. 6 and 7). In this manner the heel is not too mobile, and the flap adheres to the cancellous bone surfaces. No attempt is made to trim any redundant

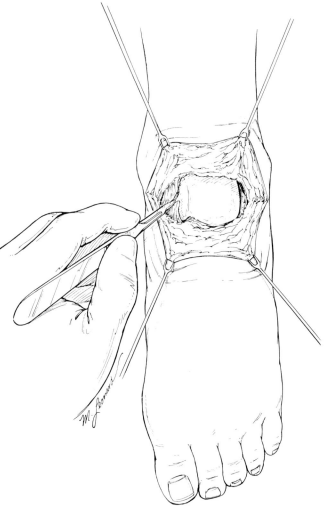

Figure 6 The talus is dissected free from its ligamentous attachments.

skin or corners of the flaps during the first stage of the procedure, because this may jeopardize the posterior skin flap. The wounds are closed in layers with thick absorbable sutures to preserve fascial layers, and the skin is closed with nonabsorbable sutures without any tension (Fig. 8). A continuous irrigation drain is used postoperatively as described previously. The wound usually is stable enough so the patient can commence walking in a well-padded cast at about 2 weeks.

The second stage of the Syme amputation is performed at about 6 weeks (Fig. 9). Medial and lateral incisions are made directly over the dog-ears, and the malleoli are osteotomized flush with the ankle joint, leaving the articular cartilage intact.

PRINCIPLES OF POSTOPERATIVE CARE

It is important that the limb is in a protected position postoperatively. Patients are encouraged to remain at

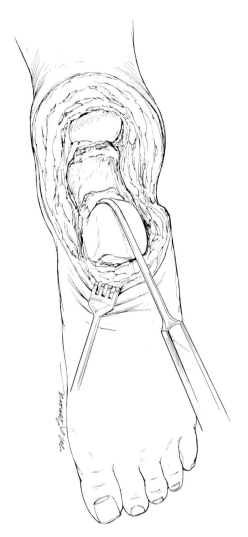

Figure 7 The calcaneus is removed by careful subperiosteal dissection.

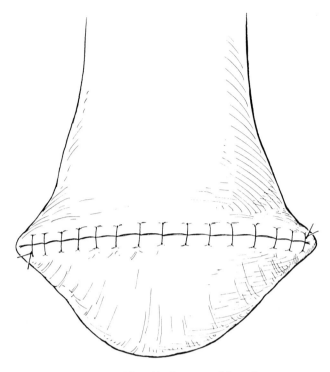

Figure 8 The skin is apposed loosely.

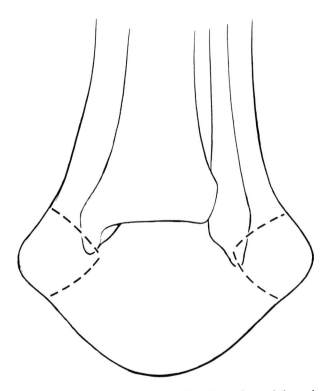

Figure 9 The second-stage procedure is performed through elliptical medial and lateral incisions.

bed rest with the limb elevated for approximately 3 weeks postoperatively. I have found that diabetic wounds take much longer to reach full maturation and healing, and it is advisable to leave sutures in for about 3 to 4 weeks when there is uncertainty about the healing of incisions. Systemic antibiotics are continued postoperatively until wounds are healing. There are no absolute criteria that I follow regarding the use of postoperative antibiotics, and these should be prescribed on an individual basis. I usually continue intravenous antibiotics for approximately 10 days postoperatively, followed by oral agents as required. Once the wounds are healing, patients may commence partial weight bearing depending on the circumstances of the amputation and the frequently use a plaster cast. Non–weight-bearing casts are applied initially for 2 weeks. The initial cast is changed between 4 days and 1 week and the wound inspected. After the second week, a well-fitted total-contact cast is applied, and the patient begins ambulation. Some patients require crutches or other ambulatory assistance until independent, but most patients are full weight bearing after a few days in this walking cast. The cast is discontinued as soon as maturation of the wound has occurred. The use of the total-contact cast has been an immense improvement to our postoperative management of these patients. It helps mobilize the patient rapidly, preventing many of the problems associated with prolonged bed rest. The cast also helps control postoperative edema, distributes the load on the plantar weight-bearing surface of the foot, and most important can support the surgical wound postoperatively. The presence of edema, local increases in temperature, and tenous wound edges are all indications for continuing total-contact cast treatment.

The Lisfranc amputation stumps usually are long enough to suspend a shoe, but—because of the tendency to develop an equinus deformity—can make shoe fitting difficult. I have found that the wear on the plantar aspect of the distal foot can be prevented by stabilizing the ankle with a polypropylene ankle-foot orthosis. The Chopart amputations are too short to suspend a shoe, and these patients always should be fitted with an ankle-foot orthosis. The only drawback of the Syme amputation is its large bulbous stump, and the prosthesis similarly must be large to accommodate the stump, making it less attractive for use in females. Modifications of the prostheses now are available that can be fabricated from lighter materials, allowing a snug fit of the stump, and although the ankle still appears bulky, it usually is acceptable to most patients.

SUGGESTED READING

Harris RI. The history and development of Syme's amputation. Artif Limbs 1961; 6:4.

Jacobs JE. Observations of neuropathic (Charcot) joints occurring in diabetes mellitus. J Bone Joint Surg 1958; 40A:1043–1057.

Mooney V, Wagner FW Jr. Neurocirculatory disorder of the foot. Clin Orthop 1977; 122:53–61.

Srinivasan J. Symes amputations in insensitive feet. J Bone Joint Surg 1973; 55A:558.

Wagner FW Jr. A classification and treatment program for diabetic neuropathic, and dysvascular foot problems. In The American Academy of Orthopaedic Surgeons instructional course lectures. Vol 28. St. Louis: CV Mosby, 1979:143.

TRAUMA

METATARSAL FRACTURES

SHEPARD HURWITZ, M.D.

Metatarsal fractures occur for a variety of reasons and may be seen in various combinations. These fractures occur both singly and multiply, open and closed, with or without compartment syndrome, and associated with other trauma to the foot and skeleton. Little scientific understanding now exists regarding the exact mechanisms of these injuries and what is required for painless function after healing. Treatment of all the varieties and combinations of metatarsal fracture may be found in standard textbooks of orthopedics, fracture surgery, and surgery of the foot. Few standard treatments exist, reflecting a lack of prospective clinical studies with objective outcome evaluation.

My personal algorithm regarding treatment of metatarsal fractures starts with whether there is a wound of the skin (Fig. 1). I divide open wounds into two categories: penetrating trauma and bursting trauma. For both open and closed fractures, I also make a branch point in my treatment protocol for those with and without compartment syndrome. For all fractures, open or closed, I determine whether the injury is solitary or part of a much larger injury complex in a polytrauma patient. Each group contains several subdivisions, depending on the anatomic location of the fracture. I prefer to subcategorize proximal joint injuries, shaft fractures, neck fractures, and head (distal joint) fractures (Table 1; Fig. 2).

Fracture dislocation of Lisfranc's joints are treated differently from distal metatarsophalangeal (MP) joint injuries.

ANATOMY

Metatarsals have a network of strong ligaments both proximally and distally. The capsular ligaments tend to be strong on the plantar side and somewhat weak on the dorsal side. In addition to the ligaments, the interosseous muscles help bind the metatarsals to one another. The anatomic recession of the second metatar-

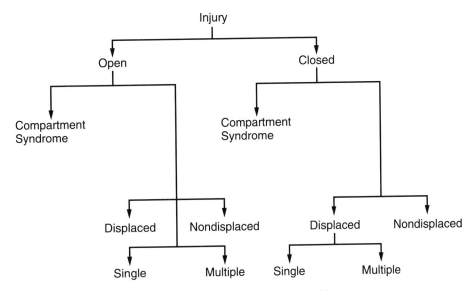

Figure 1 Metatarsal fracture algorithm.

225

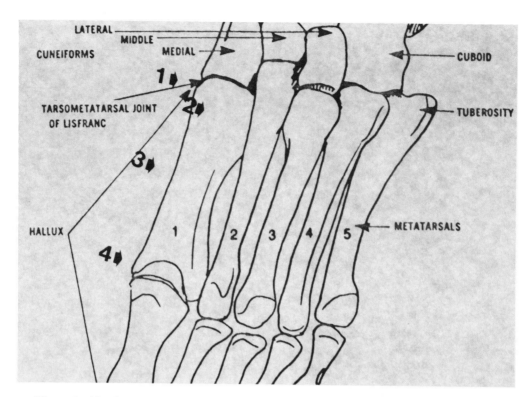

Figure 2 Numbered arrows point to the zone of fracture (see Table 1). (From Hurwitz SR, Labropoulos PA, Feffer HL, Wiesel SW. Foot and Ankle Pain. Charlottesville: Michie Company, 1988; with permission.)

Table 1 Classification of Metatarsal Fractures

Type I	Proximal/Lisfranc's
Type II	Base (nonarticular)
Type III	Shaft
Type IV	Neck/head

sal base adds medial and lateral stability to the entire forefoot-midfoot junction. There is greater dorsal and plantar mobility of the first and fifth metatarsals than of the central second, third, and fourth metatarsals. The second, third, fourth, and fifth metatarsals are partially or completely covered dorsally by the short extensor muscle group. The terminal portion of the anterior tibial artery plunges into the plantar aspect of the foot in the recess between the basis of the first and second metatarsals. Pronation and supination of the forefoot at Lisfranc's joints should not occur clinically. These anatomic points, I believe, lay the foundation for observations that affect treatment. The goal in treating shaft and Lisfranc's fractures is stability of the forefoot. Fractures of the neck of the metatarsal are reduced to decrease the likelihood of malposition of a toe. Metatarsal head fractures are similarly treated to preserve alignment of the toe, but also to minimize the likelihood of post-traumatic arthritis.

MECHANISM OF INJURY

Little is known about the mechanism of injury in traumatic fractures and fracture-dislocations of the metatarsals. I believe that isolated fractures of the base or shaft of the fifth metatarsal usually result from indirect trauma such as a twisting injury to the foot. Single fractures of the second, third, and fourth metatarsals most commonly are the result of a direct blow of an object falling on the foot or the foot being caught and pressed between objects. Fractures of the first metatarsal singly are for the most part thought to be a result of blunt injury, but also may result from twisting (pronation and dorsiflexion). The mechanism of injury comes under the broader topic of history of injury, which in turn clues the treating physician as to the degree of energy absorbed by the foot before fracture and whether other areas of the foot or lower extremity should be examined more carefully. Such would be the case of a styloid fracture of the fifth metatarsal, in which case one should look for all the associated injuries with an inversion "ankle sprain."

TREATMENT

Open Fractures

In those injuries from indirect trauma or massive crushing blows in which the skin bursts open, initial treatment is as for any open fracture, which includes irrigation and the appropriate debridement. Antibiotic coverage for the contamination is started and is based on whether the wound is massively contaminated (e.g., farm or field injury) or is simply a result of local contamination from sock and shoe. A higher degree of contamination requires multiple antimicrobials.

In addition to wound management, with suspected high-energy absorption to fracture, compartment syndrome should be ruled out by the appropriate measurements. Open wounding is not necessarily a guarantee that plantar or interosseous muscles cannot sustain excessive swelling within closed spaces. Operative treatment should continue within the overview of the surgeon's judgment of how to fixate these bony injuries, after the soft tissue component has been addressed. Options consist primarily of temporary wire fixation with transcutaneous Kirschner (K-) wires or Steinmann pins versus compression screw fixation. In those patients with large open wounds and moderate contamination, I prefer minimal fixation with large Steinmann pins for proximal or shaft fractures, with delayed wound closure and fixation for multiple K-wires. For distal fractures I use K-wires for metatarsal neck fracture and debride large fragments of bone and cartilage from the metatarsal head if it is involved with an open joint injury.

Temporary fixation of the toe is helpful, by way of a crossed K-wire to an adjacent toe or metatarsal, thus preventing excessive shortening following metatarsal head debridement (Fig. 3).

Patients with large wounds and moderate-to-advanced contamination require a second debridement 24 to 48 hours postoperatively and possibly multiple debridements thereafter. Skin closure should be planned and be done in conjunction with the appropriate service if flap coverage is needed. I prefer to place a splint with a posterior plaster or fiberglass mold on the foot and ankle until the wound is closed, followed by casting for the duration of the desired period of immobilization. I enforce strict elevation until 48 hours after the last surgical procedure. The patient is kept non–weight bearing until the fracture heals.

Rehabilitation may be started before metatarsal and/or joint fractures have healed. Primarily the goal is to start knee and ankle movement, and possibly even subtalar motion, depending on the progress made at the metatarsal site and whether other foot injuries exist. I avoid any strengthening of the lower extremity until the fractures heal and then progress activity to weight bearing as tolerated, encouraging physical therapy with a strengthening program started proximally and working down to the foot and toes.

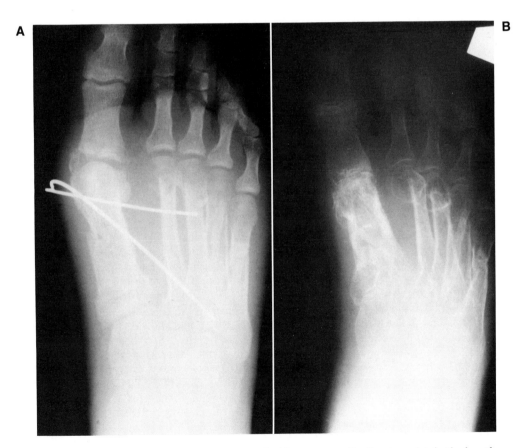

Figure 3 *A,* An open bursting wound treated with temporary fixation to maintain the length of the first metatarsal. *B,* Two year result of great toe alignment and metatarsal length.

Swelling of the foot is a difficult problem and should be addressed in conjunction with physical therapy. The treatment may include compression stockings, pneumatic compression (roughly 1 hour daily, 5 days a week), elevation and ice, high-voltage electrical stimulation, and diuretic medication. Occasionally the patient needs venous studies to rule out thrombosis.

Closed Fractures

The isolated nondisplaced fracture of the shaft of the second, third, or fourth metatarsals can be treated with compression and elevation for several days, followed by application of a posterior foot-ankle splint until the patient can place the foot painlessly on the ground. Then weight-bearing protection continues with cane or crutch until there is radiographic evidence of healing. With fracture of the fifth metatarsal shaft or multiple metatarsal shaft fractures, patients use a posterior foot-ankle splint with elevation for 1 week, then a short-leg cast for another 4 to 6 weeks, and yet another short-leg cast fully weight bearing until radiographs show the fractures have healed.

There is great latitude for surgical judgment regarding when to allow the patient to bear weight. If early weight bearing is started, radiographs are obtained within the first 2 weeks and again 2 weeks after the splint change to observe any change in position, which would require a change in treatment plan. Once patients are walking painlessly in a cast, I believe they can remain in a short-leg walking cast until healed. Fracture near the base of the second metatarsal with soft tissue injury to the ligaments around the Lisfranc joints may be treated in a closed manner similar to multiple metatarsal fractures. In the otherwise healthy person, I prefer to insert K-wires across the first and fifth tarsometatarsal joints and to keep this patient non–weight bearing for 4 weeks, with repeat radiographs at 4 weeks and 8 weeks (Fig. 4). The K-wires are removed after 4 weeks and a new short-leg cast is applied, with 2 weeks of non–weight bearing and 2 weeks of weight bearing before repeat radiographs. If the midfoot is not tender, the patient can use a custom-molded insole to support the arch, with weight bearing to tolerance, and begins rehabilitation exercises of the ankle and leg. With Lisfranc's injury, the patient should not have any inversion or eversion exercises postinjury for 6 months.

A closed, isolated, nondisplaced fracture of the first metatarsal should be elevated in a splint for several days, followed by use of a well-molded short-leg cast to support the medial arch, with the patients kept non–weight bearing until they can rest the foot painlessly on the ground. This then becomes a walking cast for 6 weeks. Custom-molded medium-firmness arch support should be worn until radiographs show the fracture has healed. Sometimes a bunion splint is helpful after the cast is removed if the patient is tender over the first metatarsal head medially. I have found an incidence of post-traumatic hallux valgus associated with first meta-

tarsal fracture, and the bunion splint may be treating a ligamentous injury that occurred at the time of fracture.

Repeat radiographs and examination are necessary for closed nondisplaced metatarsal fractures to see if deformity is developing. The most likely problem with multiple shaft fractures is that one of the metatarsal heads finds a more plantar location than others. The goal is to maintain an even distribution of pressure across the ball of the foot with treatment of these shaft fractures.

Displaced Fractures

For displaced fractures of the metatarsal, the first rule of alignment is not to allow the foot to widen from splaying or to allow dorsal or plantar deformity to interfere with foot pressure or the position of the toe within a shoe. The goal of treatment with displaced fractures is to try to reduce the displacement and then to hold the alignment while the fractures heal. I prefer to try closed reduction and repeat radiographs without traction. If the alignment is reasonable, and the reduction appears stable, a short-leg cast is applied and the radiograph is repeated. If the radiographs still are acceptable, repeat the radiographs in 2 weeks after non–weight-bearing activity and convert to a weight-bearing cast sometime between the fourth and sixth week. Total time in a cast is about 2 months, followed by rehabilitation for the foot and ankle.

For those fractures that either do not reduce or are not stably reduced, fixation with K-wires is needed. The irreducible fracture needs to be opened, with a reasonable restoration of length and alignment before fixation. Closed reduction and transcutaneous K-wire fixation are required for fractures that reduce well closed but show evidence of deformity as soon as the traction is let off. The foot then should be splinted and elevated for approximately 2 days, followed by a short-leg non–weight-bearing cast that remains non–weight bearing until the pins are removed at about 6 weeks. A short-leg fiberglass walking cast then is worn until radiographs show healing. With multiple shaft fractures that have been reduced, I find a custom insole orthotic relieves pressure on the metatarsal heads. This orthotic is used after the cast treatment and should be fabricated before full unrestricted weight bearing is permitted. Fractures of the metatarsal neck, usually are angulated and are difficult to reduce closed. If they can be reduced closed, I pin them transcutaneously; if they do not reduce I open them by way of dorsal incision and have the wire exit distally on the plantar surface of the toe and then fit the wire into the medullary canal at the metatarsal in a retrograde fashion. This then is followed with a soft bulky dressing over which a non–weight-bearing cast is applied in approximately 2 days and remains until the pins are removed.

In patients with severely comminuted metatarsal head fractures who are otherwise healthy, I open the joint and remove the fragments. Elderly patients, who often have stiff joints, are treated nonoperatively. For

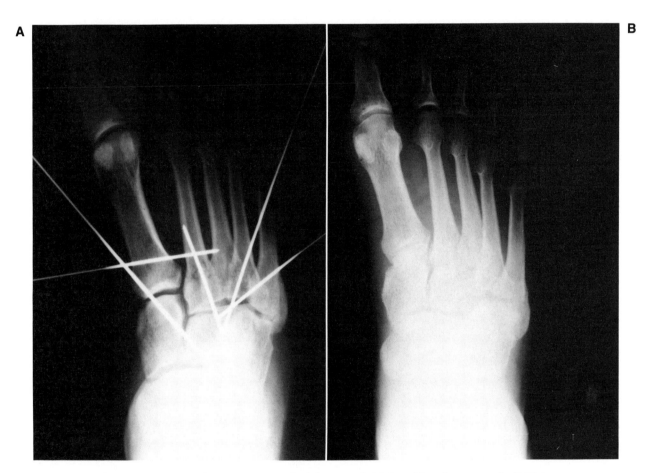

Figure 4 *A,* K-wire fixation of fractures of the second, third, and fourth metatarsals. *B,* Three year follow-up in an asymptomatic patient.

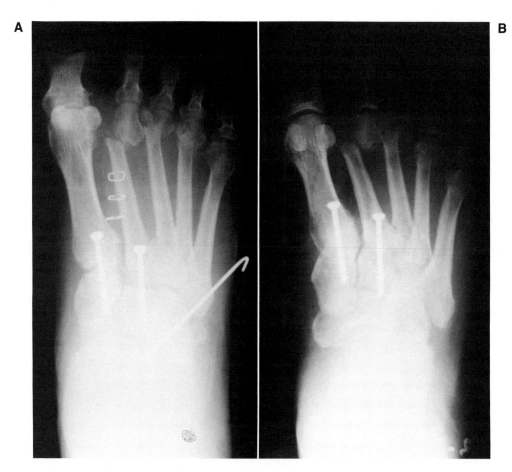

Figure 5 *A,* Fixation of Lisfranc's injury with open metatarsal neck fractures left without fixation after debridement. *B,* Two year follow-up with healed fractures, painless hardware, and the need for a custom insole for metatarsalgia.

metatarsal head fractures that are in two large pieces with moderate displacement, I open the joint and internally fixate the pieces and then apply a non–weight-bearing long-leg cast in approximately 2 days.

The problem with open reduction and fixation is the number of incisions that the foot tolerates. If the patient has a Lisfranc fracture dislocation plus metatarsal head and neck fractures, I often fix the Lisfranc fracture operatively and address the most severely displaced metatarsal head or neck injury by extending one of the dorsal incisions. I then wait several weeks for the wounds to heal before performing open reduction of other severely displaced neck and head fractures (Fig. 5). In the interim the patient has been in a cast and is non–weight bearing.

Fractures of an isolated metatarsal involving the proximal joint are treated by reduction and percutaneous K-wire pinning or open reduction, especially if there is a dorsal dislocation. Fracture at the base of the second metatarsal should be treated as a Lisfranc injury. Isolated subluxation of the first or fifth metatarsal base may occur and should be treated with open reduction and K-wire fixation. The K-wires may be removed at 6 weeks, after the patient has been mobilized in a non–weight-bearing short-leg cast.

Fractures of the styloid process at the base of the fifth metatarsal are common, and despite what may be several millimeters of displacement, heal regardless of the treatment modality. For those with more than 1 cm of displacement, I prefer open reduction and K-wire fixation plus repair of the peroneal tendon insertion. This then requires non–weight-bearing immobilization in a short-leg cast until the wire is removed. On occasion a minimally displaced fracture becomes a greatly displaced fracture with a painful prominence by the base of the metatarsal and is by definition a joint injury. Excision of the bony fragment and reinsertion of the tendon is the best salvage procedure for a progressive displacement of the styloid process or in cases in which the patient presents late with a chronic finding of bony displacement.

A Jones fracture is a fracture of the proximal shaft of the fifth metatarsal caused by indirect trauma. Much has been written about the increased incidence of nonunion of this fracture, particularly in the high-demand athlete. I prefer, in all patients other than high-demand athletes, to treat this nonoperatively with rest and elevation with non–weight bearing until resolution of the immediate fracture pain, followed by either a wooden-sole postoperative shoe in the more elderly group or a short-leg cast in younger, more active age groups. The internal fixation of choice for injured high-performance athletes is an axial compression screw passed through the styloid into the medullary canal. This must be of sufficient length to give compression across the fracture site. This fracture then is treated in a cast, non–weight bearing for a minimum of 6 weeks, followed by rehabilitation of the ankle and continued protection either with a brace or a postoperative shoe. Occasionally further surgery is required for symptomatic nonunion.

For patients with an asymptomatic nonunion, further treatment rarely is indicated.

Stress Fractures and Pathologic Fractures of the Metatarsals

The most common nontraumatic fractures of the foot involve the central metatarsals. The fracture usually occurs distally near the neck, but may also occur at the base. These usually are in solitary bones and are not found commonly in prior pathologic lesions.

Occasionally there may be an underlying pathologic lesion such as an enchondroma. Prior metatarsal fracture with angulation may also predispose an adjacent metatarsal to fracture by way of chronic repetitive loading. On rare occasion an osteomyelitis may exist in the bone, which could lead to fracture.

The problem with stress fractures of the metatarsals initially is pain and swelling. These fractures almost always heal unless there is a destructive process or a mechanically unsuitable condition. Osteomyelitis may require acute intervention to treat the infection, whereas the condition created by an enchondroma may require excision (and bone grafting) at a later date. After any stress fracture of the metatarsal may come a slight or even moderate shift in alignment of that metatarsal, creating an angular deformity and/or pressure on the adjacent metatarsal heads. If there is marked dorsal displacement of a healed stress fracture, the first treatment should be to support the other metatarsal heads to prevent further fractures. If symptoms develop in the dorsal displacement of the metatarsal, primarily in the dorsum of the toe, it may be helpful to perform an osteotomy and realignment of that particular metatarsal. My suggestion is to add cancellous bone graft and firm fixation with multiple K-wires to try and fill the medullary space. Nonunion of a stress fracture is common; if it occurs and is symptomatic, a bone biopsy and bone culture would be helpful to determine whether there is a pathologic process that requires treatment. If the fracture does not heal, I advocate internal fixation with bone graft and the appropriate period of immobilization and protection until union. My experience with electrical stimulation to heal nonunited fatigue fractures is limited because this may delay the diagnosis of a treatable condition.

Gunshot Wounds

A special category of penetrating wounds of the foot are those caused by gunshot wounds that penetrate the metatarsal area. The most problematic are close-range shotgun blasts or high-velocity rifle rounds—both of which commonly occur in hunting accidents. The low-velocity handgun round or small-caliber .22 rifle slug does not create great difficulty in management. The shotgun blast needs fairly thorough debridement and redebridement. Often there is bone loss and a good deal of swelling. The high-velocity rifle round from close range creates a massive soft tissue lesion and may have a deceptive low-energy fracture pattern if the bullet did not strike a metatarsal directly. Of the two wounds, the high-velocity rifle wound may require more aggressive treatment in that soft tissue coverage may be required by way of free tissue transfer. The shotgun wound probably heals secondarily or with the addition of skin grafting after a suitable period. Both types of wounds may require delayed bone grafting or joint fusion. Serious neurologic injury usually does not result from gunshot wounds to the foot; the proximal half of the foot should have normal plantar sensation and most distal-plantar sensation is intact.

A single principle vital to salvage of the foot injured by a high-energy missle or blast is to estimate the amount of contamination and soft tissue damage. Also, when wounding of the foot occurs in addition to multiple gunshot injuries, care of the foot may have a low priority in the first few days of patient care. This now is becoming more common in inner city hospitals treating patients with multiple wounds resulting from close-range, high-energy injury. The role of the person caring for the foot wound, however, is to become part of the trauma team and maintain adequate viability of the foot and plan late reconstruction.

SUGGESTED READING

DeLee JC. Fractures and dislocations of the foot. In: Mann RA, ed. Surgery of the foot. 5th ed. St. Louis: CV Mosby, 1986:729.

Hansen ST. In: Mueller NE, ed. Manual of internal fixation-techniques recommended by the AO-ASIF Group. 3rd ed. New York: Springer Verlag, 1990:616.

Heckman JD. Fractures and dislocations of the midpart of the foot. In: Evarts CM, ed. Surgery of the musculoskeletal system. New York: Churchill Livingstone, 1990:4278.

Heckman JD. Fractures and dislocations of the foot. In: Rockwood CA Jr, Green DP, Bucholz RW, eds. Fractures in adults. 3rd ed. Philadelphia: JB Lippincott, 1991:2140.

Mann RA. Complications of treatment of fractures and dislocations of the foot. In: Epps CH Jr, ed. Complications in orthopaedic surgery. 2nd ed. Philadelphia: JB Lippincott, 1986:671.

Myerson MS. Injuries to the forefoot and toes. In: Jahss MH, ed. Disorders of the foot and ankle. Philadelphia: WB Saunders, 1991:2239.

LISFRANC INJURIES

SAUL G. TREVINO, M.D.
JUDITH FORD BAUMHAUER, M.D.

The tarsometatarsal joint or the Lisfranc joint involves the articulation of the forefoot with the midfoot. Injuries to this area include joint dislocations or subluxations with or without an associated fracture. The incidence of a Lisfranc injury is common and has been under-represented in literature because of the difficulty in diagnosis and the complex anatomy of the multiple involved joints. Up to 20 percent of the Lisfranc joint injuries are missed on initial presentation. Appropriate treatment of these injuries is dependent on a thorough understanding of the structural and neurovascular anatomy.

The Lisfranc complex is composed of bony and ligamentous elements that give structural support in forming the transverse arch of the midfoot. The first through third metatarsals articulate with the corresponding cuneiforms. The fourth and fifth metatarsals articulate with the cuboid. The "keystone" to the transverse arch is the second metatarsal, which is recessed and bordered by the first and third metatarsals. The ligamentous support is composed of the Lisfranc ligament and the intercuneiform ligaments, which are the primary stabilizers. The secondary stabilizers include the accessory ligaments, the dorsal capsule, and intermetatarsal ligaments (metatarsals 2 through 5). Recognizing that there is no intermetatarsal ligament between the first and second metatarsals stresses the importance of the Lisfranc ligament in maintaining the anatomic relationship between the medial metatarsal and lateral metatarsal groups.

THERAPEUTIC ALTERNATIVES

Treatment options include closed reduction and casting, closed reduction and percutaneous fixation, open reduction and internal fixation (ORIF), open reduction and external fixation (OREF), and arthrodesis. The goal of treatment is to maintain an anatomic reduction of the Lisfranc joint complex. Closed reduction and casting do not maintain an adequate reduction in the acutely injured patient, and therefore for the majority, surgical stabilization with Kirschner (K-) wires or screw fixation is preferred. Criteria for judging the adequacy of reduction have been suggested by Myerson. The space between the bases of the first and second metatarsals and medial and middle cuneiforms must be 2 mm or less. The talometatarsal angle should not be greater than 15° and there should be no displacement of the metatarsals in the dorsal-plantar plane (Table 1).

OREF is used in severe crush injuries with marked comminution of the joint complex and in open fractures with or without soft tissue degloving. Closed reduction and pinning versus ORIF is the treatment of choice in all other acute injuries at our institution. Arthrodesis has its role as a salvage procedure only.

PREFERRED APPROACH

Patient Selection

Without adequate and maintained anatomic reduction, the probability of a good result is poor with frequent high morbidity. The main contraindications for surgery are pre-existing dysvascular disease, if the injury is more than 6 weeks old, or a neuropathic foot. Surgery on the neuropathic foot is a relative contraindication, depending on the experience of the surgeon.

Timing of Surgery

Because of the traumatic mechanism of these injuries, extensive soft tissue swelling can result. Surgical treatment is preferred within the first 24 hours after injury. The attempt at closed reduction at a later point becomes difficult secondary to local swelling. In addition, operating through a compromised soft tissue envelope is ill-advised. Good results have been obtained with open reduction up to 6 weeks postinjury. This is easy particularly when the articulation is subluxated or dislocated without fracture. We attempt an open reduction and internally fix these injuries up to about 1 month postinjury if the deformity is mild. If the patient presents later than 1 month, we continue with closed treatment and treat the symptoms as they arise. For severe deformities we attempt a reduction up to 6 weeks.

Preoperative Preparation

The radiographic findings may vary. In high-energy trauma such as a motor vehicle accident, a wide displacement is obvious. In lower-energy injuries, such as a fall, the radiographic findings may be more subtle. Routine non–weight-bearing anteroposterior (AP) and lateral views may be inadequate for these subtle injuries.

Table 1 Surgical Indications in Lisfranc Injuries

Operative indications
  Widening between first ray and second and middle cuneiform
    > 2 mm
  Talometatarsal angle >15°
  Dorsal-plantar displacement of metatarsals
  Inability to maintain reduction by casting
  Vascular compromise
Contraindications
  >6 weeks since injury
  Pre-existing dysvascular foot
Relative contraindications
  Neuropathic joint
  Severe swelling or fracture blisters

It is helpful to obtain bilateral weight-bearing AP and lateral films, although this may be difficult because of pain. A 45° medial-oblique view evaluates the lateral aspect of the foot. If the diagnosis still is unclear, polytomography may delineate the injury pattern further. Computed tomographic (CT) scans are less helpful because of the need for sagittal cuts. However, if the CT scan is performed with three-dimensional (3D) reconstruction, it is extremely helpful in determining the position of the metatarsals. Radiologic evidence of subtle Lisfranc's injuries can include a number of specific findings: (1) a flake fracture off the base of the second or lateral aspect of the first cuneiform; (2) loss of the smooth articulation of tarsometatarsal joints; (3) subtle widening between the first and second metatarsal shafts; (4) associated compression fractures medially of the navicular or laterally of the cuboid.

Choice of Procedure

Acute injuries may have one to two attempts made at a closed reduction. If an anatomic or near-anatomic reduction (within 2 mm) can be obtained, a stabilization procedure is performed. If an anatomic reduction cannot be obtained closed, an open reduction is performed.

Closed Reduction

To obtain maximum muscle relaxation, the patient is given a spinal or general anesthetic. The foot is prepped and draped in a sterile fashion. Modified finger traps are applied to the great toe and one or two child-size finger traps are necessary on the lesser toes. Longitudinal traction along the foot is applied with the weight of the leg for 5 minutes. The deformity is reduced with either a supination or pronation motion. It is rare to note a palpable or audible reduction. Often a large AO reduction clamp is necessary to assist with the reduction of a diastasis between the second metatarsal and the first ray. Radiographic confirmation of the reduction is a necessity. We have found fluoroscopy to be unreliable and therefore perform routine radiographs out of traction to confirm proper reduction. K-wire and screw fixation have been used to stabilize the reduction. Maintaining a reduction with K-wires alone may be difficult, and we prefer to use the 4.0 mm cannulated screw system developed by Richards. This has the advantage of placing definitive lag screw fixation directly over the guide pins, which act as provisional fixation. It is important to insert the screw in a lag mode, otherwise the advancing edge of the screw causes distraction of the articulation. Provided they are used in a lag fashion, 3.5 mm cortical screws also are satisfactory.

Open Reduction

If an anatomic reduction cannot be obtained closed, an open reduction is performed. Using an extensile approach to the anteromedial aspect of the midfoot has been helpful for orientation and prevention of skin necrosis and prevention of neuromas (Fig. 1). The patient is positioned so that the ipsilateral hip is elevated to facilitate placement of the foot in a neutral and plantigrade position for intraoperative fluoroscopy and permanent radiographs.

After proper positioning, the leg is exsanguinated with an Esmarch bandage. A curvilinear incision is started over the midportion of the navicular and extended over the medial aspect of the third metatarsal base and to the distal third of the first metatarsal. This provides an extensile approach to the middle two-thirds of the midtarsal area. The path of the incision avoids the dorsal prominence of the foot, thus minimizing sensitive scars. It also avoids multiple small incisions that lead to inadequate exposure and skin necrosis.

With the use of 2.5× magnification and the extensile incision, one easily can identify the multiple fine extensions of the medial and intermediate branches of the superficial peroneal nerve. Divide the fascia lateral to the extensor hallucis longus tendon and retract the tendon medially. The dorsalis pedis artery and deep peroneal nerve are located inferior to the musculotendinous junction of the extensor hallucis brevis tendon. By subperiosteal dissection the neurovascular structures can be mobilized laterally. The surgeon should be careful of the perforating branch of the dorsalis pedis artery between the bases of the first and second metatarsals. Stability should be checked at this point. Stress the articulation between the first and second cuneiforms and lateral rays to rule out any occult instability. The affected joints should be irrigated to remove hematoma and osteochondral fragments. If it becomes necessary, the exposure can be extended to include adjacent intercuneiform and naviculocuneiform joints.

The lateral portion of the second and third metatarsals are approached by way of a deep fascial incision lateral to the dorsalis pedis artery. Again, a subperiosteal dissection is carried out to expose the affected joints. For lateral exposure, a straight longitudinal incision is made between the fourth and fifth metatarsals. A small lumina spreader is useful to see the inferior surface and allow adequate debridement. Use this instrument for the exposure of the intercuneiform region as well. A similar form of debridement of the affected joints is carried out.

Although there are multiple classifications and variations of Lisfranc's injuries, some general ORIF guidelines can be followed. The steps described subsequently belong to three broad categories.

Step I: Stabilization of the First Ray. The first ray includes the first metatarsocuneiform joint and the naviculocuneiform joint. Stabilization is required of both joints. In this particular illustration (Fig. 2A), the naviculocuneiform joint is considered to be stable. After reduction of the first metatarsocuneiform, a pin is used for temporary fixation. The pin is inserted 1.5 cm from the articulation and directed in a plantar-proximal

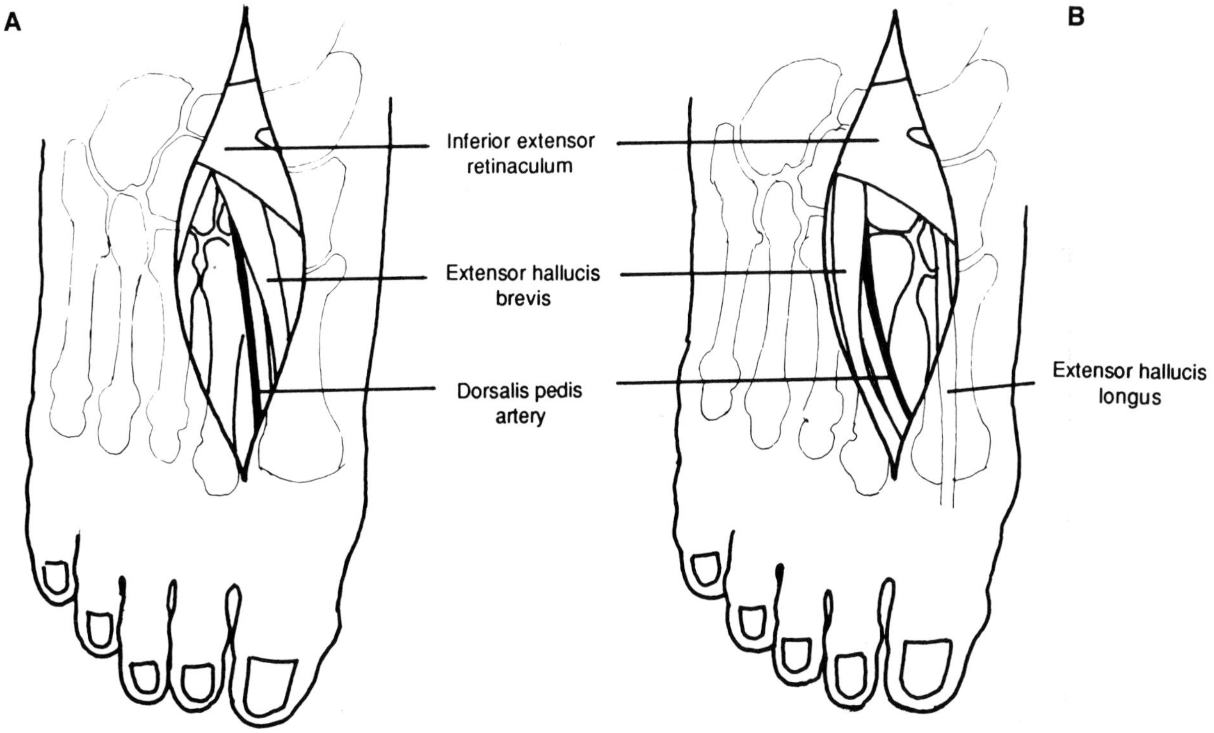

A
B

Inferior extensor
retinaculum

Extensor hallucis
brevis

Dorsalis pedis
artery

Extensor hallucis
longus

Figure 1 Extensile dorsal-medial approach to the midfoot. Universal incision. A curvilinear incision centered over the medial base of the third metatarsal. The incision originates at the lateral third of the tarsonavicular and extends up to the neck of the second metatarsal (not shown). Deep exposure. *A,* Dorsal-lateral approach to the second and third metatarsal. The extensor hallucis brevis tendon and neurovascular bundle have been retracted medially. The lateral base of the second metatarsal and the entire third metatarsal base are exposed. *B,* Dorsal-medial approach to the first and second metatarsal. The extensor hallucis brevis tendon and neurovascular bundle have been retracted laterally. The medial base of the second metatarsal and the entire first metatarsal base are exposed, providing access to the Lisfranc region.

plane. Once the preliminary fixation is accomplished, attention is directed to the Lisfranc ligament complex.

Step II: Stabilization of the Lisfranc Ligament Complex. The second part of the procedure is stabilization of the Lisfranc ligament complex—that is, the alignment between the medial cuneiform and its adjacent second metatarsal. A thorough debridement of any loose fragments is performed before any attempt at reduction. A temporary reduction is performed with the use of a reduction clamp between the medial cuneiform and the base of the second metatarsal, thus establishing the medial portion of the keystone configuration. If radiographs at this time reveal adequate reduction, 4.0 cannulated screws are inserted in proper sequence (Fig. 2B). Countersinking of the drill hole is recommended at the bases of the metatarsals so as to prevent fracture to an adjacent joint. Care is taken not to overtighten the lag screw. Supplemental fixation between the medial and middle cuneiform is used if indicated.

Step III: Stabilization of the Third Through Fifth Metatarsal Rays. Sequential reduction is performed by using fixation from the base of the individual metatarsals into adjacent tarsal bones (Fig. 2C and D). Supplementary procedures may be needed if there is comminution or compression of the navicular or cuboid bone.

In summary, this approach allows the surgeon to treat the varied presentations from simple diastasis (Fig. 3A) to divergent or partial incongruity injuries in a logical fashion (Fig. 4). Supplemental fixation may be needed for proximal tarsal fractures or distal metatarsal fractures as indicated.

Postoperative Care

Patients are immobilized for 8 weeks in plaster. Weight bearing is begun at 6 weeks. Hardware is removed at 12 to 16 weeks. Since these are primarily capsuloligamentous injuries, the articulation is not stable until the third or fourth month. If screws are removed prematurely, diastasis may recur. Removal of hardware before commencing weight bearing is considered important by other authors. After cast removal, our

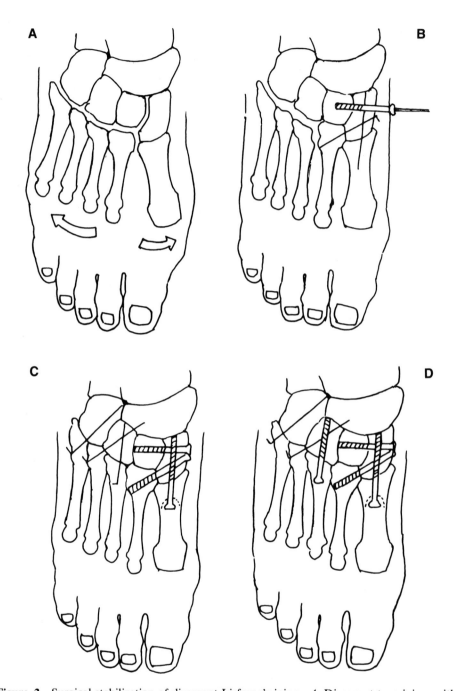

Figure 2 Surgical stabilization of divergent Lisfranc's injury. *A,* Divergent-type injury with medial subluxation of first ray, interruption of the Lisfranc complex, and lateral subluxation of the second through fifth metatarsals. *B,* Medial and lateral column fixation. Step 1: Temporary K-wire fixation of the first metatarsocuneiform joint. Step 2: Temporary K-wire fixation of the medial intercuneiform joint. Step 3: Temporary K-wire fixation of the second metatarsal medial cuneiform joint. Step 4: Cannulated cancellous screws have replaced temporary K-wire fixation of the medial column to lateral column. *C,* Temporary lateral column fixation. Temporary K-wire fixation of the third through fifth metatarsal tarsal articulations. *D,* Permanent lateral column fixation. Cannulated cancellous screw fixation is used only for the third metatarsal and lateral cuneiform joints.

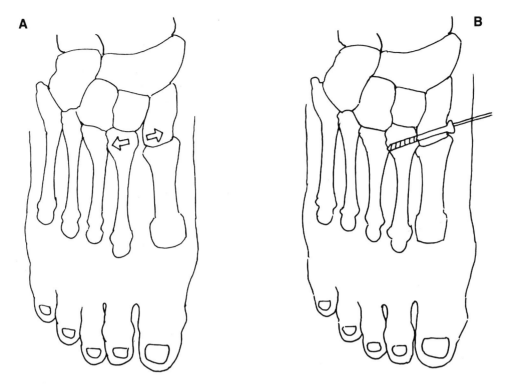

Figure 3 Surgical stabilization of simple diastasis. *A,* Widening between the medial cuneiform and second metatarsal base as a result of rupture of the Lisfranc ligament. *B,* Stabilization of the Lisfranc ligament by cannulated screw technique. The path of the screw is parallel to the origin and insertion of this ligament.

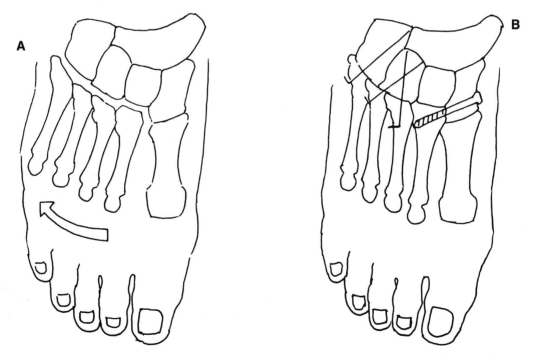

Figure 4 Surgical stabilization of partial incongruity. *A,* Lateral partial incongruity type of injury with lateral subluxation of the second through fifth metatarsals. *B,* Operative fixation with lag screw stabilization of the Lisfranc ligament complex; K-wire fixation of the third through fifth metatarsal tarsal articulation.

patients wear a removable walking splint for an additional month. A shoe with a flexible steel shank is used for 1 year postoperatively.

COMPLICATIONS

Post-traumatic Osteoarthritis

Many patients develop postoperative arthritis despite adequate reduction. The evidence of arthritis does not appear to correlate with poor results.

In symptomatic patients and those with a missed initial diagnosis, reconstructive surgery is necessary. Reduction of deformities along with arthrodesis is the appropriate treatment. This is discussed further in the chapter *Tarsometatarsal Arthrodesis.*

Devascularization

Important neurovascular structures surround the Lisfranc joint complex. The deep peroneal nerve and branch of the dorsalis pedis artery pass through the first web space between the first and second metatarsal bases. Injuries to this complex can involve damage to these structures with entrapment, denervation, and even devascularization requiring amputation.

Although documented to represent less than 2 percent of all the Lisfranc fracture dislocations, damage to the perforating branch of the dorsalis pedis artery can be combined with damage to the posterior tibial artery, resulting in an ischemic foot. Vascular injury or evidence of ischemia is an indication for an open reduction and exploration of the involved vessels.

Infection

With the use of prophylactic antibiotics, the risk of infection in closed cases approaches that of elective procedures. With a severely compromised soft tissue envelope, visualization of the skin incisions during the early postoperative course is recommended.

Skin Compromise

Skin necrosis can occur with crush injuries. Observation in the initial postoperative course is required to recognize the need for any additional soft tissue procedures including muscle or skin flap coverage for skin slough.

Compartment Syndrome

Compartment syndrome of the foot is a recognized entity because of the high energy involved in these injuries. Any suspected compartment syndrome of the foot must be evaluated with compartment pressures and fasciotomies as needed.

Neuropathic Joint

Lisfranc's injuries may occur in neuropathic joints. The most common cause of a Charcot joint is diabetes mellitus. A swollen, warm, erythematous foot in a diabetic requires a radiograph. The midfoot may show the typical Charcot changes of erosion and subluxation of the Lisfranc complex. This may occur without any recognized antecedent trauma. Our approach to these Lisfranc injuries is somewhat different than described previously. An aggressive operative approach is not used. Our goal is to maintain a functional plantigrade foot. Non–weight bearing until swelling and warmth have decreased is the rule. Total-contact casts are used in the compliant patient. Patients are followed at 2 week intervals to monitor for signs of active inflammation. Patients are weaned from total-contact casting into a short-leg brace or PTB brace and maintained in this until 1 year postinjury.

SUGGESTED READING

Arntz CT, Veith RG, Hansen ST. Fractures and fracture-dislocations of the tarsometatarsal joint. J Bone Joint Surg 1988; 70A:173–181.
Brunet JA, Wilen JJ. The late results of tarsometatarsal joint injuries. J Bone Joint Surg 1987; 69B:437–439.
Licht N, Trevino S. Lisfranc injuries. Tech Orthop 1991; 6:77–83.
Myerson MS. The diagnosis and treatment of injuries to the Lisfranc joint complex. Orthop Clin North Am 1989; 20:655–664.
Sangeorzan BJ, Veith RG, Hansen ST. Salvage of Lisfranc's tarsometatarsal joint by arthrodesis. Foot Ankle 1990; 10:193–200.

NAVICULAR AND CUBOID FRACTURES

BRUCE J. SANGEORZAN, M.D.

Fractures involving the tarsonavicular joint can be direct or indirect. Direct injuries generally are displaced minimally because of the dense network of surrounding ligaments. Indirect injuries, on the other hand, occur as the scaphoid is compressed between the talus and the cuneiforms. When displaced, these injuries involve the talonavicular joint as well as the cuneiform joint. They often are accompanied by shortening of the medial column of the foot and frequently are accompanied by occult injuries in the lateral column of the foot, in either the anterior process of the calcaneus or the cuboid.

Similarly, injuries of the cuboid are uncommon. Most often these are avulsion fractures, but indirect injury by compression between the metatarsal and calcaneus also can occur. As in the navicula, the bone is surrounded by dense ligaments with attachments to multiple tarsal and metatarsal bones. Displaced fractures may involve the calcaneocuboid joint and the cuboid metatarsal joint, and may lead to a shortening of the lateral column and secondary forefoot abduction. In both navicular and cuboid fractures, nondisplaced fractures are treated with a short-leg non–weight-bearing cast. For displaced fractures operative treatment is selected with the hope of restoring articular congruity, as well as neutral alignment of the foot. The function of Chopart's joint depends on the integrated motion of the subtalar, talonavicular, and calcaneocuboid joints. If any of these joints are misaligned, ankylosed, or incongruous, the others are affected.

NAVICULAR FRACTURES

Patient Selection

Indications for operative treatment of a navicular fracture include displacement of an articular surface, shortening of the medial column, or detachment of a major soft tissue structure. Avulsion of the tuberosity may occur without intra-articular displacement. Under these circumstances, the main issues dictating treatment are the functional integrity of the tibialis posterior tendon and of the calcaneonavicular ligament. The literature suggests small amounts of displacement of the tuberosity will most likely heal and leave the soft tissue structures in a functionally acceptable condition. When the tuberosity is displaced 5 mm or more, I assume that the soft tissue structures are incompetent. In addition, this distance may increase during healing because of tension in the posterior tibialis muscle. Tuberosity avulsions are treated by open reduction through medial

incision. A soft tissue washer may be helpful in securing the tuberosity, with its overlying tibial tendon insertion, in a secure fashion.

Selection of patients with displaced navicular body fractures is more straightforward. If the fracture is displaced in the talonavicular joint, on the anteroposterior (AP) or lateral view, open reduction is selected. An oblique view is in the central part of the radiographic evaluation of all midfoot injuries and often detects the more subtle injuries. It also may obviate the need for cross-sectional imaging such as computed tomography (CT). If CT is used, it should be done in two planes. One plane should be parallel to the plantar surface of the foot and the other perpendicular to the plantar surface of the foot. These sections should be 3 mm deep with a 3 mm field to allow adequate sagittal reconstructions without missing small fragments.

Patients are placed in a posterior splint at the time of examination to attempt to hold the foot in a neutral position. In addition to helping with comfort, this standardizes the imaging studies. The foot is elevated until swelling begins to diminish. The swelling need not resolve completely; it is diminished adequately when the skin begins to wrinkle. Surgery is performed either acutely at the time of presentation or 5 to 10 days after injury when the swelling has begun to subside.

Surgical Technique

Navicular fractures are reduced through a medial incision and a dorsal incision. The medial incision parallels the posterior tibial tendon, but is superior to it. The dorsal incision parallels the extensor digitorum longus tendon, and of necessity may go through the extensor brevis or medial to it, depending on the fracture pattern. After exposure of the fracture through these incisions, a small distractor is placed on the medial border of the foot. Terminally threaded 2.5 mm pins are used: one is placed in the talus and one into the cuneiforms. It is placed dorsomedially so as to not obstruct the view into either of the surgical incisions. The distractor is used to lengthen the medial ray longer than its usual position to allow visualization into the talonavicular joint and the navicular cuneiform joint. The clot is evacuated, and any small pieces of cartilage and bone in the joint are removed. Using this technique of visualization, the navicula is reduced and provisionally held with Kirschner wires. In the ideal circumstance, when sufficient bone exists laterally to allow purchase of the cortical lag screw, two 3.5 mm cortical lag screws are used to lag the medial fragment into the lateral one. Commonly, there is insufficient bone in the medial-plantar side to allow screw purchase, and the screws may be directed into the cuboid or into the cuneiform. AP, lateral, and oblique views are performed interoperatively to establish the adequacy of reduction. The goals of reduction are to restore congruity of the talonavicular and the navicular cuneiform joints and to re-establish normal length of the medial column. At times, the articular surface is depressed much like a fracture of the tibial plateau. Under these circumstances, elevation of the cartilaginous surface with a dental pick or Freer elevator may be performed and the defect packed with cancellous bone from the iliac crest or tibia. With the internal fixation in place, the foot is taken through a range of motion. This maneuver should establish satisfactorily that the fixation is rigid and that joints function as they should. Because the navicula is a concave bone, screws that begin too proximally in the tuberosity may cross the talonavicular joint. This should be prevented by placing the screws under radiographic guidance. When reduction and placement of internal fixation of devices are documented satisfactorily both radiographically and clinically, the fixator is removed and the wounds are closed. Postoperatively, the patient is kept in a short-leg non–weight-bearing cast for 6 weeks. AP, lateral, and oblique views are obtained at 6 weeks. If early bridging of the fracture is apparent, the patient is placed in a short-leg walking cast for approximately 3 weeks and then is allowed to weight bear in a regular shoe. When the swelling has abated, patients are fitted with a custom-molded, full-length, rigid sole. Patients are told to expect continued swelling for 6 to 12 months and that symptoms will continue to improve for more than a year. Radiographically, most will have narrowing of the talonavicular and navicular cuneiform joints and lose at least 50 percent of their hindfoot motion. Both stiffness and swelling are apt to be symptomatic in the majority of patients.

Complications

The most common complications are loss of fixation as a result of poor bone quality or premature weight bearing, and avascular necrosis of the navicula. When the navicula appears densely white on radiographs, the patient should be warned that this is a fairly serious problem. However, vascularization is slow, and patients are allowed to continue weight bearing their custom-molded orthotic. Should collapse occur, fusion of the medial border of the foot is performed. A tricortical bone graft from the iliac is used to fill the defect in the talus and cuneiforms after debriding the avascular bone of the navicula.

Many of the symptomatic complaints are aided by the custom-molded insole. If the shoe is inadequate, the next alternative is to place a steel shank in the shoe to diminish across the midfoot or add a rocker-bottom sole with the same goal in mind.

CUBOID FRACTURES

Patient Selection

Healthy patients with intact blood supply to the foot and significant deformity or intra-articular displacement are selected for surgical treatment. Relative contraindications include smokers of advancing age, diabetics with peripheral neuropathy or history of infection, or patients with significantly impaired ambulation. At the time of injury, patients are placed in a short-leg posterior splint and elevated until the swelling begins to abate. Radiographic evaluation includes AP, lateral, and oblique films. If the fracture anatomy remains uncertain, this can be supplemented with two-plane CT scans as in other midfoot injuries. Timing of treatment is based on timing of presentation, the mechanism of injury, the viability of

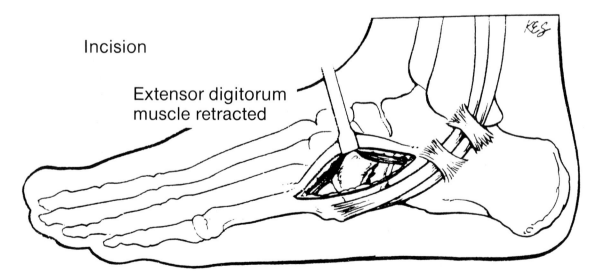

Figure 1 The surgical approach is made superior and parallel to the peroneus brevis tendon. Both the calcaneocuboid and cuboid metatarsal joints may be visualized through this approach. If the lateral border is shortened, a distractor is applied to the calcaneus and the fourth and fifth metatarsal and lengthened. When the contours of the foot have been restored and the impacted joint may be visualized, lengthening is stopped.

the soft tissue envelope, and other more practical considerations. In general, these procedures are done 2 to 10 days after injury.

Surgical Technique

Fractures are approached through longitudinal incision, dorsal to the peroneus brevis and longus tendons (Fig. 1). The fracture generally is compressed, with either the proximal or distal-articular surface impacted into the substance of the cuboid. At times, other fracture patterns may be present that are amenable minimally to lag screws. When this is true, lag screws are placed across the fracture after reduction, and the cast is applied. More commonly, the fractured and impacted articular surface is treated like any other intra-articular fracture. First, the length of the lateral border is restored and the fracture is disimpacted. The articular surface is restored, bone graft is used, and some type of internal fixation is required. The lateral border of the foot is lengthened using a small distractor with 2.5 mm pins into the calcaneus and into the fourth and fifth metatarsals. If the cuboid still is impacted with the lateral border distracted, 0.045 inch Kirschner wires are placed into the cuboid, one beneath the distal-articular surface and one beneath the proximal. These are teased apart gently using a lamina spreader until the articular relationships of the cuboid and the metatarsals are restored (Fig. 2). The size of the defect then is measured, and tricortical bone graft from the iliac crest is placed in the defect. A one-quarter tubular plate can be used to span this defect and 3.5 mm screws placed proximal and distal and through the bone graft (Fig. 3).

Postoperatively, patients are placed in a posterior splint. This is maintained for 2 weeks. The patients then go into a short-leg non–weight-bearing cast for 4 weeks and are allowed to bear the weight of the limb in this cast. At the end of 6 weeks, radiographs are obtained. Depending on the appearance of the fracture at that point, the patients then may go into a walking cast or a removable commercial walking brace.

Complications

Complications of this procedure are relatively uncommon. The sural nerve is in danger with the incision, and the patient should be warned preoperatively of the potential for some hypertension in the lateral border of the foot. The lateral column seems to be more forgiving and does not seem to cause as much stiffness or swelling as injuries of the medial column. Arthrodesis has not been required as a result of this injury.

DISCUSSION

Fractures of the tarsal bones are uncommon and most often are caused by a direct blow. When displaced, open reduction and internal fixation are recommended. The evaluation should include an AP, a lateral, and an oblique radiograph of the foot. Treatment by open reduction and internal fixation should restore the articular anatomy, as well as the alignment of the foot. Fixation should be sufficiently rigid to maintain this position until healing. Postoperative symptoms can be diminished by the use of custom-molded, full-length, semirigid insole.

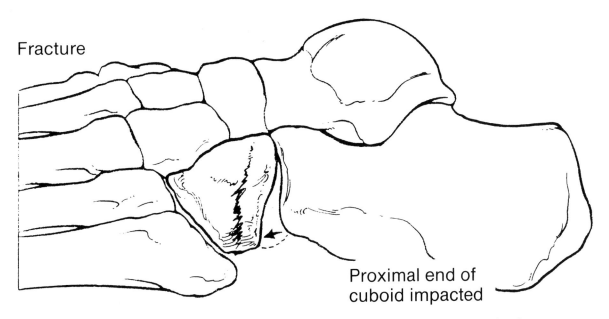

Figure 2 The length of the cuboid is restored, and the articular surface is templated against the calcaneus or the metatarsal bases. Sometimes it is helpful to place a Kirschner wire in the proximal and distal parts of the cuboid and spread them with a lamina spreader.

A

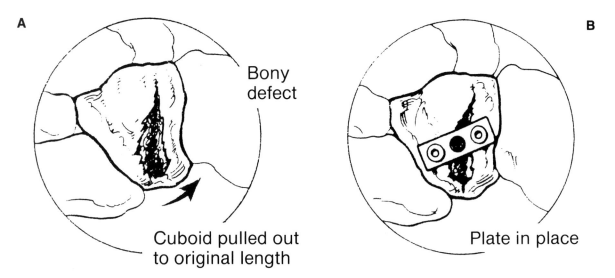

Bony
defect

Cuboid pulled out
to original length

B

Plate in place

Figure 3 *A,* When the cuboid is restored to its normal length, a cap remains from impaction in the central part. This space is filled with bone graft. *B,* A small plate, usually a one-quarter tubular or mini "t" buttress plate, is used to buttress the restored length of the cuboid.

SUGGESTED READING

Eichenholtz SN, Levine DV. Fractures of the tarsal navicular bone. Clin Orthop 1964; 34:142–157.

Leyman EP, Eskeles IH. Fractures of the tarsal scaphoid with notes on the mechanism. J Bone Joint Surg 1928; 10:108–113.

Main BJ, Jowett RL. Injuries of the mid-tarsal joint. J Bone Joint Surg 1975; 57B:89–97.

Sangeorzan BJ, Mosca V, Benirschke SK, et al. Displaced intraarticular fractures of the tarsal navicular. J Bone Joint Surg 1989; 71A:1504–1510.

Sangeorzan BJ, Swiontkowski MF. Displaced fractures of the cuboid. J Bone Joint Surg 1990; 72B:376–378.

TALAR NECK FRACTURES

RICHARD G. ALVAREZ, M.D.

Successful treatment for fractures of the neck of the talus depends on the amount of displacement, the remaining blood supply to the talus, the precision of reduction, and the adequacy of fixation.

Several surgical approaches have been proposed, and the anteromedial approach often is regarded as least damaging to the vascular supply of the talus. Unfortunately this approach not only disturbs the vascularity, but also prevents placement of a screw through the center of the head into the body of the talus at the most advantageous angle to the plane of the fracture. The posterior approach minimizes damage to the talar vascular supply and has the advantage of allowing excellent internal fixation by a screw or screws that can be placed perpendicular to the fracture plane into the head of the talus. This biomechanical advantage of compressive, rigid internal fixation allows for early range of motion and provides improved results in management of the subtalar dislocation, which is a highly important component of type II, type III, and type IV talar neck fractures.

Another added advantage of the posterior approach is in type III fractures with the body extruded posteriormedially, hinged by the deltoid ligament and sitting behind the sustentaculum tali on the medial side of the calcaneus. After unsuccessful manipulation using a calcaneal pin for distraction, the surgical recommendation is to osteotomize the medial malleolus. Reduction always is difficult, even with an extensive anteromedial approach. With the posterior approach, however, an external fixator can be applied through the incision into the distal tibia and calcaneus. The ankle can be distracted and the fracture manipulated to reduce the body, without further compromising the vascularity of the talus or performing a medial malleolus osteotomy.

PREFERRED APPROACH

The anesthetized patient is placed in the side-lying position with the uninjured side down on the image table, with the foot and ankle extending slightly beyond the table edge. With type II fractures, the foot is manipulated into maximal plantar flexion and the forefoot is everted. This brings the talar head and neck down to the plantar-flexed body and at the same time reduces the body of the talus onto the subtalar joint. (Neutral or slight dorsiflexion causes the talar body to be slightly subluxed posteriorly.) The fracture position is checked by the lateral and anterior views using the image intensifier. It is important to roll the anterior image, checking the neck reduction. Eversion of the foot should

align the cortices of the neck. The fracture should be reduced to less than 5 mm of displacement and 5° of angulation.

The foot, ankle, and leg are prepped and draped. Under tourniquet control, a 6 to 8 cm curvilinear incision is made lateral to the Achilles tendon down to the lateral tubercle of the calcaneus (Fig. 1). (A straight incision causes less exposure and possibly a contracture later.) The sural nerve is identified, protected, and retracted laterally. The adipose tissue is dissected down to the posterior aspect of the ankle and the subtalar joints.

The flexor hallucis longus is identified and retracted medially, and the lateral tubercle of the talus is palpated just lateral to this tendon. Once these two important landmarks are identified, the subtalar joint is opened just lateral to the lateral tubercle (in type III fractures this already is exposed). The foot is held in the corrected position, and the reduction is confirmed by the image intensifier. Using the lateral border of the tubercle as a landmark, two 2.0 pins are drilled across the fracture, using the AO three-hole guide if available. If not, two 2.5 pins are drilled as parallel as possible. Using image control, the pins are drilled into the head from the posterior aspect of the talus body. The pins are replaced

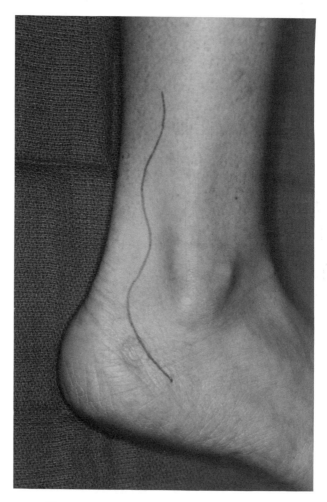

Figure 1 Posterolateral curvilinear incision.

243

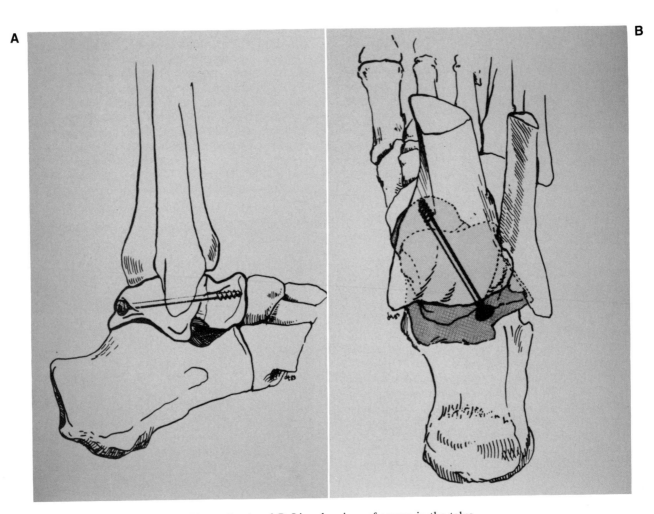

Figure 2 *A* and *B*, Line drawings of screws in the talus.

one at a time with a short-thread cancellous screw (4.5 mm AO canulated screws work well), after determining length and tapping. Both screws should be countersunk to avoid obstruction to plantar flexion (Fig. 2). After wound closure a well-padded short-leg cast or a posterior-medial-lateral splint is applied with the foot at 90°. After 3 to 5 days the wound is inspected and a new short-leg cast is applied. To allow some healing of the extensive soft tissue injury that occurs with these fractures, ankle and subtalar motion is started at approximately 3 weeks postoperatively. Minimum weight bearing is allowed at 8 weeks, progressing to full weight bearing by 12 weeks postoperatively if sufficient fracture union is documented.

To identify aseptic necrosis of the body of the talus, a technetium-99 bone scan (using a pinhole collimator) or magnetic resonance imaging (MRI) is performed at 8 to 12 weeks postoperatively.

TYPE III FRACTURES

Type III fractures require special considerations, since the entire body has rotated from the ankle and subtalar joints. Closed reduction is tried first by having the anesthetized patient supine and the foot and leg off the end of the operating table so the knee is flexed 90°. After the heel area is prepped, a large Hoffmann or Steinmann pin is placed from medial to lateral and a traction bow applied. Longitudinal traction is applied for 5 to 10 minutes (approximately 10 to 15 pounds). While

maintaining traction, the calcaneus is everted and the foot is dorsiflexed as much as possible, thus recreating the violence that caused the injury. The thumb is placed on the talar body, which lies on the medial calcaneus (Fig. 3). By pushing the body, it can be engaged in the mortise. With continuing traction the foot is plantar flexed gently, and the talar body is squeezed back into the mortise by the calcaneus and tibia closing together posteriorly as that foot is plantar flexed. This converts a type III to a type II fracture, which then is handled as previously mentioned.

If the talar body does not reduce after no more than two attempts, an open reduction is necessary. The posterolateral approach is used, with the patient placed on the image table in the side-lying position with the sound side down. Dissection is carried out as previously described, with or without the calcaneal pin still in place. The reduction again is attempted under direct visualization by the method just discussed. One can see that the talar body must be rotated and engaged under the mortise. After one unsuccessful attempt, the incision is extended proximally enough to place one or two half-pins into the distal tibia. A half-pin is placed into the lateral calcaneus in the distally exposed internal surface of the calcaneus, or the same calcaneal pin placed previously can be used for the external fixator (Fig. 4). Once the distraction-compressor external fixator is applied, gradual lengthening is carried out slowly, taking advantage of the viscoelastic properties of the tight tissue. Once distraction has been carried out enough to allow the body to be engaged by pressing it into the mortise with the thumb,

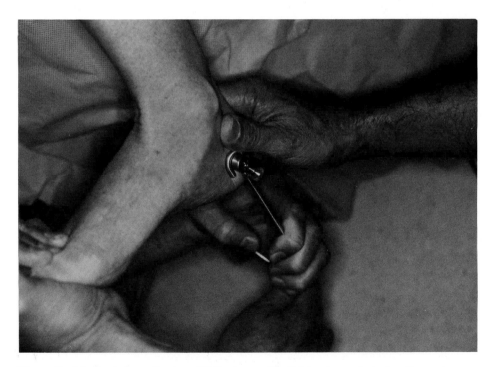

Figure 3 Manipulation of a type III fracture with distal calcaneal pin traction, calcaneus eversion, foot dorsiflexion, and the thumb pushing the talar body back into mortise.

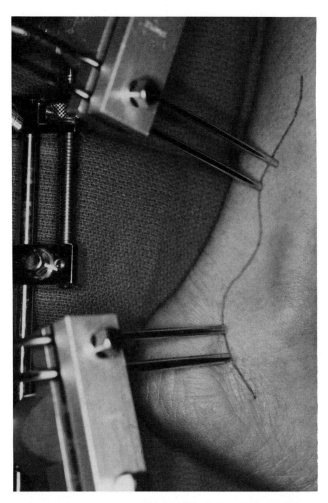

Figure 4 External fixator position with the Hoffman compressor-distractor. (The incision can be extended distally and proximally to allow for pin placement.)

the fixator is loosened as the foot is dorsiflexed. Then plantar flexing causes the talar body to be pinched back into the ankle joint by the calcaneus and tibia coming together posteriorly. Remember, a rotatory motion of the talar body that is hinged by the deltoid ligament is a highly important part of this reduction. Once the body is reduced, the fracture is converted from a type III to a type II fracture. One then proceeds as discussed previously for type II fractures, using the two-screw method of fixation (Figs. 5 and 6).

POSTOPERATIVE CARE AND SEQUELAE

Thirteen talar neck fractures have been treated by this method. Nine were type II and four were type III fractures. The age range of the patients was 13 years to 36 years, with an average age of 29 years. Time spent immobilized ranged from 19 days to 38 days (mean 23 days). This was to allow the soft tissues to heal. A removable cast substitute such as a Bledsoe was used. The physical therapist saw the patient three to five times per week, working on ankle range of motion and subtalar range of motion. Ambulation was initiated after radiographic evidence of fracture union. If aseptic necrosis was documented, a PTB brace was used with partial weight bearing allowed. Talus revascularization can take 2 years or more. Malunion, which is the most frequent problem of this type of fracture, did not occur with less than 5° of angulation and less than 5 mm of displacement criteria for reduction.

Two of the type II fractures had a fair result, defined as having no pain and only limited motion of the subtalar joint compared with the contralateral side. One type II fracture had a poor result, defined as having pain and presence of aseptic necrosis. There was only a trace subtalar motion, and ankle range of motion was reduced by half compared with the contralateral side. Three type III fractures had a good functional result by the above criteria, and one type III fracture had a poor result with the presence of the aseptic necrosis and pain.

PROS AND CONS OF TREATMENT

Vascular supply of the talus comes from three main arteries: anterior tibial artery, posterior tibial artery, and perforating peroneal artery. Only two-fifths of the surface of the talus can accommodate a blood supply, because the remaining three-fifths is covered by articular cartilage. There is minimal vascularity at its posterior capsular attachment. For this reason, the posterior approach to these fractures disturbs the remaining vascular supply less than the anteromedial approach.

Operative management of talar neck fractures has several advantages: it avoids immobilization of this type of fracture in equinus for more than 8 weeks, it can achieve fracture stability, and it can initiate early mobilization.

The posterior approach respects the vascular supply of the talus, which already has been compromised by the trauma, and it affords exact placement of the screw into the head of the talus perpendicular to the fracture plane. Unfortunately this form of treatment does not protect the talus from aseptic necrosis. Another shortcoming of this technique is lack of direct visualization of the fracture site. However, use of the image intensifier and a closed reduction to within 5 mm of displacement and 5° of angulation are mandatory if this approach is used and malunion prevented.

Type III fractures can be reduced through the posterior approach. However, an understanding of the mechanisms of injury, anatomy, and external fixature for distraction is necessary for a reduction.

Normal subtalar motion after type II and type III fractures compared with the contralateral side may be unlikely. Pain-free ambulation is obtainable if there is a fracture union and no aseptic necrosis.

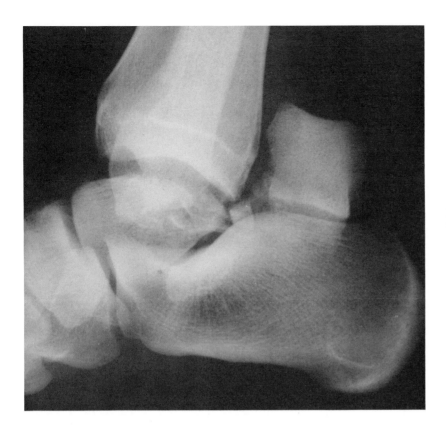

Figure 5 Posterolateral dislocation with comminution and dorsal bone loss.

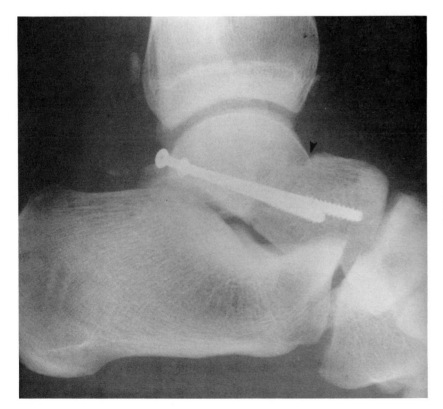

Figure 6 Cannulated 4.0 mm screw fixation. Note the slight dorsal angulation *(arrow)* as a result of bone loss.

DISCUSSION

A posterior approach for reduction and internal fixation of talar neck fractures should be considered part of the treatment approach for talar neck fractures, because it respects the compromised vascularity of the talus and allows for early mobilization.

SUGGESTED READING

Canale TS, Kelley FB. Fractures of the neck of the talus. J Bone Joint Surg 1978; 60A:143–156.
DeLee J, Curtis R. Subtalar dislocations of the foot. J Bone Joint Surg 1982; 64A:433–437.
Hawkins LG. Fractures of the neck of the talus. J Bone Joint Surg 1970; 52A:991–1002.
Watson-Jones R. Injuries of the foot. In Wilson IN, ed., Fractures and joint injuries. Vol 2. 5th ed. New York: Churchill Livingstone, 1976.

FRACTURES OF THE CALCANEUS

MARK MYERSON, M.D.
HEIDI MULTHOPP-STEPHENS, M.D.

Calcaneal fractures may be of the relatively simple extra-articular or complex intra-articular type. The superior portion of the calcaneus is made up of the articular facets of the subtalar joint, which are involved in the intra-articular fractures. Extra-articular fractures generally are avulsions or nondisplaced body fractures. The tendo Achilles inserts posteriorly, the bifurcate ligament inserts on the anterior process, and the spring ligament inserts plantarly. Intra-articular fractures involve the subtalar articulation to varying degrees. Several authors have classified intra-articular fractures according to the appearance on computed tomographic (CT) scan. In this chapter intra-articular and extra-articular fractures are discussed separately because the severity, treatment, complications, and prognosis are markedly different.

EXTRA-ARTICULAR FRACTURES

Extra-articular fractures are either avulsion fractures by way of the tendo Achilles or bifurcate ligaments or are associated with compression and shearing, which fractures the sustentaculum tali when landing in hindfoot inversion. Displaced body fractures may occur that do not involve the subtalar joint, but do cause shortening and widening of the calcaneus.

Treatment of extra-articular calcaneal fractures consists of cast immobilization with closed reduction if necessary. Open reduction and internal fixation (ORIF) may be required for an anterior process fracture if it is displaced more than 2 mm, large, and not comminuted. If comminuted, the fragments probably are best excised acutely. An Essex-Lopresti tongue-type fracture should be treated with ORIF with 4.0 cancellous screws if the fracture is displaced more than 6 to 8 mm. We do not recommend the Essex-Lopresti technique using percutaneous pins because of complications including pin infection, potential osteomyelitis, and the need for cast immobilization. A compressive splint and elevation should be used initially to allow swelling to subside. A short-leg cast or walker boot then is applied. If the patient is compliant, a short-leg walker allows active range of motion before allowing weight bearing. Toe touch weight-bearing status should be maintained for 6 weeks or until there is radiographic evidence of union. Progressive weight bearing then is permitted, and range of motion of the ankle and subtalar joints is maximized with physical therapy.

Complications of extra-articular fractures of the calcaneus include stiffness of the ankle and subtalar joint, widening of the heel, and nonunion. Nonunion generally occurs with displaced avulsion fractures and can be treated with ORIF, if large and amenable to fixation, or by excision of the ununited fragment and reinsertion of the ligament or tendon. In general the prognosis for extra-articular calcaneal fractures is good with closed treatment. There is minimal or no long-term disability, and complications are rare and treatable.

INTRA-ARTICULAR FRACTURES

Intra-articular fractures result from compressive forces. The lateral process of the talus acts as a wedge, causing the primary fracture and producing the major anteromedial (sustentacular) and posterolateral (tuberosity) fragments. Further force causes secondary fractures, compressing and rotating the posterior facet as much as 90° anteriorly. Although many classifications of intra-articular calcaneus fractures have been proposed, the most useful for planning treatment is based on the number of fragments on a coronal and oblique CT scan view through the sustentaculum and the posterior facet. Management options include closed treatment, ORIF, or primary subtalar arthrodesis.

The clinical findings of an acute calcaneal fracture include severe swelling, pain, and ecchymosis. Severe burning pain and sensory deficits also may be present if associated with a compartment syndrome. After 1 to 2 days, fracture blisters may involve the hindfoot, and ecchymosis may extend to the knee. These fractures are associated with high energy, and the patient's general medical condition, lumbar spine, and lower extremities must be evaluated carefully. Anteroposterior, lateral, oblique, and axial radiographs of the foot are obtained. If there is uncertainty about involvement of the posterior facet, particularly if comminuted, a CT scan is obtained, which is essential for preoperative planning.

If a compartment syndrome is suspected because of increasing pain, paresthesias, or pain on passive dorsiflexion of the toes, compartment pressures must be measured. In a series of 98 intra-articular fractures at our institution, 13 percent had compartment pressures greater than 30 mm Hg. We recommend fasciotomy if the pressure is greater than 40 mm Hg; the technique is discussed in the chapter *Crush Injuries and Compartment Syndromes*. We now routinely evaluate these patients for evidence of myoneural ischemia, admit them to the hospital, and schedule a CT scan. Elevation, ice, and bulky compressive dressing are used immediately following examination to control swelling. We also use an intermittent compression pump device applied to the foot to reduce edema rapidly in selected patients. This pump is particularly useful in patients who present late and are markedly swollen.

TIMING OF SURGERY

Surgical planning and timing are critical. The skin should regain its normal turgor with the fine surface

249

wrinkles before surgery. A useful test is to pinch the skin on the lateral aspect of the foot; if wrinkling occurs, the tissues are less likely to be compromised. Generally, we prefer to wait 5 to 7 days following injury before performing ORIF. Although the fracture ideally is treated 6 to 8 hours following injury, we seldom have completed imaging studies at this stage. An open fracture or compartment syndrome necessitates emergent operative treatment, but not necessarily definitive fracture treatment. Authors differ on whether fracture blisters should be debrided as they appear or left intact until the time of surgery; we leave them and have no problem operating through blisters provided swelling has resolved and skin turgor is normal.

INDICATIONS FOR SURGERY

ORIF is indicated in a medically fit patient with mild-to-severe comminution. A two- or three-part fracture should be fixed if displaced more than 3 mm. Severely comminuted fractures seem impossible to fix correctly and obtain secure fixation. Yet it is precisely these severe fractures, in which the lateral process of the talus is driven through the floor of the calcaneus, which must be reduced and fixed. Severely comminuted and depressed fractures also should be fixed. Although these are technically difficult, it is important to restore normal alignment including height and width of the hindfoot. In these comminuted fractures, anatomic restoration of the joint surfaces is difficult. However, we always are able to restore the height and width of the calcaneus, and once alignment is restored, a subsequent salvage procedure

(i.e., arthrodesis) is simplified. The surgeon *must* consider whether or not he or she can improve the prognosis with surgery. Patients have approximately a 65 percent chance of having reasonable function if treated conservatively. In our own hands, we are able to improve on this with open treatment of grade II injuries, with 80 to 85 percent of patients doing well. For grade IV injuries or worse, the prognosis without surgery is poor, with more than 60 percent requiring subsequent salvage surgery. Here again we can improve on this significantly, and although this reflects a personal philosophy, it also greatly reduces long-term disability.

SURGICAL TECHNIQUE

The patient is positioned on a beanbag, and a pneumatic thigh tourniquet is applied. Following induction of a general anesthetic, the patient is placed in a lateral decubitus position with the involved extremity up. It is essential that the foot lies perfectly lateral and is not falling away from the surgeon during the procedure. The leg and the ipsilateral anterior iliac crest are prepped and draped. Prophylactic antibiotics are administered.

We use an extensile lateral approach with a long J- or L-shaped incision, with the apex inferior and posterior to the peroneal tendons and sural nerves as they pass behind the lateral malleolus (Fig. 1). The apex of the incision is curved gently to prevent tip necrosis of the flap. A medial approach rarely is necessary and is used only if there is an extruded medial fracture fragment inaccessible from the lateral side. The flap then is elevated directly off the lateral wall of the calcaneus and

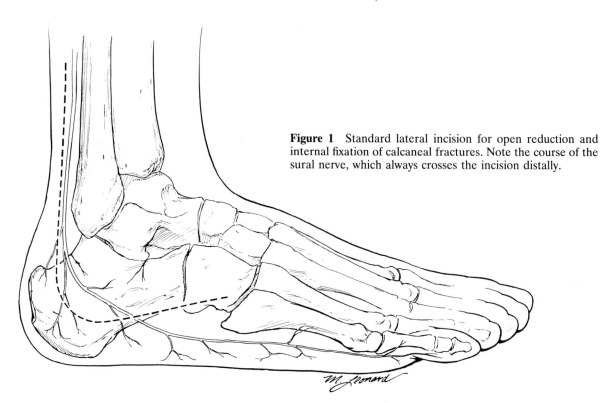

Figure 1 Standard lateral incision for open reduction and internal fixation of calcaneal fractures. Note the course of the sural nerve, which always crosses the incision distally.

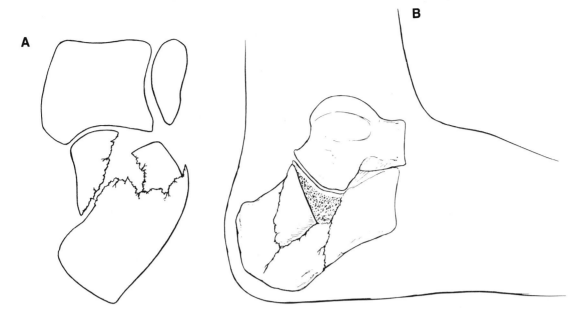

Figure 2 *A,* Coronal, and *B,* lateral views of a two-part intra-articular calcaneal fracture. Note on the lateral view that the articular surface of the posterior facet is rotated and impacted and oriented almost vertically. The varus position of the calcaneus is typical *(A).*

includes the peroneal tendons with their sheath intact. It is important to dissect the flap sharply. The sural nerve is not visualized in the main part of the flap and should not be looked for except in the distalmost part of the incision, where the nerve crosses over the peroneal tendons. Subperiosteal dissection is continued along the lateral calcaneus, and the calcaneofibular ligament is dissected free or excised. Once the subtalar joint is identified, short 0.045 inch Kirschner (K-) wires are inserted into the fibula posteriorly and the talus anteriorly and are bent to retract the skin flap without constant manual retraction of the skin. The skin flap is kept moist throughout the procedure. The dissection is carried anteriorly to the level of the calcaneocuboid joint, which is exposed only if the fracture extends distally. Using this incision the distal dissection over the peroneal tendons is difficult, and one may need to work both dorsal and plantar to the tendons. The lateral wall is exposed fully, and the lateral portion of the tuberosity or posterior facet is retracted away from the body of the calcaneus (Figs. 2 and 3). This fragment is often free of soft tissue attachments and can be exteriorized and placed in saline-soaked gauze on the back table.

Once this fragment is removed, the primary fracture line extending toward the medial aspect of the subtalar joint can be visualized. The rotated posterior facet fragment is identified and gently disimpacted by inserting a large periosteal elevator or osteotome under the anterior aspect of the fragment. A Schantz pin is inserted into the posteroinferior and lateral aspect of the calcaneus to aid in the reduction (Fig. 4). The pin should not be inserted percutaneously, but through the exposed bone at the apex of the incision. The combined force

applied to this pin is distraction and valgus while one visualizes the medial subtalar joint and palpates the medial wall of the calcaneus. It takes some time to learn to palpate the medial wall displacements. Try to appreciate the varus and shortened position of the tuberosity fragment while placing your index finger over the fracture line. It is easy to feel the shift in this fracture

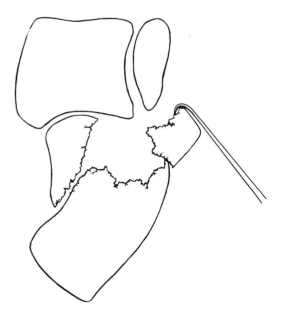

Figure 3 Once exposed, the first step is to disimpact the lateral wall fragment, which is best accomplished with a small bone hook.

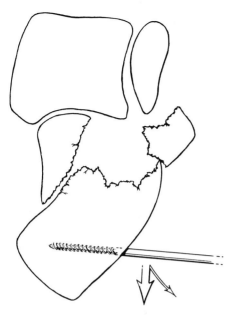

Figure 4 Disimpaction is achieved with longitudinal and valgus traction to reduce the anteromedial and posterolateral fragments.

line, which actually is the most posterior edge of the sustentacular fragment.

Once the primary fracture is reduced and heel height and valgus restored, 0.062 or 0.045 inch K-wires are inserted from plantar and posterior across the primary fracture into the talus as provisional fixation (Fig. 5). These K-wires restore the height and concavity of the medial wall. When inserting them, try to avoid

placing them into the defect created by the fractured tuberosity, since they block reduction of the posterior facet if they are not intraosseous. The midportion of the posterior facet now is aligned and held reduced with K-wires introduced from lateral to medial (Fig. 6). These should be positioned to avoid interfering with the permanent fixation. We therefore try to angle them slightly so that the lateral screw fixation does not necessitate immediate removal of the K-wires.

We generally try to restore the height of the tuberosity using a vertically oriented H-plate (Figs. 7 and 8). This can be planned to include the fixation of the facet through the superior three holes of the plate. The articular facet then is reduced and fixed provisionally including the fragment that was removed; 3.5 mm cortical screws are used to lag the subchondral bone just beneath the articular facet and hold the articular reduction. The correctly sized H-plate is selected and applied to the lateral wall as a buttress and secured with 3.5 mm screws. These screws are inserted in a lag fashion for the facet, preferably by triangulating the three superior screws through the plate. The rest of the screws are not inserted width a gliding hole. If there is involvement of the calcaneocuboid joint, this is reduced and fixed temporarily with K-wires and then with 3.5 mm cortical or 4.0 mm cancellous screws. Bone grafting of the defect rarely is necessary if correct fixation technique is used, but may be performed if it is thought to increase the stability of the reduction. This depends to a large extent on the type of fixation used and the pattern of bone loss under the posterior facet. With the vertical H-plate, the entire lateral wall is spanned; the defect under the plate is irrelevant since the facet is held elevated, supported, and reduced. There is no fixation,

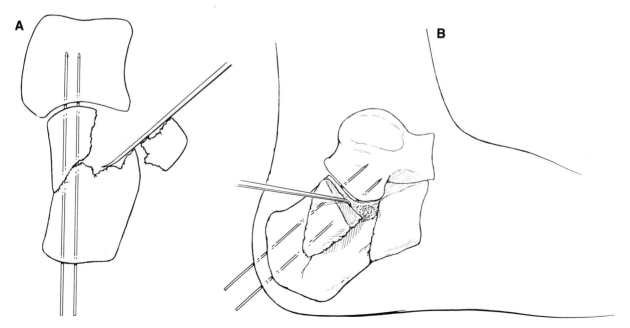

Figure 5 *A* and *B*, 0.045 inch K-wires are used for provisional fixation of the anteromedial and posterolateral fragments, following manual reduction. These provisional fixation pins are driven across the subtalar joint.

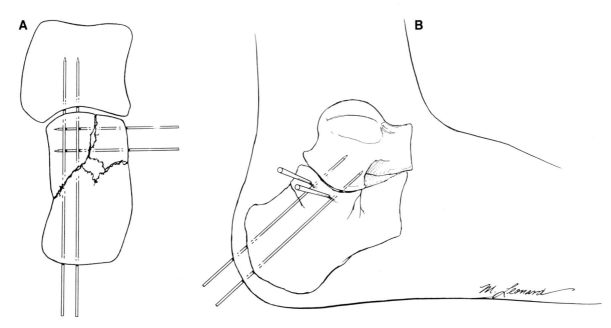

Figure 6 *A* and *B,* The lateral wall fragment is reduced with additional K-wires, which provisionally fix the lateral wall fragment and hold the subtalar articular congruency during screw placement.

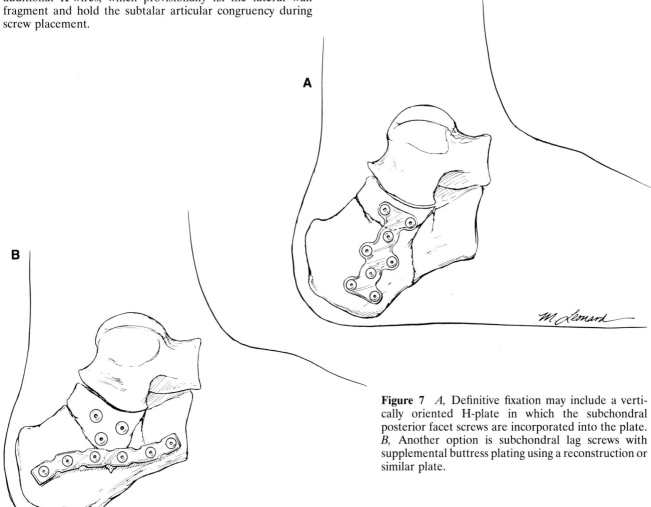

Figure 7 *A,* Definitive fixation may include a vertically oriented H-plate in which the subchondral posterior facet screws are incorporated into the plate. *B,* Another option is subchondral lag screws with supplemental buttress plating using a reconstruction or similar plate.

A

B

C

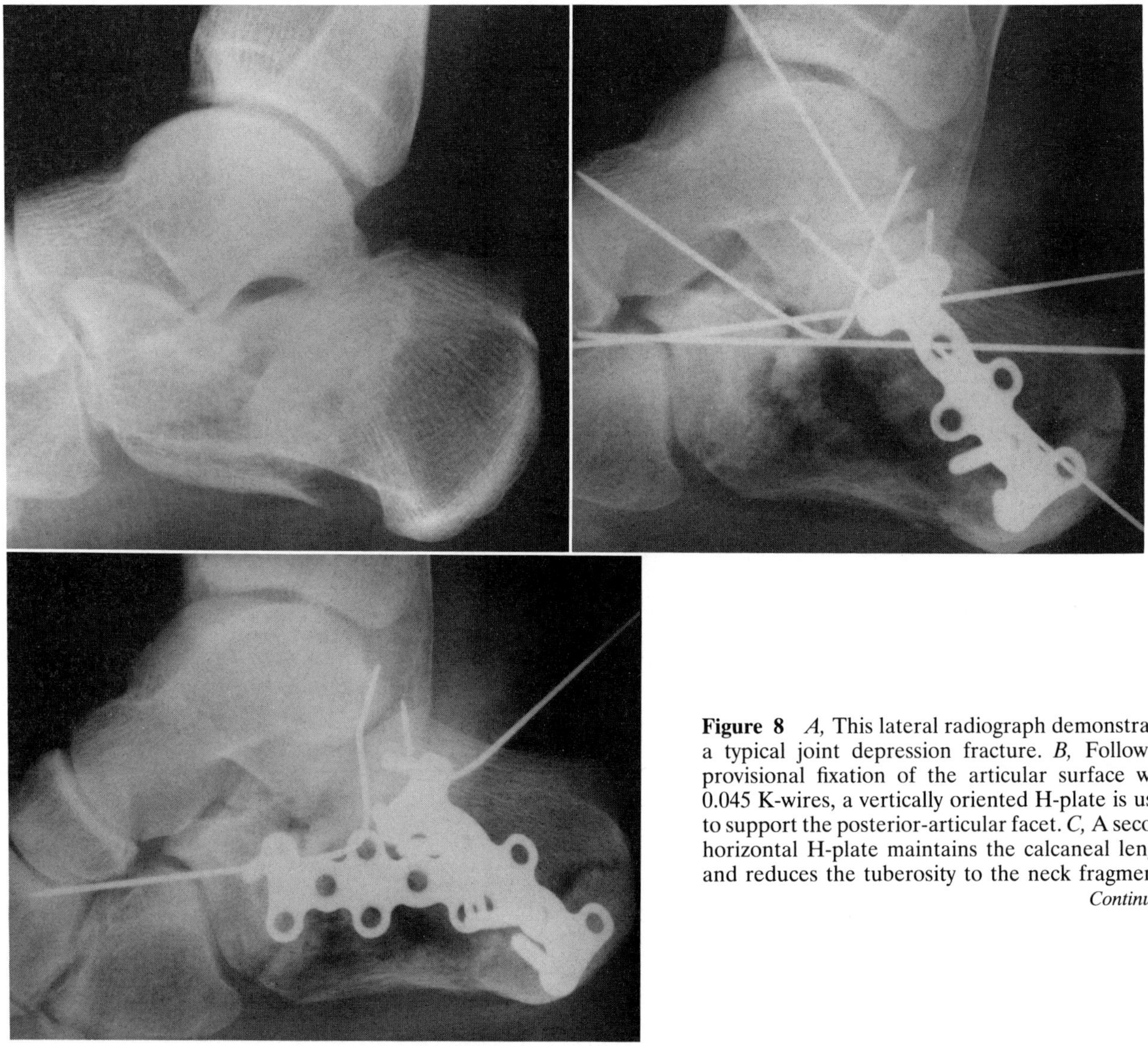

Figure 8 *A,* This lateral radiograph demonstrates a typical joint depression fracture. *B,* Following provisional fixation of the articular surface with 0.045 K-wires, a vertically oriented H-plate is used to support the posterior-articular facet. *C,* A second horizontal H-plate maintains the calcaneal length and reduces the tuberosity to the neck fragments. *Continued.*

however, using the H-plate system between the tuberosity and the neck across the primary fracture line, which has to be supported with additional rigid fixation. If a longitudinal reconstruction plate is used, the primary fracture is held rigidly, but the posterior facet may not be supported adequately (see Fig. 7*B*). This depends on the size of the facet, which also is called the thalamic fragment. If the fragment is large, the inferior edge may be secured by the dorsally curved portion of the plate. Occasionally more than one plate system is necessary for fixation, including the vertical H-plate and a second H- or reconstruction plate longitudinally.

The subcutaneous tissue does not require suture, and the skin is closed using modified vertical mattress nylon sutures over a suction drain. Bulky compressive dressing is applied postoperatively and early range of motion commenced once the sutures are removed. ORIF is performed to retain motion, so it is senseless to immobilize the foot for a prolonged period. If the patient

is reliable, a walker boot allows range of motion of the ankle and subtalar joint before weight bearing. The patient is kept non–weight bearing for 3 months, but toe touch weight-bearing and swimming pool exercises are commenced at 6 to 8 weeks.

Intra-articular fractures of the calcaneus treated conservatively are complicated by loss of calcaneal height, lateral wall extrusion, subtalar arthritis, and hindfoot varus. Anatomic reduction and internal fixation restores the normal alignment, the bony architecture, and the joint surface. This preserves motion and prevents sequelae such as peroneal impingement and arthritis.

PRIMARY ARTHRODESIS

In fractures with severe comminution and bone loss, a primary arthrodesis often is the procedure of choice

D

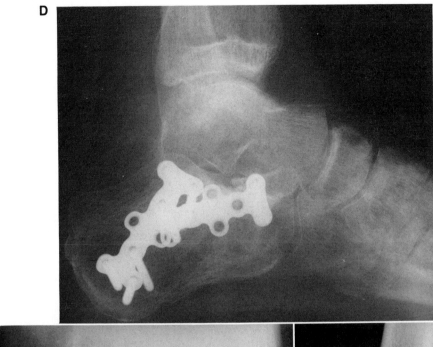

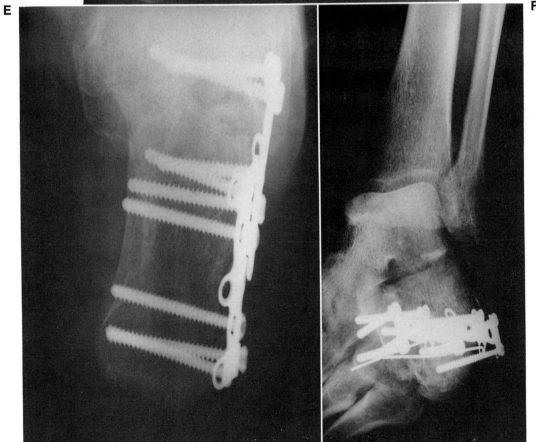

Figure 8, cont'd. Postoperative lateral *(D)*, axial *(E)*, and Broden's *(F)* views. Note the restoration of the posterior facet and Bohler's angle.

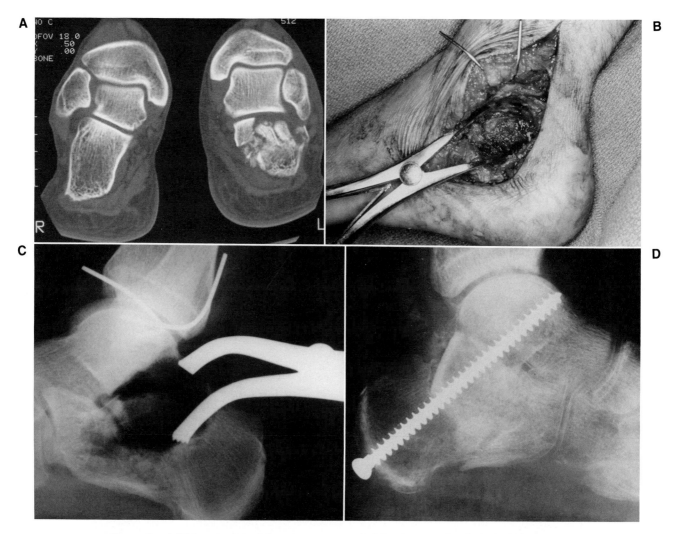

Figure 9 *A,* This comminuted fracture was treated with primary arthrodesis. *B,* The subtalar joint is distracted using a lamina spreader. *C,* Radiographs are obtained to confirm reduction. *D,* A tricortical iliac crest bone graft is harvested and placed in the defect to restore the talar declination angle, and screw fixation secures the graft.

(Fig. 9). It must be understood that the overall approach is identical to that described for ORIF. Care is taken to restore height and to decompress the lateral recess and narrow the lateral wall. When the bony architecture has been restored with plate and screw fixation, the articular cartilage is removed using either thin chisel blades or a burr. Bone graft is packed into the joint, and fixation is performed using the large AO cannulated screw system with fully threaded cancellous screws. If considerable fragmentation and comminution is present, a tricortical bone block graft is used. Care is taken to align the subtalar joint properly in neutral to slight valgus before inserting the guide pin. The screws of the calcaneal fixation may interfere with placement of the cannulated guide pins, and one should be aware of the need for subsequent pin placement for the arthrodesis when performing the open reduction and internal fixation. One or two parallel, large, cannulated screws are used to

fix the subtalar joint, and their position is checked with intraoperative imaging.

Primary arthrodesis as described gives the best functional result with a minimal period of recuperation for severely comminuted fractures that are not possible to fix anatomically.

SUGGESTED READING

Burdeaux BD. Reduction of calcaneal fractures by the McReynolds medial approach technique and its experimental basis. Clin Orthop 1983; 177:87–103.

Essex-Lopresti P. The mechanism, reduction technique, and results in fractures of the os calcis. Br J Surg 1952; 39:395–419.

Harding D, Waddell JP. Open reduction in depressed fractures of the os calcis. Clin Orthop 1985; 199:124–131.

Hermann OJ. Conservative therapy for fractures of the os calcis. J Bone Joint Surg 1937; 19:709–718.

LeTournel E. Open reduction and internal fixation of calcaneal fractures. In: Spiegel P, ed. Topics in orthopedic surgery, Baltimore: Aspen, 1984:173.

Leung K, Chan W, Shen W, et al. Operative treatment of intraarticular fractures of the os calcis. J Ortho Trauma 1989; 3:232–240.

Soeur R, Remy R. Fractures of the calcaneus with displacement of the thalamic portion. J Bone Joint Surg 1975; 57B:413–421.

Stephenson JR. Treatment of displaced intra-articular fractures of the calcaneus using medial and lateral approaches, internal fixation, and early motion. J Bone Joint Surg 1987; 69A:115–130.

PILON FRACTURES

JUDITH FORD BAUMHAUER, M.D.
SAUL G. TREVINO, M.D.

Pilon fractures are distinct ankle fractures that involve the distal-articular surface of the tibia. The management of these fractures is complicated because of the magnitude of comminution, the degree of soft tissue trauma associated with the injury, and the component of metaphyseal impaction. As a result of the high energy involved in sustaining these injuries, pilon fractures frequently are open. The mechanism of injury involves an axial load with or without a rotational element. The classification scheme by Ruedi and Allgower is cited most often in the literature and is based on the degree of comminution and displacement of the articular fragments, graded I through III. The more recent classification by Mast (Table 1) takes into account the mechanism of injury, as well as the comminution and displacement, which aid the prognosis and treatment of these injuries. Rotational-type injuries have a better prognosis than purely compressive-type injuries.

THERAPEUTIC ALTERNATIVES

Treatment options for pilon fractures are based on the degree of comminution, the amount of displacement, and the condition of the soft tissues.

Closed Reduction and Casting

Nondisplaced fractures can be treated in non–weight-bearing casts. These frequently need to be long-leg casts for rotational stability. The drawback to this mode of treatment is the potential for progressive angulatory deformity and shortening, stiffness, and loss of range of motion. In the elderly with poor bone stock or patients with metabolic bone disease, closed reduc-

Table 1 Pilon Fracture Classification

Grade I	Malleolar fractures with axial load component
	Large plafond fragments
	Posterior malleolar or anterior marginal fractures
Grade II	Spiral tibia fractures extending into the plafond
Grade III	Axial load injuries with central compression
	(Ruedi-Allgower A, B, C classification)
	A. Nondisplaced fracture
	B. Mild displacement of articular fragments
	(3 or less)
	C. Displacement of fragments (more than 3),
	metaphyseal impaction

From Mast JW, Spiegel PG, Pappas JN. Fractures of the tibial pilon. Clin Orthop 1988; 230:68–82; with permission.

tion and casting may be advisable. The key to successful closed reduction and casting management in these fractures is demonstrating that the fractures truly are nondisplaced. Tomograms in the coronal and sagittal planes aid in this determination. Displaced articular fractures treated with casting have a less than satisfactory result and should be treated operatively.

Traction

Calcaneal pin traction for definitive management of extremely comminuted pilon fractures has been suggested in the literature. The potential complications include pin track infections and inadequate reconstructions of the articular surface of the tibia. Calcaneal pin traction essentially has been replaced by external fixation. Traction has a role as a temporary option awaiting surgical intervention.

External Fixation

The indications for external fixation of pilon fractures include severely comminuted fractures not amenable to open reduction and internal fixation and grade III open fractures or a compromised soft tissue envelope such as a crush injury or burn. The basic goals of external fixation are maintenance of length and reduction using ligamentotaxis.

Multiple external fixation devices are available. The Orthofix System is a unilateral construct that is biomechanically stable. We have found it simple to use and well tolerated by patients. The Orthofix device can be articulated at the tibiotalar joint for early plantar and dorsiflexion motion. The distraction aligning the distal-articular surface of the tibia is maintained throughout the motion segment. We use two screws placed in the talus parallel to the axis of the ankle joint and two in the tibia proximal to the fracture. This avoids immobilization of the subtalar joint. Gentle active motion is begun at 4 to 6 weeks after injury.

Limited Open Reduction and Internal Fixation

The concept of key fragment fixation with limited open reduction and internal fixation (ORIF) of large articular fragments, or stabilization of the fibula alone, has not proved superior to ORIF or external fixation. Limited ORIF has similar potential complications of both ORIF and closed reduction and casting including skin necrosis, infection, and loss of reduction.

Arthrodesis

Primary tibiotalar arthrodesis for severe pilon fractures has only case-report documentation in the literature. No studies have evaluated immediate fusion versus delayed fusion. Immediate fusion risks operating through a compromised soft tissue envelope with the potential for skin necrosis and infection. We have had poor results with immediate fusions. Currently we use an external fixator in these severe cases for ligamentotaxis alignment and to maintain length. Tibiotalar fusion is reserved as a salvage procedure.

PREFERRED APPROACH

The goals of treatment include an anatomic reduction of the joint surface and early range of motion.

Patient Selection

In displaced pilon fractures, surgical intervention is the treatment of choice. ORIF is undertaken using the four operative principles dictated by Ruedi (Table 2). For severe cases with soft tissue compromise or open fractures with increased risk of infection, external fixation may be the treatment of choice.

Table 2 Four Operative Principles for Repair of Pilon Fracture

1. Restoration of the length and axis of the fibula
2. Reconstruction of the articular surface of the tibia
3. Bone grafting of the metaphyseal defect
4. Plating of the medial or anterior tibia to prevent late deformity

Timing of Surgery

Because of the axial load mechanism associated with pilon fractures and the degree of soft tissue damage, the timing of surgery is an extremely important determinant of outcome. These fractures usually occur in multiply injured patients, and treatment frequently is delayed. If more than 12 hours has elapsed since injury, we recommend waiting until the swelling has decreased. This may be as long as 7 to 10 days. In cases of open fractures in which irrigation and debridement is needed, reduction and the application of an external fixator may be indicated. Operating through compromised skin increases the risk of postoperative infection and skin necrosis.

Preoperative Preparation

An understanding of the fracture pattern and the degree of comminution and displacement of the articular surface is imperative. Good-quality plain radiographs including an anteroposterior, lateral, and mortise, with oblique views of the ankle, should be obtained. Plain films often under-represent the severity of bony injury. Tomograms in the sagittal and coronal planes add a great deal to the visualization of the fracture fragments and demonstrate the need for metaphyseal bone grafting. Computed tomographic scanning also can be helpful, but in our experience it does not add significantly to

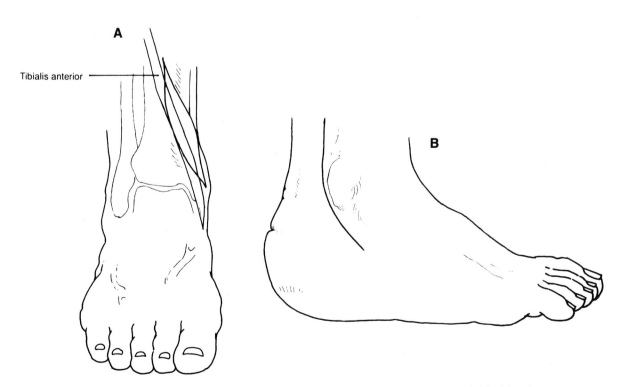

Tibialis anterior

Figure 1 Incisions for surgical stabilization of pilon fracture. *A,* Anteromedial incision for exposure of the distal tibia. *B,* Posterolateral incision for exposure of distal fibula and posterior tibia.

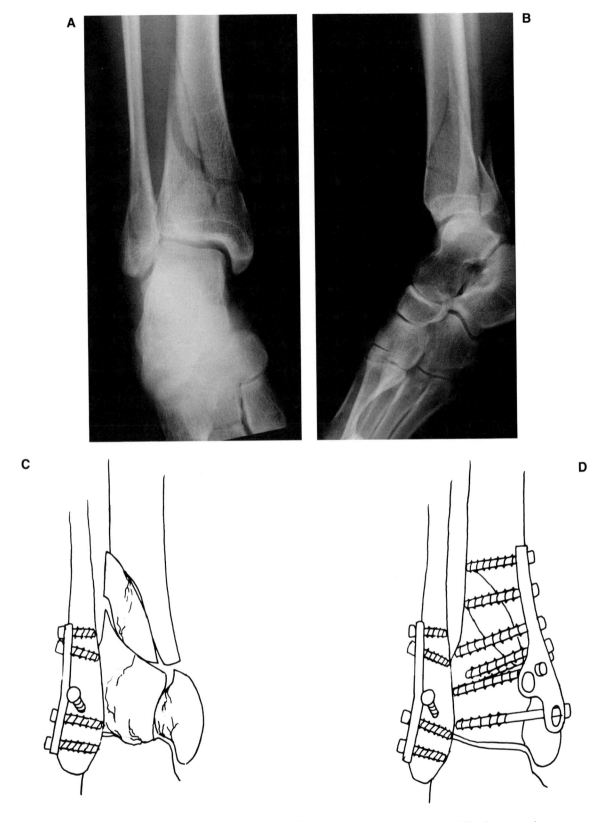

Figure 2 Radiographic and diagrammatic illustrations of pilon fracture stabilization. *A* and *B,* Anteroposterior and lateral radiographs of the right ankle at presentation. *C,* Anteroposterior illustration of fibula fixation with correction of length and rotation. *D,* Anteroposterior illustration of medial tibial buttress plate fixation with restoration of distal-articular surface.

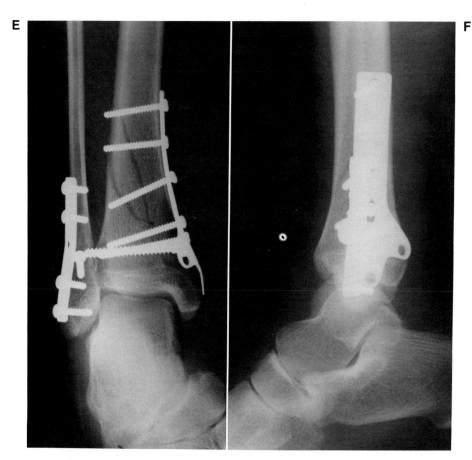

Figure 2, cont'd. *E* and *F,* Anteroposterior and lateral postoperative radiographs demonstrating anatomic reduction of the distal-articular surface of the tibia and restoration of fibula length and rotation.

the information pool after tomograms have been obtained. Preoperative planning using radiographic overlay tracings of the normal and injured ankle is helpful in preparing for these difficult cases and saves interoperative time. Staged steps are organized, and the needed equipment is ordered.

Choice of Procedure (Figs. 1 and 2)

ORIF is undertaken using the four operative principles mentioned previously. A thigh tourniquet is used. With a concurrent fibula fracture, a two-incisional approach is needed to reconstruct the ankle joint. Through a posterolateral incision to the ankle, the fibula can be brought to length and reduced. Establishing length and rotation is important in the subsequent reduction of the tibia. This incision also allows access to the posterior lip of the distal tibia for reduction and stabilization. A 3.5 mm lag screw can be placed perpendicular to oblique fibular fractures. A one-third semitubular or a 3.5 mm DC plate can be used as a neutralization plate. Six cortices proximal and distal to the fracture are recommended for stable fixation.

A second incision is made anteromedial along the medial edge of the tibialis anterior tendon. It is placed 1 cm lateral to the crest of the tibia. A minimum of 7 cm between the two incisions is recommended to prevent skin necrosis. This incision is placed off the bony prominence of the tibial crest to prevent potential skin devascularization. Meticulous handling of the soft tissues throughout the procedure is needed to prevent further skin damage. A full-thickness medial flap is raised. The periosteum is left attached to the tibia to prevent devascularization of bony fragments. An ankle arthrotomy is made. The joint is inspected for osteochondral fragments and debrided. Visualization of the fracture fragments is improved with the use of a lamina spreader or AO femoral distraction device. We use the AO device placed medially in the talus and distal tibia. The need for this instrumentation is determined on a case-by-case basis.

Often after anatomic reconstruction of the fibula is obtained, ligamentotaxis aids in the alignment of the lateral aspect of the tibial surface at Chaput's tubercle. The intact syndesmotic ligaments maintain this relationship. In the case of an intact fibula, there often is a large medial fragment with a vertically oriented fracture line. This is a result of the varus positioning of the foot at the time of the axial load mechanism. This fragment can be opened like a book to visualize the articular surface. Beginning with the larger articular fragments, each is reduced sequentially and held with 0.625 mm Kirschner wire fixation. The impacted surface of the tibia is reduced easily. A Freer elevator is placed into the metaphyseal defect, and firm pressure is applied while the articular fragment is depressed into place. The metaphysis then is bone grafted as needed. Anterosuperior iliac crest bone graft is harvested at the beginning of the procedure or by a second team to decrease tourniquet time.

Selection of the appropriate buttress plate and determination of its placement are essential before the placement of any interfragmentary screws. This prevents obstruction of plate placement. The placement of the tibial plate is based on the area of comminution and can be either anterior or medial. We use spoon plates anteriorly and T-plates medially as buttress plates. Cloverleaf plates have been reported as weaker plates and accept only 3.5 mm or 4.0 mm screws. They are used medially in only severely comminuted pilon fractures in which the additional screw holes are needed for fixation.

Intraoperative radiographs are obtained after reduction and temporary stabilization to determine the adequacy of reduction. Individual interfragmentary 4.0 cannulated cancellous screws are placed perpendicular to the plate to secure fragments not addressed by the plate-screw complex. The majority of fragments are stabilized by the interfragmentary screws placed through the plate.

Wound closure is carried out over suction drains. If swelling has progressed, which usually is the case, the medial incision only is closed. This is to protect the plate, exposed tibia, and tendon. The lateral incision is left open. The initial posterolateral placement of the incision protects the lateral plate. Wires then are placed in the skin laterally for a delayed closure at the bedside in 5 to 10 days. Procedures such as relaxing skin incisions or pie crusting of the skin are not advisable because they lead to further devascularization of the skin. The potential need for skin flaps as a result of skin complications should be recognized early and addressed. Local flaps are not recommended.

Postoperative Care

The patient is placed in a well-padded posterior splint in the operating room. The drains are removed, and incisions and skin visualized on the second postoperative day. The patient then is maintained in a non–weight-bearing, short-leg, removable splint for 8 to 12 weeks. Gentle active range of motion is begun 1 week after surgery. In cases for which the degree of comminution is extensive and the stabilization suboptimal, the patient is placed in a non–weight-bearing cast for 4 weeks. This is changed to a removable splint for an additional 8 weeks. Patient education concerning the severity of injury, potential prognosis, and non–weight-bearing status is imperative. Routine radiographs evaluating bony healing are obtained. Progressive partial weight bearing to full weight bearing is permitted with evidence of metaphyseal consolidation at 10 to 16 weeks.

Complications

A number of complications of the operative fixation of pilon fracture treatment have been alluded to in the previous section.

Skin Necrosis

Operating through compromised skin, ill-advised skin incisions, or traumatic handling of soft tissue during the procedure can lead to skin necrosis. Early recognition of this problem and appropriate flap coverage may prevent subsequent complications.

Inadequate Reduction or Loss of Reduction

Varus angulation can occur if only lag screw fixation is used without buttress plate stabilization. If needed, subsequent late reconstructive procedures or tibiotalar fusion can be undertaken.

Delayed Union or Nonunion

Delayed union or nonunion is relatively common in severely comminuted fractures with rates of approximately 25 percent nonunion and 25 percent malunion, respectively, in a recent study by Bourne. Additional bone grafting or hardware stabilization with external fixation may be indicated.

Infection

Superficial. Because of the degree of soft tissue compromise, wound cellulitis is not an uncommon complication. Prompt recognition and antibiotic treatment are needed to prevent deep infection.

Osteomyelitis. Because of the high level of trauma, infection frequently is mentioned as a complication. In our experience over the past 5 years, several cases of osteomyelitis have occurred with type III C open pilon fractures. Two of these patients underwent multiple operative procedures and subsequently opted for below-knee amputations.

Osteoarthritis

With incongruities of the tibiotalar joint, post-traumatic osteoarthritis is likely to occur. Meticulous reconstruction of the joint surface during the initial open reduction gives the best chance of preventing osteoarthritis. Even with anatomic reduction of the articular surface, the initial trauma to the cartilage may result in the development of osteoarthritis. This should be explained to the patient early in the course of fracture treatment.

SUGGESTED READING

Bourne RB, Roraback CH, MacNab J. Intra-articular fractures of the distal tibia, the pilon fracture. J Trauma 1983; 23:591–596.

Mast JW, Spiegel PG, Pappas JN. Fractures of the tibial pilon. Clin Orthop 1988; 230:68–82.

Ovadia DN, Beals RK. Fractures of the tibial plafond. J Bone Joint Surg 1986; 68A:543–551.

Ruedi TP. Fractures of the lower end of the tibia into the ankle joint: Results nine years after open reduction and internal fixation. Injury 1973; 5:130–134.

Ruedi TP, Allgower M. Fractures of the lower end of the tibia into the ankle joint. Injury 1969; 1:92–99.

Ruedi TP, Allgower M. The operative treatment of intraarticular fractures of the lower end of the tibia. Clin Orthop 1979; 138:105–110.

CRUSH INJURIES AND COMPARTMENT SYNDROMES

MARK MYERSON, M.D.
WILLIAM C. McGARVEY, M.D.

This chapter outlines the diagnosis and treatment of crush injuries of the foot used at our institution. We present the pathogenesis of compartment syndromes of the foot and outline an approach to fasciotomy based on the compartmental anatomy and the injury sustained.

PATHOGENESIS

Compartment syndrome of the foot results from local tissue pressure elevation in a closed osseofascial space leading to compression of local tissues, myoneural ischemia, and neurovascular compromise. Following a crush injury, fracture, or dislocation, bleeding occurs within closed spaces in the foot. With an increase in transudate, interstitial fluid pressure rises. In the face of inelastic osseofascial compartments, this rise in pressure is not dissipated easily and leads to a decrease in capillary perfusion followed by local venous hypertension. Any increase in venous pressure causes reduction of the arteriovenous gradient and obstruction of capillary flow. Once this gradient is compromised, the capillary flow either ceases or is not substantial enough to meet local metabolic demands. This may happen concurrently with sustained arterial flow and palpable pedal pulses.

Several descriptions of the osseofascial compartments exist. By and large, however, there are only five functionally significant compartments and most other accounts are of anatomic interest only. There are four primary compartments—medial, lateral, central, and interosseous—and a fifth calcaneal or deep central compartment (Fig. 1). For a detailed description of these compartments, we suggest referring to previous reports on this subject.

DIAGNOSIS

There are *no* absolute signs nor symptoms consistent with a diagnosis of compartment syndrome in the foot. Diagnosis relies on overall impressions, including the history of the injury, as well as a constellation of signs and symptoms consistent with myoneural ischemia.

Generally the foot is extremely swollen, and light digital pressure gives a "feel" of tension. The hallmark of a compartment syndrome is pain. Although this typically is severe, relentless, and unremitting, it may not appear out of proportion to the type of injury sustained.

It also may be difficult to discern the pain arising from myoneural ischemia from that of multiple fractures and direct nerve trauma. Gentle passive dorsiflexion of the hallux and toes causes agonizing pain if the intrinsic muscles are ischemic. Sensory losses are not reliable in the setting of acute foot trauma associated with massive swelling. Two-point discrimination and light touch, particularly of the plantar aspect of the foot and the toes, probably are more reliable indicators of neural compromise than pinprick. One should never rely on circulatory compromise to diagnose myoneural ischemia. The pulse notoriously is unreliable, particularly since massive swelling usually is present, obscuring palpation. However, a thorough vascular examination is both prudent and helpful in the management of these injuries. Patients at high risk, i.e., following crush injury, should be monitored frequently to ensure that a compartment syndrome does not evolve. Repeated manipulations of fractures are contraindicated because this may stimulate further swelling, cause further bleeding, and generally potentiate the development of a compartment syndrome. Circumferential constrictive dressings or casts have no place in the acute management of a crush injury. Instead, a large, soft, bulky dressing should be applied to allow for further swelling, easy inspection, and better patient comfort. The foot should be placed in a position at about heart level to allow for venous drainage, and not be elevated maximally because this impedes arteriolar perfusion and probably contributes to further tissue compromise.

If the initial examination of the foot is equivocal, catheterization of the involved compartments should be performed routinely (Fig. 2). We measure these compartments whenever a patient presents with an extensive crushing injury, whether open or closed, with significant swelling. Beware of the open injury, since the compartments are not decompressed automatically by the skin wound. We use a portable, self-contained monitor based on the slit catheter system to measure the pressures. It is small, hand-held, not cumbersome, and has a digital display as well as a hydrostatic pressure system built in to clear the needle tip before each reading. The medial and central compartments are measured using the abductor hallucis and first metatarsal as surface landmarks. To measure the central compartment the 18 gauge needle is advanced through the abductor hallucis muscle, recording the medial compartment pressure in doing so. The needle is advanced about 3.0 cm into the central compartment, 0.3 ml of saline is injected, clearing the needle, and the reading is recorded. The interosseous compartments are measured in two positions by introducing the needle through the second or third intermetatarsal spaces. The first dorsal interspace should not be punctured to prevent inadvertent injury to the neurovascular bundle. The deep central or calcaneal compartment is measured proximally at the level of the medial malleolus, 2 inches inferior to it, midway between the malleolus and the plantar skin. Several readings may be needed at each point to ensure accuracy and reproducibility.

Text continued on p. 269.

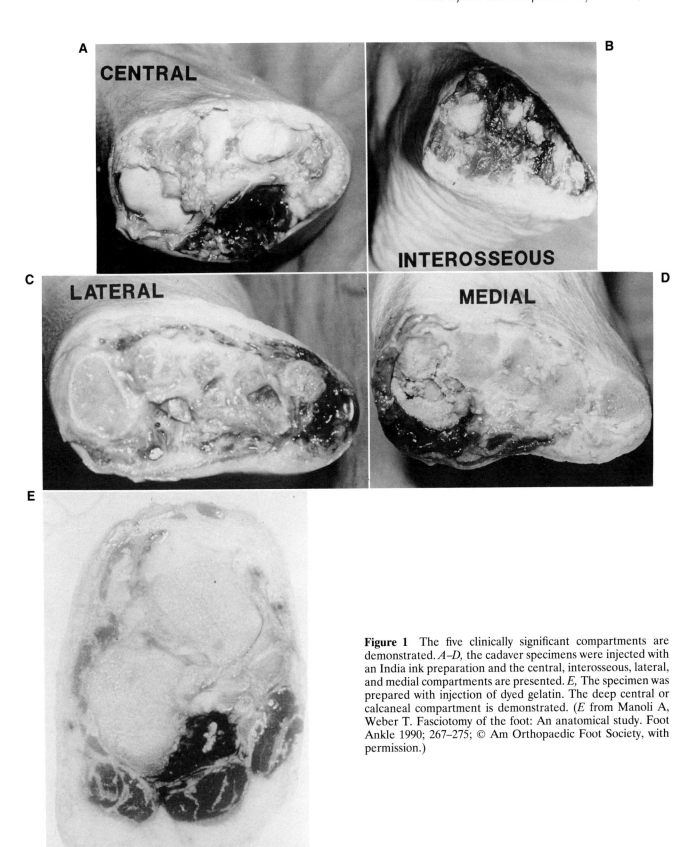

Figure 1 The five clinically significant compartments are demonstrated. *A–D,* the cadaver specimens were injected with an India ink preparation and the central, interosseous, lateral, and medial compartments are presented. *E,* The specimen was prepared with injection of dyed gelatin. The deep central or calcaneal compartment is demonstrated. (*E* from Manoli A, Weber T. Fasciotomy of the foot: An anatomical study. Foot Ankle 1990; 267–275; © Am Orthopaedic Foot Society, with permission.)

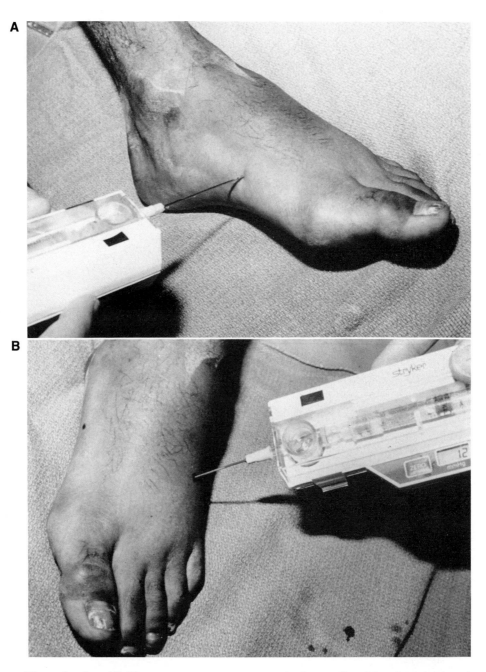

Figure 2 *A*, and *B*, The compartments are measured using needle-stick catheterization of the affected compartments.

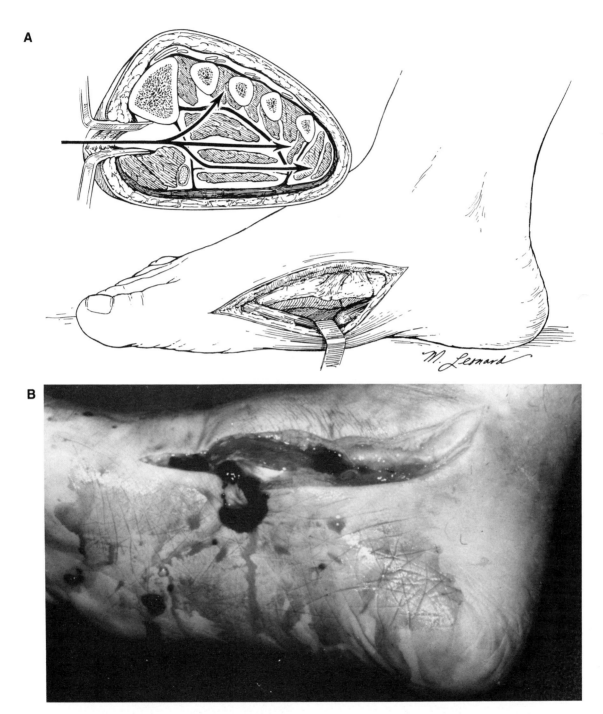

Figure 3 *A,* The medial fasciotomy incision parallels the inferior border of the first metatarsal, and the compartment is entered by retracting the abductor hallucis muscle inferiorly. *B,* Bulging of the abductor muscle following fasciotomy is common.

A

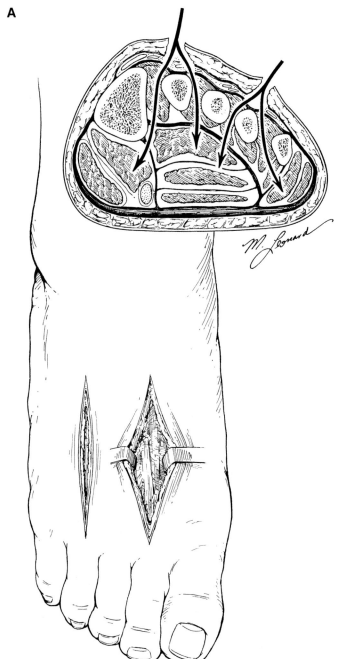

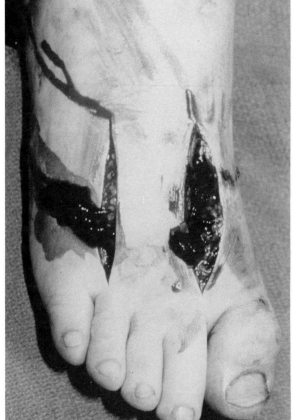

Figure 4 *A,* The dorsal approach to fasciotomy is illustrated. *B,* Following fasciotomy, hematoma typically is present in the interosseous compartments.

THERAPY

The treatment of an established compartment syndrome of the foot is expeditious fasciotomy, which we recommend if the pressure in any compartment is greater than 40 mm Hg. Many authors recommend 30 mm Hg as the threshold for fasciotomy, based on laboratory and clinical experience. However, it is difficult to know precisely when the onset of pressure elevation with subsequent symptoms began without the benefit of continuous pressure monitoring, and we therefore recommend fasciotomy for any pressure over 40 mm Hg. (These are not absolute criteria for fasciotomy since some patients become symptomatic at lower pressures while others do not.) The essence of many of these injuries is that the fracture or dislocation often requires definitive treatment, and the operative approach is modified easily to include the fasciotomy incisions. For this reason, our threshold for performing fasciotomy may be lower in an operable midfoot fracture. The principles of fasciotomy in the foot are standard. No tourniquet is used, generous incisions are made, subcutaneous fasciotomy is avoided, and the skin *never* is sutured following fasciotomy.

The approach to fasciotomy depends on the clinical setting and the associated injuries. The medial incision is a utilitarian approach originally described for use in drainage of severe plantar fascial space infections (Fig. 3). This parallels the inferior surface of the first metatarsal and provides access to the medial compartment by entering it between the metatarsal and the abductor hallucis longus muscle. After retracting the abductor inferiorly, blunt fingertip or hemostat dissection is carried out gently to prevent injuring the neurovascular bundle, and the central compartment is entered. Realistically the lateral and interosseous compartments cannot be decompressed fully with this approach. If needed the medial incision can be extended proximally to decompress the entire posterior tibial neurovascular bundle.

The dorsal approach uses two longitudinal incisions centered over the second and fourth metatarsals placed slightly medial to the second and just lateral to the fourth, to maintain as wide a skin bridge as possible (Fig. 4). Although narrow, this bridge routinely does well and does not slough if care is taken to prevent tranverse subcutaneous dissection (Fig. 5) Blunt dissection is carried out longitudinally, in line with the metatarsals with a hemostat as atraumatically as possible. Care should be taken to try to prevent perforating the subcutaneous venous plexus. Dissection is carried out down to bone and then into each interosseous compartment by proceeding medial and lateral to the metatarsal shaft. Access is obtained by piercing through the interosseous fascia. The central, medial, and lateral compartments may be entered by perforating the deep fascial layers with a curved hemostat clamp. Careful attention must be paid to this dissection so that proper planes are divided and entry is made into the appropriate compartments.

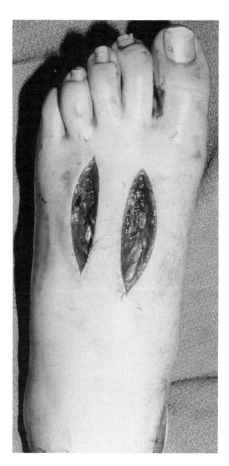

Figure 5 The skin bridge may appear narrow following fasciotomy but seldom undergoes necrosis.

The hematoma and copious edema fluid usually drain following the skin incision. We repeatedly have found that following the skin incision, once the superficial fascia is pierced the hematoma is released. Further dissection occasionally, but not always, yields more transudate and hematoma. Therefore, for practical purposes the dorsal incisions are essential, but tearing of the limiting fascial membranes probably occurs with injury, making dissection into each compartment less important.

Following fasciotomy, the skin may be covered with porcine allograft or a semisynthetic skin substitute to minimize postoperative wound edema and provide a bacteriostatic barrier. The allograft should be changed every 48 hours and the synthetic graft every 24 hours. Definitive closure or coverage can be accomplished between 5 and 7 days following fasciotomy with delayed primary closure or a split-thickness skin graft. The stickiness of the biologic dressing may be used as an indicator of the readiness of the wound for the latter form of treatment. Closure of dorsal wounds is possible at this stage, but should be avoided if the edges are tenuous because suturing may necrose the already compromised dorsal skin edges. The medial incision

A   **B**

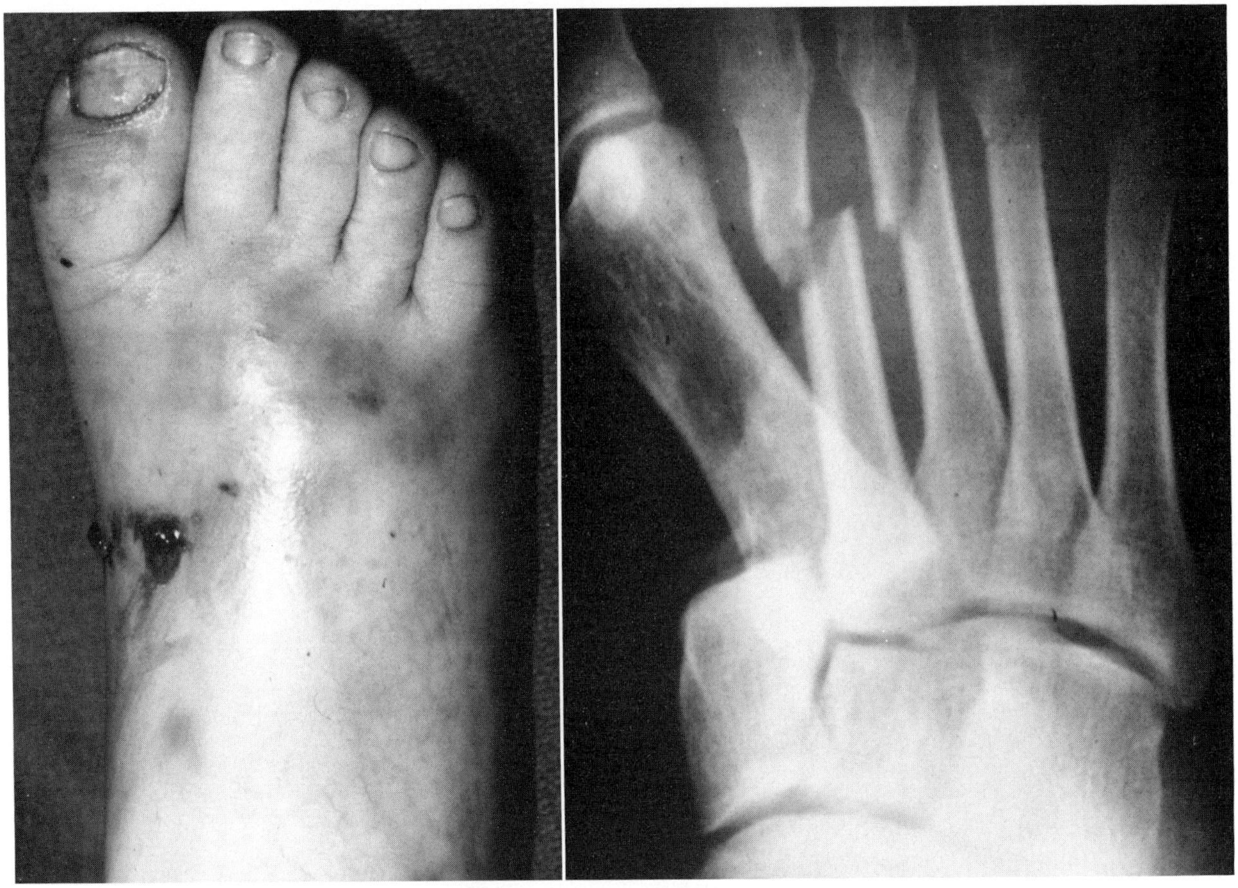

Figure 6 *A* and *B*, Compartment syndrome may be present in open fractures as demonstrated in this severe forefoot crush injury.

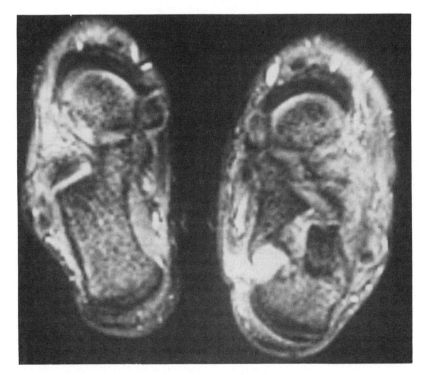

Figure 7 This oblique magnetic resonance imaging section through the posterior facet of a patient with a calcaneus fracture clearly demonstrates the large hematoma over the medial wall. This corresponds to the deep central or quadratus compartment.

A

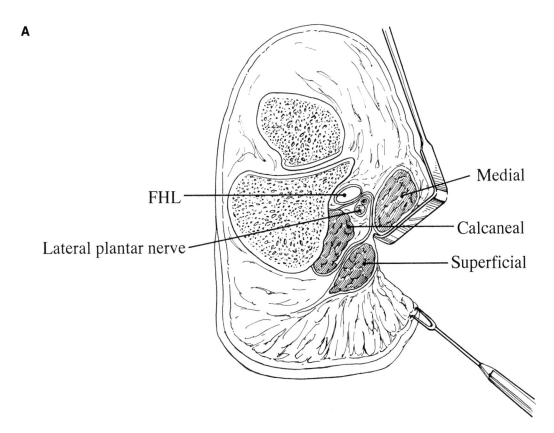

B

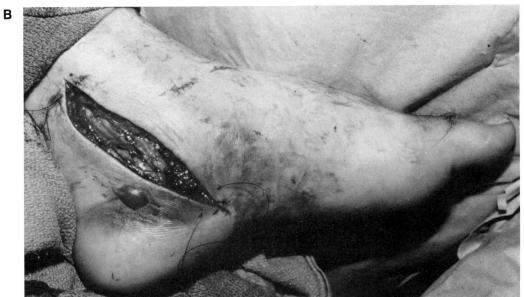

Figure 8 The surgical approach to fasciotomy for compartment syndrome associated with calcaneus fracture. *A,* The compartment is approached by elevating the abductor hallucis muscle and piercing the deep fascia overlying the quadratus muscle. FHL = flexor hallucis longus. *B,* This incision may be extended proximally to decompress the tarsal tunnel as was performed in this patient.

usually is closed secondarily, since the tissues are less thin and tenuous medially.

The decision as to which type of fasciotomy should be used is based on the clinical findings and the pattern of fracture or dislocation (Fig. 6). Both approaches provide excellent exposure and satisfactory decompression. The dorsal approach, however, is simpler to perform and avoids the more complicated anatomy of the plantar aspect of the foot. Compartment syndromes of the foot frequently are associated with fractures of the forefoot and midfoot, commonly the tarsometatarsal joint. In this setting the dorsal approach is preferable, because it offers direct access for open reduction and fixation with less trauma to the soft tissue envelope.

The medial approach provides excellent exposure and is our preference in the absence of bony injury or the need for fracture stabilization. This incision is versatile because it is easily extended proximally to decompress the posterior tibial neurovascular bundle in the presence of an acute tarsal tunnel syndrome, which occurs occasionally following calcaneus fractures.

COMPARTMENT SYNDROME AND CALCANEUS FRACTURE

It has become more obvious that bony and ligamentous injuries are not the sole culprits in either acute or residual impairment after calcaneal fractures. Soft tissue injury, particularly following compartment syndromes, causes significant chronic pain and dysfunction if untreated.

The deep central or "calcaneal" compartment is the one directly affected in this setting. As the hematoma expands and interstitial fluid accumulation escalates, the osseofascial attachments of the plantar aponeurosis remain tight, preventing penetration of blood and fluid into surrounding subcutaneous tissues (Fig. 7). Intracompartmental pressures rise and the deep plantar muscle group, particularly the quadratus plantae, is the first affected. The lateral-plantar nerve courses though this compartment. The combination of muscular and neural involvement gives rise to the findings of pain with passive dorsiflexion of the toes, burning in the toes and plantar foot, particularly in the distribution of the lateral-plantar nerve.

The fasciotomy incision is inferior to the medial malleolus, between it and the plantar skin (Fig. 8). It is carried anteriorly for about 6 cm and down to the medial fascial wall. Flaps are raised both superiorly and inferiorly (Fig. 9). Following this, a longitudinal fascial splitting incision is made 4 cm from the inferior border of the plantar aponeurosis. The abductor hallucis muscle is retracted superiorly, exposing the lateral fascial wall of the medial compartment. The muscle is stripped from the fascial attachments, and then the fascia lying superior to the plantar fascia is elevated and incised, taking care to prevent injury to the lateral-plantar neurovascular bundle. The incision is carried distally and thereby decompresses the calcaneal compartment. Fur-

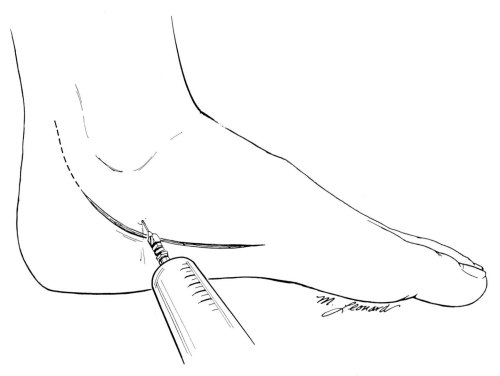

Figure 9 The position for insertion of the needle to measure the deep central or calcaneal compartment is demonstrated with the surface marking for the fasciotomy incision.

ther compartmental decompression may be carried out through either this incision or the dorsal incisions as previously discussed.

Fasciotomy is the standard of care for treatment of this problem and is true irrespective of whether treatment of the fracture is to be closed or open. Failure to address this problem may result in plantar muscle contractures and rigid painful clawing of the toes. Recent reports indicate that over 50 percent of unresolved compartment syndromes proceed to these deformities, which almost invariably are recalcitrant to all forms of conservative therapy.

At present we recommend performing fasciotomy immediately on diagnosis. If the calcaneus fracture warrants treatment by open reduction and internal fixation, this is best performed simultaneously by turning the patient for a lateral operative approach. Many patients are not prepared adequately for surgery, and since adequate imaging including a computed tomographic scan seldom is available immediately, and we often defer operative fracture care 5 to 7 days following fasciotomy, when the medial incision is closed.

SUGGESTED READING

Heckman JD, Champine MJ. New techniques in the management of foot trauma. Clin Orthop 1989; 240:105–114.

Myerson MS. Acute compartment syndromes of the foot. Bull Hosp Joint Dis 1987; 47:251–261.

Myerson MS. Split thickness skin excision: Its use for immediate wound care in crush injuries of the foot. Foot Ankle 1989; 10:54–60.

Myerson MS, Burgess AR. Initial evaluation of the traumatized foot and ankle. In: Jahss, MH, ed. Disorders of the foot. Philadelphia: WB Saunders, 1992.

Omer GE, Pomerantz GM. Initial management of severe open injuries and traumatic amputations of the foot. Arch Surg 1972; 105:696–698.

SPLIT-THICKNESS SKIN EXCISION AND GRAFTING

JOHN A. PAPA, M.D.

Degloving and crush injuries involving the foot and ankle represent a challenging management problem. The unique function and limited bulk of overlying protective subcutaneous tissue and intrinsic muscle mass render a multitude of vital structures vulnerable to injury. The final results of treatment of open or crush injuries of the foot are highly dependent on the initial management of the all-important soft tissue envelope.

PRINCIPLES OF TREATMENT AND THERAPEUTIC ALTERNATIVES

Several basic principles should be carried out in the management of all injuries associated with soft tissue compromise. Deep cultures should be obtained in the presence of open wounds and broad-spectrum intravenous antibiotics administered. Careful examination for the presence of a compartment syndrome should be performed routinely and fasciotomies done when indicated. Markedly displaced fractures or dislocations should be reduced acutely and internal or external fixation devices used to provide stability of osseous and soft tissue structures.

The treatment of compromised soft tissues is associated with the greatest controversy. Several options exist for the initial management of crushed or avulsed soft tissue flaps. One option is to reapproximate avulsed flaps and leave crushed skin alone, allowing devitalized tissues to declare themselves and thus "demarcate." This wait-and-see approach has several important disadvantages. By leaving nonviable tissue in a compromised area, bacterial proliferation with potential extension of the zone of injury can occur. In addition, increased tissue hypoxia and an increased concentration of free radicals and lysosomal proteases also are associated with delayed debridement and may further compromise the injured foot and ankle. A second approach involves the aggressive initial debridement of all nonviable portions of crushed skin or degloved flaps. Debridement includes associated underlying subcutaneous tissue and relies on the accurate initial differentiation of viable from nonviable tissue. Inaccurate determination of viability has presented the most common barrier to the routine employment of aggressive early debridement. Clinical signs including color, consistency, turgor, capillary refill, and bleeding frequently have proven unreliable.

A variety of techniques are employed to differentiate viable from nonviable tissue. Fluorescein testing is a useful tool to assess the viability of crushed skin or avulsed flaps. Fluorescein is a phenolphthalein dye, which when subjected to ultraviolet lights results in temporary electron excitement. The return of the fluorescein molecule to a stable energy state is associated with photon emission that produces a gold-green fluorescence. The intensity of the clinically observed fluorescence is proportional to the extracellular concentration of fluorescein in the injured skin and therefore allows a means to access the skin's effective capillary perfusion accurately. Following a test dose to identify idiosyncratic reactions, fluorescein is given intravenously in doses of 20 to 30 mg per kilogram of body weight. Viable skin fluoresces and can be distinguished from adjacent nonviable nonfluorescent areas. Compared with clinical appearance, fluorescein assessment of injured skin and subcutaneous tissue viability is superior. However, this technique unfortunately is not always reliable. The presence of peripheral arterial venous shunting following acute injury may impair fluorescein-aided assessment of viability. The presence of ecchymosis and dark skin pigmentation in African American patients obscures fluorescence and therefore also limits the usefulness of this technique.

PREFERRED APPROACH

Split-thickness skin excision (STSE) is a technique that was developed in an effort to improve the accurate determination of skin viability acutely. It has proven to be a reliable and accurate means of precisely defining the zone of injury and allows an aggressive approach to early debridement of nonviable tissue.

STSE does not require highly specialized instruments or prolonged intraoperative delays. Once obvious nonviable tissue has been debrided, avulsed skin and subcutaneous flaps are sutured temporarily back to their original bed (Figs. 1 and 2). Areas of crushed skin likewise are left in place. A split-thickness skin graft (0.012 to 0.015 inch thick) then is harvested from both the area of crushed skin or avulsed flap and a portion of the immediately adjacent normal-appearing skin. Careful inspection of the donor surface then is performed in an effort to identify evidence of dermal capillary bleeding. Such bleeding is a reliable and accurate indicator of skin and subcutaneous viability. Nonviable areas are identified by their lack of punctate bleeding and then are debrided sharply. Debridement includes the skin, the subcutaneous tissue, and occasionally the underlying muscle. An effort is made to preserve paratenon and periosteum, which provide well-vascularized surfaces and enhance eventual wound coverage.

Once all nonviable tissue has been removed, consideration must be given to the appropriate timing of wound coverage. Delayed coverage following an interval of several days to 1 week traditionally has been employed in hopes of minimizing the risk of subsequent infection. Such a delay in coverage is probably advisable when dealing with injuries associated with gross contamination or potentially nonviable muscle or in patients with farm

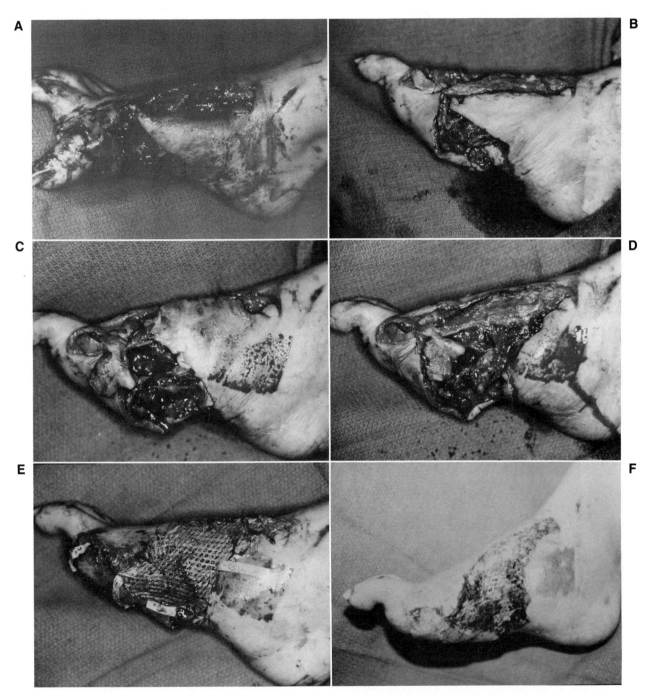

Figure 1 *A,* Initial appearance of the foot following a degloving injury. Note the partially avulsed flap (proximally based). *B,* The partially avulsed flap sutured temporarily back to the original bed. *C,* A split-thickness skin graft is harvested from a flap of questionable viability and an adjacent more normal-appearing area. Punctate capillary bleeding allows accurate differentiation of viable from nonviable tissue. *D,* Appearance following sharp debridement of nonviable tissue. *E,* The previously harvested split-thickness skin graft is meshed and applied to provide early soft tissue coverage. *F,* The apperance of the same foot several weeks later shows excellent take of split-thickness skin graft.

A, B   **C**

D, E

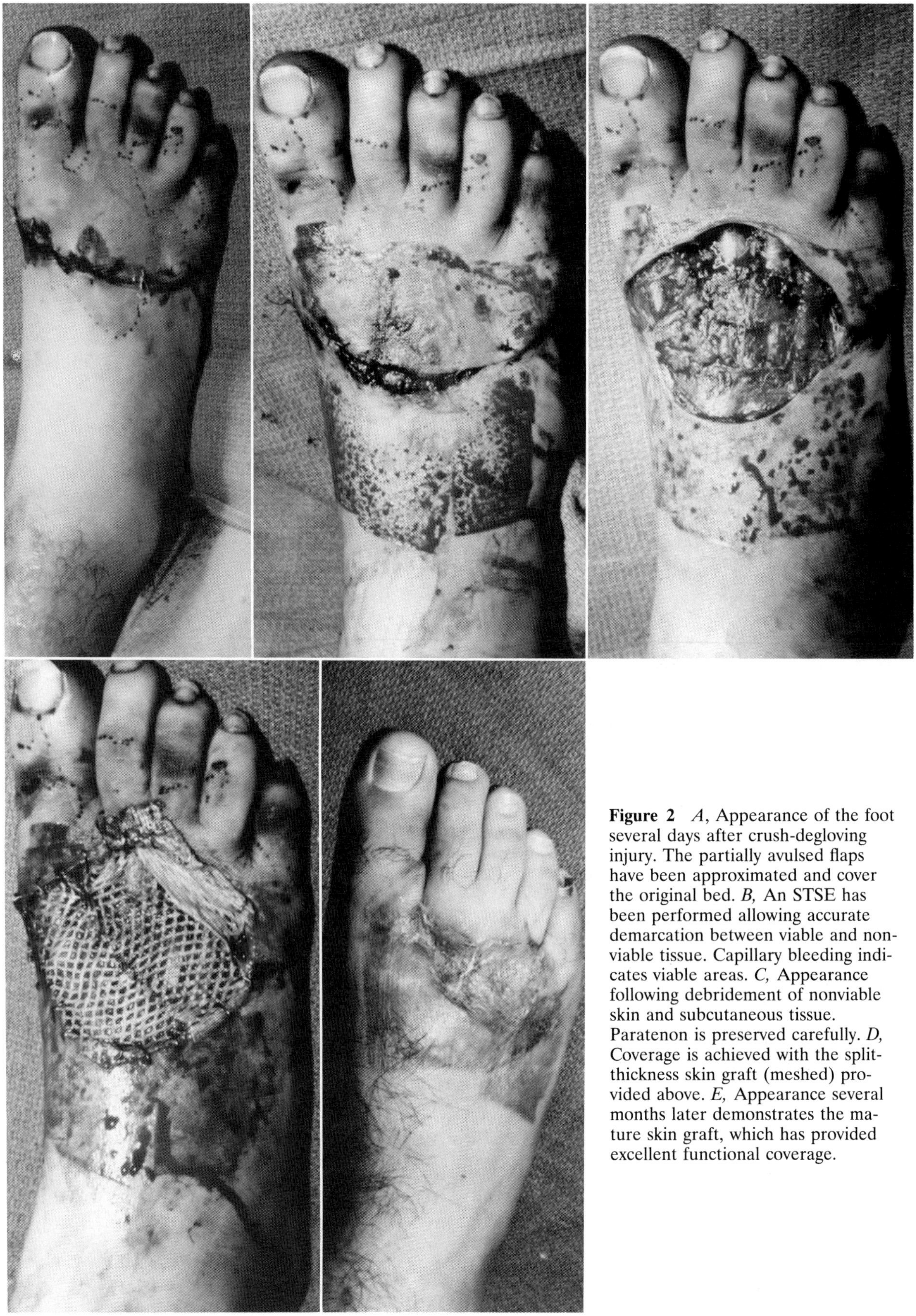

Figure 2 *A*, Appearance of the foot several days after crush-degloving injury. The partially avulsed flaps have been approximated and cover the original bed. *B*, An STSE has been performed allowing accurate demarcation between viable and nonviable tissue. Capillary bleeding indicates viable areas. *C*, Appearance following debridement of nonviable skin and subcutaneous tissue. Paratenon is preserved carefully. *D*, Coverage is achieved with the split-thickness skin graft (meshed) provided above. *E*, Appearance several months later demonstrates the mature skin graft, which has provided excellent functional coverage.

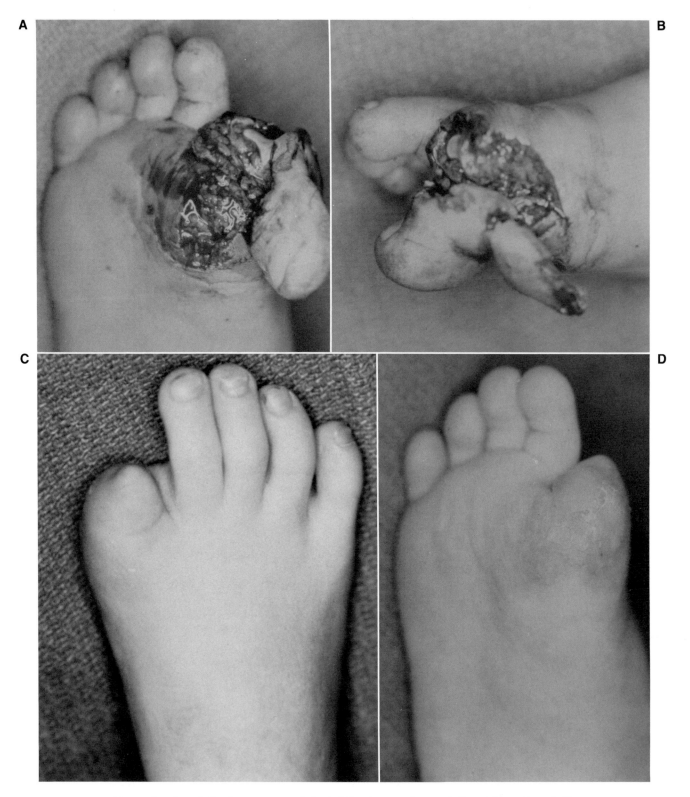

Figure 3 *A* and *B*, Appearance of foot following crush-amputation injury. *C* and *D*, Appearance several months later following primary amputation and application of split-thickness skin graft harvested from the amputated part. Skeletal shortening is minimized by the use of the split-thickness skin graft.

injuries. Delays in coverage, however, result in increased hospitalization time and potential colonization of open wounds.

The immediate coverage of a variety of wounds involving the foot and ankle can be performed successfully. STSE is uniquely suited to achieve immediate coverage. When performed acutely, the cells in the split-thickness skin graft harvested from compromised skin remain viable and survive when placed on a well-nourished bed. The harvested graft is meshed 1:1.5 and loosely applied to the open wound. It then is secured with 5-0 chromic catgut sutures and/or staples. A petroleum-based gauze (Adaptic) is used to cover the graft before applying a bulky gauze compression dressing moistened with sterile saline. The extremity then is splinted in a neutral position. The initial dressing change is performed carefully at 48 hours, then daily thereafter until good adherence of the graft to the underlying bed. For large wounds following degloving or crush injuries, additional split-thickness skin graft may be harvested from a distant site as needed.

Concern with the potential development of infection is justified when associated with the practice of immediate coverage of an open traumatic wound. In fact, wounds with potentially nonviable muscle or those associated with gross contamination or farm injuries are not thought to be appropriate for immediate coverage. However, this technique is highly effective and associated with a low infection rate when employed for most crushing or degloving injuries of the foot and ankle. Meshing of the harvested split-thickness skin graft not only provides increased coverage potential, but probably also allows adequate drainage in keeping with the traditional practice of open wound management.

STSE also can be effectively used in the treatment of crush amputation injuries involving the foot. The zone of injury can be determined accurately, and a source of split-thickness skin graft is provided for coverage. Superior functional results can be obtained by alleviating the skeletal shortening usually required for primary local flap coverage. This allows maximal preservation of stump length, which has been shown to be associated with improved function. Skin graft harvested through STSE or from a distant site then can be used to provide immediate coverage of the partially amputated foot (Fig. 3).

Survival of transplanted skin grafts is dependent on diffusion of nutrients from the underlying bed. Optimal results are achieved when grafts are placed on a well-vascularized bed without exposed bone, cartilage, or tendon devoid of paratenon. When these conditions are not present, consideration of other means of soft tissue coverage should be made. In children, however, split-thickness skin grafts adhere to almost any bed including bone with intact periosteum or bare tendon. In addition, split-thickness skin grafts often adhere to cancellous bone surfaces in adults.

Although split-thickness skin grafts may adhere and remain viable when placed on a variety of wound locations, their long-term durability may be a significant shortcoming. This is important especially when considering coverage of specialized plantar weight-bearing areas. In addition, coverage with skin grafts does not provide an effective envelope through which future reconstructive surgery can be carried out. Finally, skin grafts frequently undergo hyperpigmentation and hyperkeratosis, particularly at the junction of the graft with normal adjacent skin, which cosmetically can be suboptimal and occasionally a source of discomfort.

Despite these limitations, split-thickness skin grafting is a simple and valuable treatment option in the care of soft tissue deficits involving the foot and ankle. Likewise, STSE is highly effective in the management of degloving and crush injuries of the foot and ankle. STSE provides a means to determine skin viability accurately and a source of split-thickness skin graft, allowing an aggressive management approach to crush and degloving injuries. Using these techniques, patient morbidity is minimized and soft tissue coverage is provided.

SUGGESTED READING

Entin MA. Roller and wringer injuries: Clinical and experimenal studies. Plast Reconstr Surg 1955; 15:290.

Kudsk KA, Sheldon GF, Walton RL. Degloving injuries of the extremities and torso. J Trauma 1981; 21:835.

McGrouther D, Sully L. Degloving injuries of the limbs: Long-term review and management based on whole-body fluorescence. Br J Plast Surg 1980; 33:9.

Myerson M. Split thickness skin excision: Its use for immediate wound care in crush injuries of the foot. Foot Ankle 1989; 10:54.

Papa J, Myerson M. Soft tissue coverage in the management of foot and ankle trauma — part I. Contemp Orthop 1991; 22:509.

Ziv I, Zeligowski A, Mosheiff R, et al. Split-thickness skin excision in severe open fractures. J Bone Joint Surg 1988; 70B:23.

NERVE REPAIR

MICHAEL J. BOTTE, M.D.
SUE C. BODINE-FOWLER, Ph.D.
FIONA L. DULBECCO, B.A.
REID A. ABRAMS, M.D.

GENERAL CONSIDERATIONS AND PREFERRED APPROACHES

Nerve Traction and Crush Injuries

Nerve trauma from *closed traction* or *crush injury* can cause either neurapraxia (in which axons and microtubules remain intact, i.e., those injuries occuring from sleep palsies), axonotmesis (in which axons are disrupted but microtubules remain intact, i.e., from concussion injury caused by gunshot wound in the nerve's vicinity), and less frequently, neurotmesis (in which both axons and microtubules are disrupted and there is complete loss of nerve continuity, i.e., nerve avulsion from talus dislocation). Neurapraxia and axonotmesis have favorable prognoses for recovery since microtubules remain intact and axons can regenerate through the original tubes. Neurotmesis from traction has a poor prognosis, even with operative repair. The poor prognosis is related to the extent of the longitudinal injury that occurs in avulsion injuries. Since many nerve lesions caused by traction or blunt trauma result in neurapraxia or axonotmesis, the favorable recovery of these lesions warrants initial observation. Operative exploration usually is reserved for neuropathies that fail to demonstrate evidence of recovery by 3 to 6 months postinjury. Since neurotmesis lesions from traction have such a poor prognosis even with operative repair, initial observation before exploration usually does not alter the prognosis or outcome.

Nerve compression injury secondary to compartment syndrome warrants special attention. Obviously the initial treatment of compartment syndrome is fasciotomy with or without specific nerve exploration for decompression. If Volkmann's ischemic contracture subsequently develops in the following weeks or months, further nerve compromise can ensue from additional nerve compression within the constricting cicatrix. Nerve exploration, decompression, and possibly neurolysis usually are indicated in these cases.

Nerve Laceration Injuries

Nerve injury from laceration, in contrast with traction and blunt trauma, involves neurotmesis lesions with a localized area of nerve damage. Compared with neurotmesis from avulsion, sharp transection may have a favorable prognosis following neurorrhaphy or graft reconstruction. Primary nerve repair usually is recommended for acute, clean injuries within 8 hours of injury.

Early operative exploration (within 6 weeks postinjury) usually is recommended if the initial wound involved contamination, infection, or crushed soft tissues. In addition, early exploration is performed if the patient presented subacutely or if the diagnosis was in question or missed at the time of initial examination.

Prognostic Factors

Many factors influence the outcome of peripheral nerve repair. Favorable factors include young age (especially in children less than 10 years old); clean nerve laceration with sharp objects (without crush or traction components); relatively early repair (primary repair performed within the first 5 to 7 days having a better prognosis than secondary repair occurring later than 7 days, and neurorrhaphy occurring after 6 months having significantly poorer outcomes); distal lacerations (i.e., closer to the motor end plates or sensory organelles) as opposed to proximal lacerations; injury to a nonmixed nerve (i.e., primarily sensory or primarily motor nerves having better prognoses than nerves with large amounts of both motor and sensory components); involvement of a nerve with a better functional recovery (the tibial nerve usually having better functional recovery than the peroneal nerves); and end-to-end repair without tension (as opposed to the need for nerve grafting or suture under tension). These factors are listed in Table 1. Poor prognostic factors include increased age, longitudinal injury or segmental lacerations to the nerve, need for delayed repair or nerve grafting, proximal nerve injuries, and lacerations to mixed motor and sensory nerves.

Although variation exists, injured axons regenerate a length of approximately 1 mm per day. This is dependent on reconstitution or presence of microtubules so that the regenerating axon has a pathway to follow. Therefore regeneration proceeds following nerve repair or following an axonotmesis lesion. There usually is an initial delay of a few days or weeks following injury before regeneration commences. This rate of axon regeneration can be used to predict roughly when motor or sensory function should return by noting the distance between the injury site and the corresponding muscle or innervated skin.

Patient Selection

Based on prognostic factors, optimal patients are relatively young and healthy, without a history of peripheral neuropathy or myopathy from other causes. Primary neurorrhaphy generally should be performed in clean nerve lacerations with acute wounds less than 8 hours old. If a wound is contaminated heavily or has remained open for an extended period, bacterial colonization becomes more of a concern, and a delayed nerve repair is preferable. In these cases the wound should be irrigated and debrided thoroughly, and depending on contamination, either packed open or closed over a drain. When the wound has healed successfully and infection avoided (preferably within 2 weeks of original injury), the neurrorhaphy can be performed in a sterile environment.

Timing of Nerve Repair

As outlined above, the timing of surgery depends on the type of injury, condition of the wound, time of presentation, and condition of the patient. Primary repair is most desirable if wound and patient status permit. We prefer to repair clean lacerations that present within 8 hours acutely as an emergency procedure.

Advantages of primary repair include one surgical procedure; easier nerve alignment aided by topograpphy such as surface vessels, unscarred fascicular arrangement, relatively unchanged nerve cross-sectional shape; and the position of the nerve usually has not changed, migrated, or retracted as much as in delayed repairs. The dissection is easier without adhesions and avoids the need for secondary exploration of scarred neurovascular bundles, which is difficult, time-consuming, and risks further neurovascular injury. Electrical stimulation (within 72 hours) of the nerve ends can be performed in the awake patient for identification of motor (distal stump stimulation) and sensory (proximal stimulation) fascicles. Nerve alignment is aided in the acute situations by visible surface vessels present on both distal and proximal stumps.

For contaminated wounds, neurorrhaphy is performed as soon as the wound has healed without infection (preferably within 7 to 14 days) and a sterile environment is anticipated. Repair of crushed or avulsed nerves is performed at approximately 2 to 3 weeks to allow for both wound healing and for the proximal end of the nerve to demarcate between viable fascicles and scar tissue. For patients who present late with a healed wound (i.e., weeks or months postinjury), delayed end-to-end repair can be carried out as long as undue tension is not present. Although the upper limits of timing for nerve repair are not well established, it is known that results are significantly worse 6 months following injury. However (depending on the other prognostic factors), nerve repair or graft has been performed with limited success on pure sensory nerve lacerations at 3 years and pure motor nerve injuries at 2

years. Degradation of the motor end plates, muscle degeneration, and fibrosis are the limiting factors for successful repair or graft of motor nerves. Most information on timing of repair has become available from reports of neurorrhaphy in the upper extremity. Advantages of delayed or secondary repair of nerves include less potential for infection and improved ability of the surgeon to discern viable fascicles from scarred tubules, thickened epineurium (for easier repair), and commencement of wallerian degeneration. In addition, neurotrophic factors from the distal stump may assist the regenerating axons in finding the proper microtubules, and the nerve cell body may be metabolically more primed for regeneration.

Preoperative Preparation and Required Equipment

Suggested necessary equipment and materials include (1) an operative microscope with $10\times$ to $40\times$ magnification; (2) $2.5\times$ to $6\times$ loupe surgical telescopes; (3) a set of microsurgical instruments for the surgeon and assistant; (4) 7-0 to 11-0 fine, atraumatic, monofilament nylon or Prolene sutures; and (5) bipolar electrocautery, background contrast material, and microsponges. Other helpful instruments include a nerve stimulator for localization of lesion or verification of nerve and a demagnetizer for the microinstruments. Equipment is listed in Table 2.

The initial nerve dissection is performed with surgical telescope (loupe) magnification. Loupes of

Table 1 Favorable Factors Influencing Results of Peripheral Nerve Repair

Young age of patient
Distal level of injury
Specific nerve involved
   Predominantly motor or sensory vs. mixed nerve
   Tibial vs. peroneal nerves
Sharp laceration vs. traction or crush
Early time to repair (within 5–7 days)
End-to-end repair vs. grafting
Primary repair vs. secondary repair

Table 2 Recommended Equipment for Primary Nerve Repair

Surgical microscope
   $10\times$–$40\times$ magnification
   Motorized foot-controlled zoom and focus
   $6°$ of adjustment
   High-intensity fiber-optic lighting
   Movable solid base
   Beam splitter for observer
   Camera mounting for medical teaching
Operating surgical loupe telescopes
   Used for nerve exploration and initial preparation
   $2.5\times$–$6\times$ magnification (we prefer $3.5\times$ wide field)
Microsurgical instrument set
   Adson forceps ($\times3$)
   Small dissecting scissors
   Small straight scissors
   Jeweler's forceps ($\times4$)
   Circular microforceps
   Microneedle holders (curved, spring-handled, nonlocking preferred)
   Microscissors (spring-handled, curved or straight)
   Nonglare contrast background material
Microsuture
   Monofilament
   Nylon or Prolene
   Sizes 7-0 to 11-0 (10-0 and 9-0 most commonly used)
   70–100 μm needles (Ethicon BV-75 or BV-50)
Microsponges
Nerve stimulator
Bipolar electrocautery
Demagnetizer

2.5× to 4.5× seem to be most versatile, since depth of field and field of view are inversely proportional to amount of magnification, and higher magnification limits depth of field. The authors prefer 3.5× wide-field loupes for most applications of nerve exploration or dissection.

The final nerve preparation and neurorrhaphy are performed with the operative microscope. Desirable features of the operative microscope include motorized foot-controlled focus and zoom capabilities, 6° of excursion, magnification up to 40×, high-intensity fiber-optic lighting, a movable but solid base, and a beam splitter for medical teaching and photography.

A microinstrument set for neurorrhaphy should include small dissecting scissors; small rat-tooth forceps (×3); jeweler's microforceps (×4); spring-handled microneedle holders with curved or straight tips; spring-handled microscissors; small, straight, sharp surgical scissors; circular nerve-holding forceps; and nonglare contrast background material (3 × 3 cm).

The most commonly used suture for neurorrhaphy is 8-0 through 11-0 monofilament nylon. The 10-0 nylon is satisfactory for most sensory and small motor nerves (up to approximately 3 mm in diameter) and 9-0 for slightly larger nerves (up to 5 mm). For larger nerves, such as the sciatic nerve, a pair of 7-0 or 8-0 sutures can be used in the initial approximation of nerve ends. The 70 to 100 μm ⅜ circle needles are used most often. We commonly use Ethicon nylon monofilament 10-0 or 9-0 sutures with BV-75 or BV-50 size needles.

When planning primary end-to-end neurorrhaphy, both the surgeon and the patient must be prepared for possible nerve grafting. Therefore proper preoperative counseling, discussion, and surgical consent forms must be addressed.

Choice of Procedures

The choices for repair of peripheral nerve lesions are primary versus secondary repair, as discussed earlier. Nerve grafting is considered when a large gap is present that cannot be overcome with nerve mobilization and that places a repaired nerve under greater than physiologic tension. Benefits versus risks and donor site morbidity are weighed, and when a decision is reached, the repair or graft usually is performed by end-to-end epineurial repair and/or group fascicular repair.

End-to-end epineurial repair is the most common and universal type of nerve repair (Fig. 1). The ends of the nerve are debrided and the epifascicular epineurium (the outer epineurium that surrounds the fascicles circumferentially) of one stump is sutured to the epifascicular epineurium of the other stump using simple interrupted nylon sutures. This method works well with sharply or evenly severed nerves that have primarily motor or primary sensory function (i.e., the superficial peroneal nerve or saphenous nerve within the foot). Advantages of end-to-end epineurial repair include minimal intraneural dissection, minimal vascular disruption of the nerve, and minimal inflammation from intraneural sutures. Its main disadvantage is the poten-

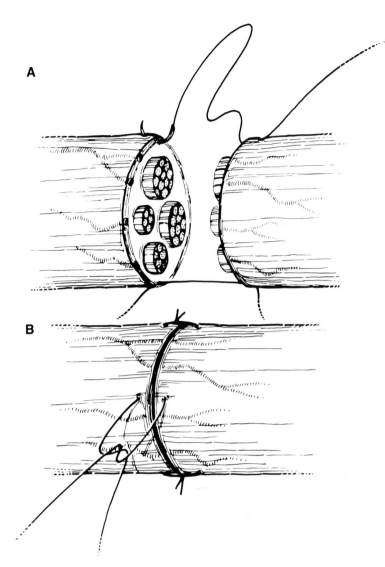

Figure 1 *A* and *B,* Diagram depicting an epineurial repair. (From Wilgis EFS. Techniques of epineurial and group fascicular repair. In: Gelberman RH, ed. Operative nerve repair and reconstruction. Philadelphia: J.B. Lippincott, 1991; with permission.)

tial for malalignment of the endoneurial tubules, an especially important consideration with repair of mixed motor and sensory nerves. Techniques used to align a nerve properly for end-to-end repair include observation of surface topography such as surface blood vessels, comparison of the cross-sectional shape and the position of the nerve ends in relation to surrounding tissues, and examination of the fascicular patterns within the nerve ends. Electrical stimulation of a nerve performed within 72 hours in an awake patient (anesthetized with local anesthetic) helps identify groups of motor fascicles in the distal stump (as noted by muscle contraction) and identification of groups of sensory fascicles in the proximal stump (as noted by the patient's verbal

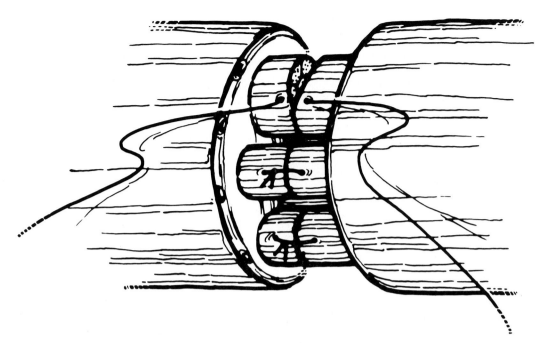

Figure 2 Diagram depicting a group fascicular repair. (From Wilgis EFS. Techniques of epineurial and group fascicular repair. In: Gelberman RH, ed. Operative nerve repair and reconstruction. Philadelphia: J.B. Lippincott, 1991; with permission.)

identification of perception of sensibility in the area previously innervated by the lacerated nerve).

When a few large groups of fascicles are identifiable (such as the tibial and peroneal portions of the sciatic nerve), a group fascicular repair can be performed (Fig. 2). Each large group of fascicles is dissected and separated as a unit. Each group of fascicles then is matched, aligned, and repaired to its corresponding group of fascicles on the opposing stump using simple interrupted nylon sutures. The sutures are placed in the interfascicular epineurium that traverses within the nerve surrounding the groups of fascicles. Group fascicular repair has the advantage of more accurate intraneural realignment. It is useful with large or mixed motor and sensory nerves, partial lacerations, uneven transections, and avulsion injuries that traumatically separate groups of fascicles. The major disadvantage of this method is that dissection to separate the groups of fascicles may disrupt intraneural vascularity further or cause mechanical trauma to the nerve. The sutures placed deep within the nerve also may cause an increase in inflammatory response or reactive fibrosis. In many cases group fascicular repair is combined with an additional outer epineurial repair.

Intraneural nerve grafting is performed electively in cases where end-to-end epineurial or group fascicular repair is not feasible. Indications for nerve grafting include a large gap (usually greater than 3 cm) or a nerve that cannot be repaired without tension or overcome with longitudinal mobilization of the nerve. Disadvantages include two suture lines that the regenerating axons must cross. Also, the procedure is longer and requires more anesthesia time, the graft is avascular, and the procedure adds another incision and the sacrifice of an additional nerve for a donor. Common donor nerves include the sural, medial antebrachial cutaneous, or lateral antebrachial cutaneous nerves.

SURGICAL MANAGEMENT OF INDIVIDUAL NERVE INJURIES

Tibial Nerve

The tibial nerve originates at the point of branching of the common peroneal nerve, approximately 10 cm proximal to the knee joint. It is vulnerable to injury anywhere along its course from the distal thigh to its terminal divisions into the medial and lateral plantar nerves. Common injury sites are the popliteal fossa (from knee dislocations or penetrating trauma) and the ankle region (from ankle fracture and/or dislocations or traction injuries from its tethered position in the tarsal tunnel). In addition, the nerve frequently is injured from grade III open tibial fractures, from partial traumatic leg amputations, and from compartment syndromes of the deep or superficial posterior compartment. The nerve and its terminal branches innervate the posterior calf muscles and most of the foot's intrinsic muscles and provide sensibility to the posterior calf and plantar foot. Muscles innervated by the tibial nerve in the calf are the gastrocnemius, plantaris, popliteus, soleus, tibialis posterior, flexor hallucis longus, and flexor digitorum longus. The nerve splits into terminal branches consisting of the medial- and lateral-plantar nerves, and more proximally, the calcaneal branch. Injury to the nerve results in loss or weakness of ankle plantar flexion, toe flexion, and weakness of ankle inversion and knee flexion. Sensibility loss occurs over the posterior calf and plantar foot. Painful dysesthesias of the foot are a perplexing and troublesome clinical problem often associated with tibial nerve injuries, especially incomplete injuries or crush injuries. These dysesthesias can develop whether the nerve lesion is treated or not treated, and the disability resulting from pain can be worse than the disability from motor paralysis or sensibility loss.

The tibial nerve enters the popliteal fossa between the deep inferior margins of the hamstring muscles. It courses superficial to the popliteal vein and artery across the popliteal fossa, giving off a contributing branch to the sural nerve, and then continues deep to the two heads of the gastrocnemius but superficial to the plantaris and popliteus. The nerve penetrates the upper margin of the soleus to continue deep to this muscle and extends distally in the superficial aspect of the deep posterior compartment of the calf. Within the deep posterior compartment of the calf, the nerve is located posterior (superficial) to the tibialis posterior and between the flexor digitorum longus (located medially) and the flexor hallucis longus (located laterally). Distally in the calf, the nerve courses medially to enter the tarsal tunnel, where it subsequently divides into the three terminal branches: the medial- and lateral-plantar nerves and the calcaneal branch. Surgical access to the nerve is not difficult in the popliteal fossa, in which the nerve is relatively superficial, lying deep to the fascia. To trace the nerve distally, however, usually requires splitting the gastrocnemius and/or soleus muscles, which can be split longitudinally in line with their fibers. In the distal fourth of the calf, the nerve becomes more superficial as it exits from the deep inferomedial margin of the soleus or Achilles tendon. The nerve can be explored by opening the tarsal tunnel and tracing the nerve proximally.

Acute, clean, complete laceration to the tibial nerve is treated by operative nerve repair on an emergency basis, as long as the wound and patient condition permit. If the laceration also is associated with a severe crush or a traction component, operative intervention is delayed for 3 to 4 weeks to allow for scar demarcation at the ends of the nerve, permitting a more accurate resection of irreversibly injured nerve ends on both the proximal and distal stumps.

Avulsion, crush, and traction injuries have relatively poorer prognoses and need to be individualized. A particularly difficult and controversial management problem is the grade III open tibial fracture or partial leg amputation, in which segmental or longitudinal injury to the nerve is noted on exploration. Recent data seem to support a less aggressive approach to salvage and reconstruction of these injuries, especially when results are compared with those of primary below-knee amputation. In addition, as mentioned earlier, incomplete injuries or traction injuries to this nerve, whether repaired or not, often lead to chronic painful dysesthesia

syndromes in the foot. In general, we have been disappointed somewhat with results of surgical repair of this nerve when a traction or crush component is suspected, when there is associated severe soft tissue injury in grade III tibial fractures, and when devascularization has required arterial repair or grafting.

Goals of repair of the tibial nerve are to provide protective sensibility to the plantar foot and restore motor function of the posterior compartment muscles of the leg. In lacerations that occur distal to the proximal tibia, many of the motor branches to the gastrocnemius and soleus are intact, and ankle plantar flexion is preserved. Prognosis for motor return in the remaining posterior leg muscles is good, because of the close proximity of the corresponding motor end plates to the nerve injury. Prognosis for the intrinsic muscle function is poor and usually not expected, except possibly in a young patient or child. If intrinsic-minus deformities subsequently develop, such as cavus foot and claw toes, these are reconstructed in a standard fashion at a later time if needed.

Traction or crush injuries usually warrant observation for 6 to 12 weeks. For penetrating injuries with nerve deficit or those thought to be a neurotmesis, acute exploration and end-to-end epineurial repair are indicated if the wound and patient condition permit. Delayed repair is performed for contaminated wounds, delay in patient presentation, and the systemically unstable patient. In the grade III open tibial fracture or severe crush injury with extensive muscle destruction or dysvascularity, especially with severe skin and soft tissue loss, a difficult decision exists between performing a primary amputation versus aggressive revascularization. Limb salvage often later requires management of subsequent infections (often requiring multiple operative procedures), soft tissue coverage procedures, and functional reconstruction with tendon transfer and or bone grafting or osteotomy.

Common Peroneal Nerve

Peroneal nerve palsy is the most common palsy of the lower extremity, accounting for up to 15 percent of all peripheral nerve injuries. The superficial course of the common peroneal nerve and its subsequent superficial and deep peroneal nerve branches render it vulnerable to direct or indirect injury from penetrating trauma, crush, compression, or traction. Most injuries occur at the level of the distal thigh or knee.

Clinical presentation depends on the level of peroneal nerve injury. Motor loss from trauma to the common peroneal nerve involves the anterior and lateral muscle compartments, resulting in loss of ankle dorsiflexion and toe extension, and loss of foot eversion, respectively. Loss of dorsiflexion causes footdrop gait. Loss of eversion results in muscle imbalance that promotes inversion deformity of the ankle or hindfoot. Sensibility loss includes the skin innervated by the superficial peroneal nerve (distal-lateral calf and dorsum of the foot) and skin innervated by the deep peroneal nerve (first dorsal web space). Proximal lesions also result in loss of sensibility function of the lateral sural cutaneous nerve (which supplies sensibility to a portion of the lateral-proximal calf) and loss of the peroneal communication branch, which joins the medial sural cutaneous nerve (from the tibial nerve) to collectively form the sural nerve.

The common peroneal nerve originates from the lateral aspect of the sciatic nerve approximately 10 cm proximal to the knee joint. It courses along the medial border of the biceps to curve around the posterior fibular neck. The nerve laterally and anteriorly is in close proximity to the proximal fibula and continues deep to the peroneus longus and extensor digitorum longus, where it divides into the superficial and deep peroneal nerves deep to these muscles and anterior to the proximal fibula. Surgical exposure to most of the common peroneal nerve is not difficult because of its superficial course. Where it enters the lateral compartment of the calf, surgical exposure may require mobilization or splitting of the peroneus longus or extensor digitorum longus.

The common peroneal nerve is at risk for injury from a variety of causes. Iatrogenic trauma has been implicated from lateral knee reconstruction, arthroscopy, meniscectomy, total joint arthroplasty, and tibial lengthening procedures. Osteotomy of the proximal tibia, such as a closing medial wedge for valgus deformity, may stretch the common peroneal nerve. Both the superficial course and its proximity to the proximal fibula (which renders the nerves at risk for compression or tethered for traction injury) contribute to the nerve's vulnerability. Fractures of the distal femur, proximal fibula, proximal tibia, and dislocation or instability of the knee dislocation have caused injury to the peroneal nerve. Compartment syndrome involving the lateral and anterior leg compartment is an additional means of nerve injury. External compression from prolonged sleep on a hard surface from drug overdose has been observed. Improper nerve protection and padding during surgical procedures with the patient in a lateral position has resulted in nerve palsy. Additionally, the peroneal nerve has been noted to have a low ratio of epineurial tissue to fascicular cross-sectional area, which perhaps places it more at risk if its connective tissue support structure is lacking.

As outlined earlier, traction injuries initially are treated with observation. Surgical exploration may be considered if there is no clinical or electromyographic evidence of recovery for 6 to 12 weeks postinjury. If an in-continuity lesion is encountered, a decision is made regarding neurolysis versus nerve resection grafting. The decision is made with the use of the microscope and nerve stimulator as dictated by the extent that fascicular detail is preserved at the injury site, as well as the presence of electrical conduction across the injured segment. If nerve injury is asymmetric, resection and grafting may be limited to the injured section only. Certainly not all peroneal traction or compression injuries warrant exploration, even with complete lesions, and many patients can be managed adequately with an

ankle-foot orthosis or tendon transfer. These are discussed in subsequent sections.

Acute, clean, complete laceration to the common peroneal nerve is treated by operative nerve repair on an emergency basis, as long as the wound and patient condition permit. If the laceration also is associated with a severe crush or a traction component, operative intervention is delayed for 3 to 4 weeks to allow for scar demarcation at the ends of the nerve, permitting a more accurate resection of irreversibly injured nerve ends on both the proximal and distal stumps.

The common peroneal nerve may exist as two separate nerves bound together, the superficial and deep peroneal nerves, which share a common epifascicular epineurium. This anatomic arrangement lends itself to a group-fascicular repair, in which a separate neurorrhaphy is performed with each of the superficial and deep peroneal nerve components, each of which is treated as a group of fascicles. The decision of neurorrhaphy versus nerve graft is made at the time of nerve exploration and based on the ease of reapproximation of resected nerve ends and presence of segmental or longitudinal damage. If the two prepared nerve ends can be reapproximated by a single 8-0 nylon suture, direct neurorrhaphy usually can be performed.

If a gap in the nerve ends is encountered that cannot be overcome with mobilization of the nerve, reconstruction using interfascicular nerve grafting is considered. The ipsilateral sural, which may be partially nonfunctional, can be harvested as a donor. If additional graft is required, contralateral sural nerve or ipsilateral superficial peroneal nerve is used. The grafts are sutured with end-to-end repair of each graft, using 10-0 nylon monofilament sutures.

Superficial Peroneal Nerve

Isolated injury to the superficial peroneal nerve is less common than to the deep peroneal nerve. The superficial peroneal nerve innervates the peroneus longus and peroneus brevis and supplies sensibility to the distal-lateral calf and to the major portion of the dorsum of the foot. Injury results in loss of active ankle eversion, which can promote an inversion deformity or tendency, and numbness to the dorsally supplied skin of the foot. Although the sensibility deficits often can be tolerated by the patient and the motor impairment usually can be controlled with an ankle-foot orthosis, nerve repair in acute sharp lacerations is thought to be indicated not only to restore the motor and sensory deficits, but also to prevent painful neuromata that often are more disabling than the motor and sensibility impairments alone.

The superficial peroneal nerve courses through the lateral compartment of the calf. The nerve originates at the bifurcation of the common peroneal nerve at or distal to the anterolateral margin of the fibular neck. The nerve continues distally in the lateral compartment near the septum that separates the superficial and anterior compartments (anterior peroneal septum). The nerve extends superficially in the anterolateral portion of the compartment, adjacent to the peroneus longus (in the proximal portion of the compartment) and adjacent to and anterior to the peroneus brevis (in the mid and distal portion of the compartment). The nerve exits the compartment and pierces the deep fascia to become subcutaneous in the distal portion of the calf. In this region the nerve usually bifurcates and continues along the anterolateral calf, passing superficial to the superior and inferior extensor retinaculi. The nerve crosses the anterolateral ankle and further branches to extend over the dorsum of the foot as far medially as the medial aspect of the metatarsophalangeal joint. Surgical access to this nerve is not difficult throughout most of its course because of its superficial location in the compartment and subcutaneous location in the distal calf and foot. However, in the proximal portion of the lateral compartment of the leg, the nerve passes deep to the peroneus longus, and surgical exposure may require mobilization, splitting, or partial detachment of the muscle.

The superficial location of the nerve on the lateral side of the calf renders it vulnerable to penetrating injuries. In addition, fractures of the fibula and tibia, compartment syndrome of the lateral compartment, traction injuries or laceration from tibial osteotomy, and the variety of causes as listed in the preceding section are possible. An unusual but frequently occurring injury in our institution has been nerve lacerations sustained by water-skiers, divers, and boat enthusiasts cut by propeller blades.

Traction injuries initially are treated with observation. Surgical exploration may be considered if there are no clinical or electromyographic signs of recovery for 6 to 12 weeks postinjury. If a lesion in continuity is encountered, a decision is made whether to perform a neurolysis or to resect the injured nerve segment and perform nerve grafting. Because many patients can be managed with orthotic devices or tendon transfer for motor dysfunction of the lateral compartment, one must weigh the risks, benefits, and prognosis to nerve grafting. It can be difficult to localize the area of injury in a traction injury to this nerve. Compression or ischemic injuries from compartment syndrome are managed acutely with fasciotomy, and for chronic compression in a constricting cicatrix, neurolysis can be performed. Nerve grafting, however, usually is not performed for injury from compartment syndrome because of the longitudinal extent of injury. Tendon transfer or orthosis management ultimately can be performed to improve function.

We prefer to treat acute laceration to the superficial peroneal nerve by emergent operative nerve repair if the wound is clean and patient condition permits. When the patient presents late (>8 hours) or the injury occurred in fresh or salt water from boat propeller blades, we have preferred delayed repair to allow the wound to heal and decrease the chance of infection following neurorrhaphy. Potential *Mycobacterium marinum* infections are worrisome problems associated with these injuries occurring in lakes or in the ocean. If the laceration also is associated with a severe crush or a traction component,

operative intervention is delayed for 3 to 4 weeks to allow for scar demarcation at the ends of the nerve, permitting a more accurate resection of irreversibly injured nerve ends on both the proximal and distal stumps.

End-to-end epineurial repair usually is the most feasible for this nerve. The size of the superficial peroneal nerve usually is between 2 and 4 mm and repair usually can be performed with 9-0 or 10-0 sutures. In the foot, 10-0 sutures are preferred.

If a gap in the nerve ends is encountered that cannot be overcome with mobilization of the nerve, reconstruction using interfascicular nerve grafting is considered. This should be considered only when both motor and sensory deficits are present in proximal lesions of this nerve. Nerve grafting probably should not be performed for sensory-only deficits, unless a painful neuroma has formed at the nerve injury site. Donor site morbidity with resultant additional areas of sensibility loss (and neuroma formation) must be kept in mind whenever nerve grafting is considered a possibility. These lesions may be appropriate for nerve grafting using non-neural donor material such as synthetic silicone tubules or vein graft conduits.

Deep Peroneal Nerve

Injury to the deep peroneal nerve results in loss of ankle and toe dorsiflexion from paralysis of the tibialis anterior, extensor hallucis longus, extensor digitorum longus, peroneus tertius, and extensor digitorum brevis. Clinically the patient displays a footdrop gait and may develop an equinus contracture from chronic muscle imbalance. In addition, injury to the deep peroneal nerve results in loss of sensibility to the dorsum of the first web space, which has little clinical significance with the exception of its diagnostic value. However, laceration of the deep peroneal nerve can lead to painful neuroma in the foot or calf. Therefore, consideration for surgical repair in acute lacerations can be made, even to the sensory-only portion of the nerve.

The deep peroneal nerve originates from the common peroneal nerve at the level of the fibular neck or proximal fibular diaphysis. The nerve enters the anterior compartment of the calf deep to the peroneus longus and extensor digitorum longus muscles. The nerve joins the anterior tibial artery, in which both structures initially lie between the extensor digitorum longus and tibialis anterior muscles. Further distally, at approximately one-fourth or one-third the proximal length of the tibia, the extensor hallucis longus takes origin and the deep peroneal nerve and anterior tibial artery come to lie between the extensor hallucis longus and tibialis anterior. The nerve continues in this plane the length of the anterior compartment and continues deep to the superior and inferior extensor retinaculum (as opposed to the superficial peroneal nerve, which courses superficial to these structures). Near the level of the ankle, the nerve, along with the anterior tibial artery, pass deep to the tendon of the extensor hallucis longus to continue between the tendons of the extensor hallucis longus and the extensor digitorum longus. The nerve courses distally in the foot, along with the artery that has become the dorsalis pedis, dorsal to and between the first and second metatarsals to bifurcate proximal to the first web space and supply sensibility to that area.

Surgical access to the nerve is not difficult, except in the proximal portion of the calf, in which nerve lies deep to the extensor digitorum longus. Throughout the remainder of the anterior calf, the nerve can be explored surgically through muscle planes. Caution is required, however, since the nerve travels in close proximity to the anterior tibial vascular structures. This is relevant especially in a delayed exploration, in which adhesions between nerve and vascular structures risk further damage to both nerve and vessels.

The deep peroneal nerve is at risk for injury from fractures of the tibia or fibula, compartment syndrome of the anterior compartment, traction injuries or laceration from tibial osteotomy, penetrating injuries, and various causes as listed in the earlier section Common Peroneal Nerve.

Traction injuries initially are treated with observation for 6 to 12 weeks. Surgical exploration may be considered if there are no clinical or electromyographic signs of recovery after that period. If an in-continuity lesion is encountered a decision is made whether to perform a neurolysis as opposed to resection of the injured nerve segment and nerve grafting. Because many patients can be managed with orthotic devices or tendon transfer to restore ankle dorsiflexion, one must weigh the risks, benefits, and prognosis to nerve grafting. Like the complexity of many traction injuries, it can be difficult to localize the exact area of nerve injury. Compression injuries from ischemic contracture can be managed with neurolysis. Nerve grafting, however, usually is not feasible because of the longitudinal extent of injury. Tendon transfer or orthosis management is the preferred treatment.

Acute lacerations to the deep peroneal nerve are treated emergently by operative nerve repair if the wound is clean and patient condition permits. Surgery usually is indicated when significant motor impairment is present. For distal nerve injuries in which sensibility deficits alone are present, surgical repair can be considered as a means of possible painful neuroma prevention. If the laceration of the deep peroneal nerve also is associated with a severe crush or a traction component, operative repair is delayed for 3 to 4 weeks to allow for scar demarcation at the ends of the nerve, permitting a more accurate resection of irreversibly injured nerve ends on both the proximal and distal stumps (see Figs. 1 and 2).

If a gap in the nerve ends is encountered that cannot be overcome with nerve mobilization, reconstruction using interfascicular nerve grafting is considered. This should be considered only when both motor and sensory deficits are present in proximal lesions of this nerve. Nerve grafting probably should not be performed for sensory-only deficits, since impairment is minimal, with the exception of problems associated with a painful neuroma at the nerve laceration site, and donor site morbidity results in an additional area of sensibility loss.

Medial- and Lateral-Plantar Nerves

Injury to the medial- or lateral-plantar nerves results in loss of respective sensibility on the medial or lateral aspect of the plantar foot, as well as motor loss to the corresponding intrinsic muscles. The patient's specific complaints are variable, from plantar numbness, intrinsic muscle palsy, and painful neuromas. Although the indications for surgical repair of these nerves is not well established, more proximal lesions should be repaired to restore plantar sensibility. More distally, repair can be considered to prevent traumatic neuroma formation. Caution must be exercised in repair of these nerves if repair requires placement or elongation of an incision on the plantar aspect of the foot, which can result in painful scar formation, especially if the incision is placed in the weight-bearing portion of the foot. Therefore risks and benefits of repair of these nerves must be weighed carefully and the treatment of each patient individualized.

The medial- and lateral-plantar nerves, the largest of the terminal branches of the tibial nerve, arise within or distal to the tarsal tunnel. These branches continue distally and plantarly coursing deep to the abductor hallucis muscle to enter the plantar aspect of the foot and continue distally between the first and second layers of plantar foot muscles. Each nerve is accompanied by its corresponding plantar artery. In the midfoot, the nerves divide into subsequent terminal sensory branches to supply the toes. Surgical access to the medial- and lateral-plantar nerves is available proximally near the origin of the two nerves (proximal to the point where the nerves course deep to the abductor hallucis brevis). Lesions deep to the abductor hallucis require mobilization or splitting of the muscle. Lesions distal to the abductor hallucis usually require fasciotomy or partial fasciectomy of the plantar fascia for exploration of the nerve between the first and second layers of muscles. In the forefoot and toes, the common digital nerves are accessible from the plantar approach. Care must be taken in the placement of incisions on the plantar foot for the operative exploration of the medial- and lateral-plantar nerves and their branches, with attempts to use the non–weight-bearing portions in the arch and base of the toes if possible. Large traumatic lacerations on the plantar foot often provide adequate exposure for exploration of these nerves.

The medial- and lateral-plantar nerves commonly are injured by penetrating trauma or crush injuries. Less frequently, hindfoot fracture or dislocation and/or iatrogenic causes including surgical exposure of calcaneas or subtalar joint, plantar fasciotomy, or partial fascietomy result in nerve injury. Traction injuries are rare, but do occur in the tarsal tunnel region in which the nerves are tethered. Crush injuries (or concomitant compartment syndrome) can cause longitudinal irreparable nerve trauma.

Traction or crush injuries of the medial- and lateral-plantar nerves initially are treated with observation for 6 to 12 weeks. Surgical exploration may be indicated if there are no clinical or electromyographic signs or symptoms of return after that period. More commonly, chronic pain from a crush injury or neuroma formation promotes surgical exploration for neurolysis or neuroma excision. As mentioned above, the risks and benefits of nerve repair must be weighed carefully, because little clinical information is available that has established the indications for repair of these nerves.

Acute lacerations or penetrating injuries to the proximal portions of the medial- or lateral-plantar nerves are treated emergently by operative nerve repair if the wound is clean and patient condition permits. Surgery usually is indicated when significant motor and sensory impairment is present. For distal forefoot nerve injuries in which sensibility deficits alone are present, repair of the nerve can be performed as a means to prevent neuroma formation. As mentioned above, caution must be exercised in the placement or elongation of incisions on the plantar foot, and risks of painful incisional scar formation must be weighed carefully against the benefits of nerve repair, especially in more distal lesions.

Sural Nerve

Laceration to the sural nerve results in loss of sensibility of the distal-lateral calf and foot. There is no motor loss. It is the nerve used most often as a source for nerve graft. Following laceration a painful neuroma may result; however, this is rare. In general, we prefer to repair the nerve if it is easily accessible and lacerated sharply; however, the indications for surgical repair of this nerve are not well established. Nerve grafting generally is not indicated, with the possible exception of treatment of a refractory neuroma.

The sural nerve is located subcutaneous just deep to the fascia of the calf. It is formed by contributions from the medial and lateral sural cutaneous nerves. The nerve courses distally and laterally and passes posterior to the lateral malleolus. It continues distally and laterally in the foot to reach the skin over the distal-lateral portion of the fifth metatarsal.

From its superficial location, the nerve is injured most often from lacerations. Iatrogenic neuroma formation can occur following harvest for nerve graft. The nerve is at risk for injury from surgical approaches to the lateral hindfoot.

Traction and crush injuries that cause disability are rare with the sural nerve. Painful neuromata can cause disability that is more disabling than sensibility loss. Traction injuries and crush injuries that cause nerve dysfunction should be treated with observation. Painful refractory neuromata are treated with neuroma excision and placement of the nerve stump in a protected environment.

Acute lacerations are treated with primary repair or with acceptance of the sensibility loss. Repair of the nerve may lessen the possibility of neuroma formation. Once formed, a neuroma is treated with neuroma resection and placement of the proximal nerve stump in a protective environment versus end-to-end repair of the nerve stumps.

SUGGESTED READING

Aldea PA, Shaw WW. Lower extremity nerve injuries. Clin Plast Surg 1986; 13:691–699.

Gorman PW, Dell PC. Instrumentation for nerve repair. In: Gelberman, RH, ed. Operative nerve repair and reconstruction. Philadelphia: JB Lippincott, 1991.

Kline DG. Operative management of major nerve lesions of the lower extremity. Surg Clin North Am 1972; 52:1247–1265.

Marsh D. Does the use of the operating microscope improve the results of peripheral nerve suture? J Bone Joint Surg 1987; 69B:625–630.

Millesi H, Terzis JK. Nomenclature in peripheral nerve surgery. Clin Plast Surg 1984; 11:3.

Wilgis EFS. Techniques of epineurial and group fascicular repair. In: Gelberman RH, ed. Operative nerve repair and reconstruction. Philadelphia: JB Lippincott, 1991.

Wood MB. Peripheral nerve injuries to the lower extremity. In: Gelberman RH, ed. Operative nerve repair and reconstruction. Philadelphia: JB Lippincott, 1991.

USE OF THE ILIZAROV FIXATOR

JASON H. CALHOUN, M.D., M. Eng.
JON T. MADER, M.D.

The Ilizarov technique, developed by Gavriil Il-izarov of Kurgan, Russia, recently has been introduced into the United States. It is a method of external fixation using gradual distraction to correct extremity deformities such as equinocavus; distal tibia nonunion, angulation, or shortening; osteomyelitis; and severe pilon fractures. Many of these problems were either difficult or impossible to manage with other techniques. This chapter discusses our use of the Ilizarov technique in the foot and ankle.

EQUINOCAVOVARUS CORRECTIONS

Mild (<20°) and moderate (20° to 40°) equinus deformities respond to the accepted techniques of

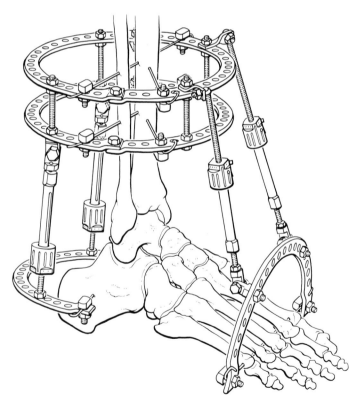

Figure 1 Ilizarov frame for equinus correction. Tibiofibular segment is secured with wires from the fibula to the tibia and the medial face of the tibia. The calcaneal wire and half-ring allows distraction of the calcaneus and the ankle joint. The metatarsal wire and half-ring (first and fifth metatarsals) allow for correction of the equinus.

physical therapy, casts, and soft tissue surgery. More severe corrections, however, have needed midfoot closing-wedge osteotomies or amputations. The causes of these deformities include burns about the foot, poliomyelitis, trauma, and congenital deformity. All frames are applied in the operating room with sterile technique and a regional or general anaesthetic. If possible, the frame is assembled preoperatively to save operating room time and to introduce the patient and the family to the fixator.

An equinus frame consists of a tibial segment, one calcaneal half-ring, and one metatarsal half-ring (Fig. 1). This frame is connected to the bone with 1.5 or 1.8 mm wires (for children and adults, respectively) that are tensioned to 110 kg-force on the full rings and 90 kg-force on the half-rings. A two-ring tibial section is preconstructed by connecting four half-rings with four small threaded rods. This is secured with two fibula to tibia–directed pins and two medial-face tibial pins at about the distal third of the leg. If preferred, half-pins can be used in place of some or all the wires for the tibial segment ("hybrid system"). The calcaneal wire is directed from the medial to lateral side to avoid the posterior tibial nerve. The calcaneal wire is located relatively proximally and posteriorly in the calcaneus to prevent wire "cut out" and increase its biomechanical advantage. The metatarsal pin also is directed from medial to lateral from the first metatarsal to the fifth metatarsal. Only these two metatarsals are pinned so a synostosis does not develop between adjacent metatarsals. Half-rings are connected to the metatarsal and calcaneal wires. The calcaneus half-ring is connected to the tibiofibular rings with distraction rods and the metatarsal half-ring is connected with compression rods. Hinges are used to allow posterior translation of the calcaneus pin and anterior translation of the metatarsal pin as the equinus deformity is corrected. The calcaneus is distracted manually in the operating room without plantar flexing the forefoot. This allows ankle joint distraction and prevents cartilage damage, as well as midfoot dorsiflexion deformity (rocker bottom).

Postoperatively deformity correction is started as soon as the patient can comfortably tolerate it (1 to 3 days). The calcaneus is pushed distally and the metatarsals are pulled proximally as rapidly as is comfortable for the patient (usually 1 to 4 mm per day). The rate of correction is slowed or stopped if traction blisters appear on the skin, which may occur with burn scars. Usually the metatarsals are moved more rapidly than the calcaneus because the metatarsal pin is farther from the ankle. Intraoperative and postoperative radiographs (1, 2, 4, and 6 weeks) are used to follow deformity correction and keep the ankle distracted 2 to 5 mm as compared to preoperative radiographs. Because the forefoot lever arm (metatarsal pin) is farther from the fulcrum (ankle) than the posterior lever arm (calcaneal pin), the metatarsals are dorsiflexed more rapidly than the calcaneus is plantar flexed. Usually the calcaneus is distracted 2 mm (0.5 mm every 6 hours), while the forefoot is dorsiflexed 3 to 4 mm per day (1.0 mm every

A

B

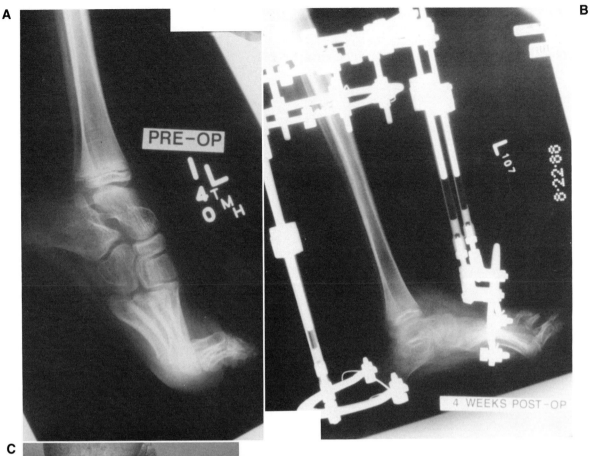

C

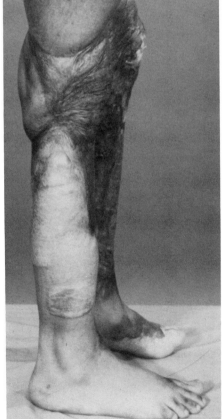

Figure 2 *A*, Radiograph of an 11-year-old boy 4 years after a burn that caused a 60° equinus deformity. *B*, Four weeks after application of the Ilizarov frame with correction of deformity. *C*, Three years after removal of the fixator, the patient's left foot (far side) is maintained in 5° of plantarflexion with the use of night splints and special shoes.

6 hours). After correction to 5° to 10° of ankle dorsiflexion, the frame is left in place for 2 to 6 weeks depending on the soft tissue rigidity. The frame is dismantled and the pins are removed, usually in the clinic with an intravenous and local anesthetic. A short-leg cast is applied for 6 weeks. Depending on the etiology and whether or not physical therapy is used, braces or orthotics as well as tendon transfer or joint fusion may be needed to prevent recurrence (Fig. 2).

Complex Equinus Deformities

More complex deformities in the foot and ankle can be corrected with modifications of this basic frame. A medial or lateral contracture (varus or valgus) with an equinus ankle makes it more difficult to correct, because the calcaneus or metatarsals "slide" on the pins until the half-ring contacts the skin. Olive or multiple wires and half-pins are used to prevent the sliding, but they increase the infection rate, risk of nerve and vessel injury, and frame complexity. Bone deformities require more complex frames, osteotomies, and longer device time. Muscle injury and nerve injury make the corrected equinus deformity difficult to maintain. Tendon lengthening, arthrodesis, casting, or a repeat Ilizarov correction may be needed to prevent or treat partial recurrence.

Cavus

Mild or moderate midfoot cavus caused by contraction of plantar tissues may be corrected with equinus correction or with the accepted techniques of a plantar fascia release or a midfoot osteotomy. Severe cavus usually has required midfoot closing-wedge osteotomies as well. Cavus is classified as severe when the metatarsal calcaneal angle is less than 120°. Mild (135° to 150°) and moderate (120° to 135°) cavus are best treated with stretching, casts, and soft tissue releases. Severe (>120°) midfoot cavus foot deformities can be corrected with the Ilizarov technique by distracting the calcaneus and metatarsal with half-rings with a medial and lateral lengthening rod (Fig. 3). The lateral rod usually is not lengthened because most of a cavus deformity is medial.

Rocker-bottom Foot

The rocker-bottom foot deformity usually is a result of dorsal contracture or overcorrection of the forefoot during equinus correction. Rocker-bottom foot deformities have been treated with midfoot osteotomies or fusions. Rocker bottom may be classified as severe when the metatarsal calcaneal angle is greater than 200°. Mild (165° to 180°) and moderate (180° to 200°) rocker-bottom deformities may respond to arch supports or dorsal soft tissue releases. The surgical technique for the Ilizarov rocker-bottom frame is similar to the cavus frame, except that a third midfoot half-ring (cuneiform to cuboid pin) is pulled dorsally to re-create the arch. A severe rocker-bottom foot with valgus, varus, external

rotation, or hindfoot problems is corrected with a more complex frame and usually requires fusions or osteotomies to maintain the correction.

Prevention

Equinocavus prevention is important if the Ilizarov technique is used for severe deformity correction above the foot and ankle. This most commonly is needed for tibial lengthening (shortness) or transport (segmental defect) of more than 4 cm. For equinus prophylaxis, a static half-ring on the calcaneus and metatarsal with the foot in the neutral position is used.

TIBIAL BONE DEFORMITY

Deformities of the distal tibia such as shortness, angulation, rotation, side-to-side translation, and nonunion can be managed with the Ilizarov technique. Usually tibial shortness is corrected by proximal lengthening. Occasionally, however, the distal tibia is lengthened for reasons of time (proximal and distal tibial lengthening), proximal tibial problems (nonunion, knee arthrodesis, infection), or distal tibia coexisting deformities (malunion).

For distal tibia malunion, the frame is similar to the equinus frame, but additional wires are placed in the talus or very distal tibia (Figs. 4 and 5). The bone is osteotomized in as gentle a manner as possible (we use a percutaneous osteotome) to prevent soft tissue injury and to speed healing. After 7 to 10 days to allow wound healing, lengthening is started. Distraction rods lengthen the tibia 1 mm per day (0.25 mm every 6 hours). Hinges are added for angular deformity correction in a manner similar to the equinus frame. Derotation and translation are done after angular and lengthening corrections have been made. Derotation is accomplished by rotating the proximal ring segment with respect to the distal ring segment. Translation is done by pushing or pulling the distal segment sideways with respect to the proximal segment.

The nonunion needs to be debrided if infected, and antibiotic therapy needs to be directed by an infectious disease specialist. The nonunion then is compressed, and bone grafting usually is used to speed healing. If an infection is present, wait 2 weeks after the debridement and the start of antibiotics before grafting. If shortness with a distal tibial nonunion is present, the tibia is lengthened proximally.

ANKLE ARTHRODESIS

We have fused 12 ankles with the Ilizarov technique (Fig. 6). This technique is helpful when internal fixation is contraindicated because of infection, bone loss, or soft tissue problems. Basically the technique is to use the same frame used for pilon fractures or distal tibia lengthening. The talus, however, is compressed into the

A

B

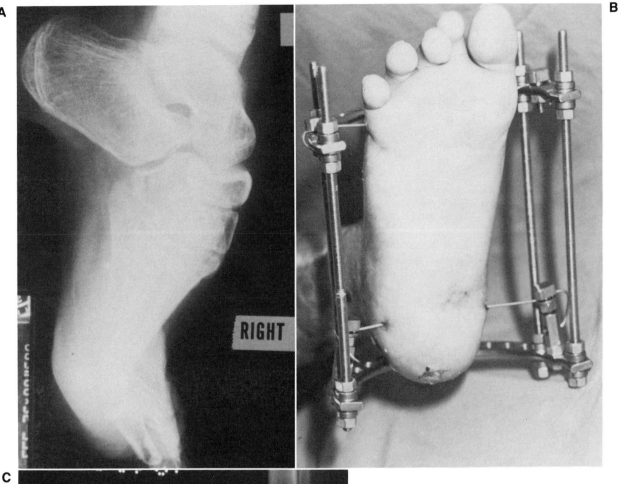

C

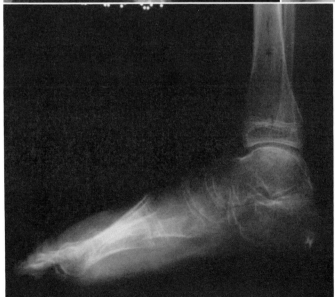

Figure 3 *A,* Preoperative radiograph of an 11-year-old boy with severe equinocavus. The equinus deformity was corrected with the same technique as the patient in Figure 2. The cavus deformity, however, required a special frame. *B,* The cavus frame. The calcaneal half-ring is distracted from the metatarsal half-ring to correct the cavus gradually. Usually most of the correction that is needed is medial. *C,* Postoperative radiograph of the corrected deformity. At 3.5 years after surgery, this patient has a plantigrade foot, normal shoe wear, and participates in all sports.

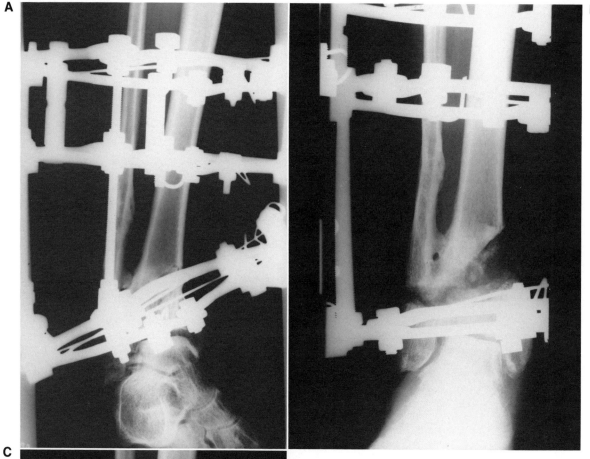

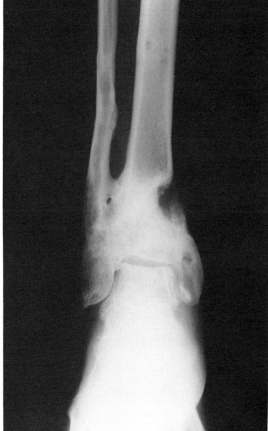

Figure 4 *A,* Radiograph of a 24-year-old white female 3 years after a motor vehicle accident with a 25° posterolateral apex malunion, 2 cm of shortness, and a tibiofibular synostosis. The frame was applied and a distal tibiofibular corticotomy was done. *B,* Two months after the frame application, the regenerate is seen to be maturing. *C,* One year after the frame was removed, the new bone has matured and the angular and shortness correction is maintained.

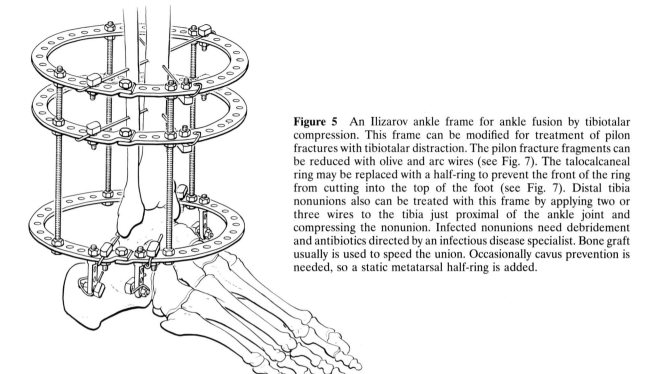

Figure 5 An Ilizarov ankle frame for ankle fusion by tibiotalar compression. This frame can be modified for treatment of pilon fractures with tibiotalar distraction. The pilon fracture fragments can be reduced with olive and arc wires (see Fig. 7). The talocalcaneal ring may be replaced with a half-ring to prevent the front of the ring from cutting into the top of the foot (see Fig. 7). Distal tibia nonunions also can be treated with this frame by applying two or three wires to the tibia just proximal of the ankle joint and compressing the nonunion. Infected nonunions need debridement and antibiotics directed by an infectious disease specialist. Bone graft usually is used to speed the union. Occasionally cavus prevention is needed, so a static metatarsal half-ring is added.

tibia by compressing the tibia frame to the foot frame 1 to 2 cm intraoperatively. Using the Doppler effect, the pulses are monitored to make sure the vessels do not collapse. Postoperatively the tibia and talus are compressed 1 mm per day until they contact, then at the rate of 1 mm per week. This weekly compression can be gradual (0.25 mm every 2 days) or all at once (1.0 mm each week). If there is significant shortness (>2 cm) from distal tibia or talar loss, the tibia is lengthened proximally. Radiographs then are used to judge fusion and proximal regenerate maturity, and the frame is removed and the leg casted.

SEVERE PILON FRACTURES

Two patients with type III (Ruedi-Allgower) tibial plafond fractures were treated with ligamentotaxis using the Ilizarov frame (Fig. 7). A calcaneotalar ring distracts the ankle. Olive wires or arch wires are used to reduce the fracture fragments. The pilon frame is left in place for 4 to 8 weeks. A short-leg cast then is applied and weight bearing is started as indicated by radiographs.

POSTOPERATIVE TREATMENT

Complications with the use of the Ilizarov fixator such as pain, infection, nerve and vessel injury, and device problems are common but manageable. Patients with pin and traction pain may need oral analgesics, often just acetaminophen (Tylenol) or nonsteroidals. Immediate postoperative oral narcotics may be needed, although older patients may need long-term analgesics.

Pin-site infection occurs frequently. This is best prevented with local pin care and by avoiding bone injury (burning) on pin insertion. During deformity corrections, patient and fixator care are important to obtain the treatment goals. Pin sponges or gauze dressings are placed around the pins in the operating room for hemostasis and sterility. These dressings can be removed after a few days, and daily bathing with soap and water is allowed. If the pin sites continue to drain or if the patients prefer, pin-site dressings are continued. Local pin-site infections are common and usually are managed with local care (hydrogen peroxide three times daily) and oral antistaphylococcal antibiotics. Pin removal, minimal debridement, deep cultures, and longer doses of antibiotics may be needed for the rare abscess or osteomyelitis.

The device problems of pin movement and breakage and contractures can be prevented by using a more stable two-ring tibial frame with wires, large (1.8 mm) wires, or half-pins with a one-ring frame. Contractures of the knee may be prevented or treated with aggressive physical therapy, a knee brace, or splint.

Adequate planning is essential for success with the Ilizarov technique in the foot and ankle. Preoperatively a thorough physical examination is necessary to docu-

A

B

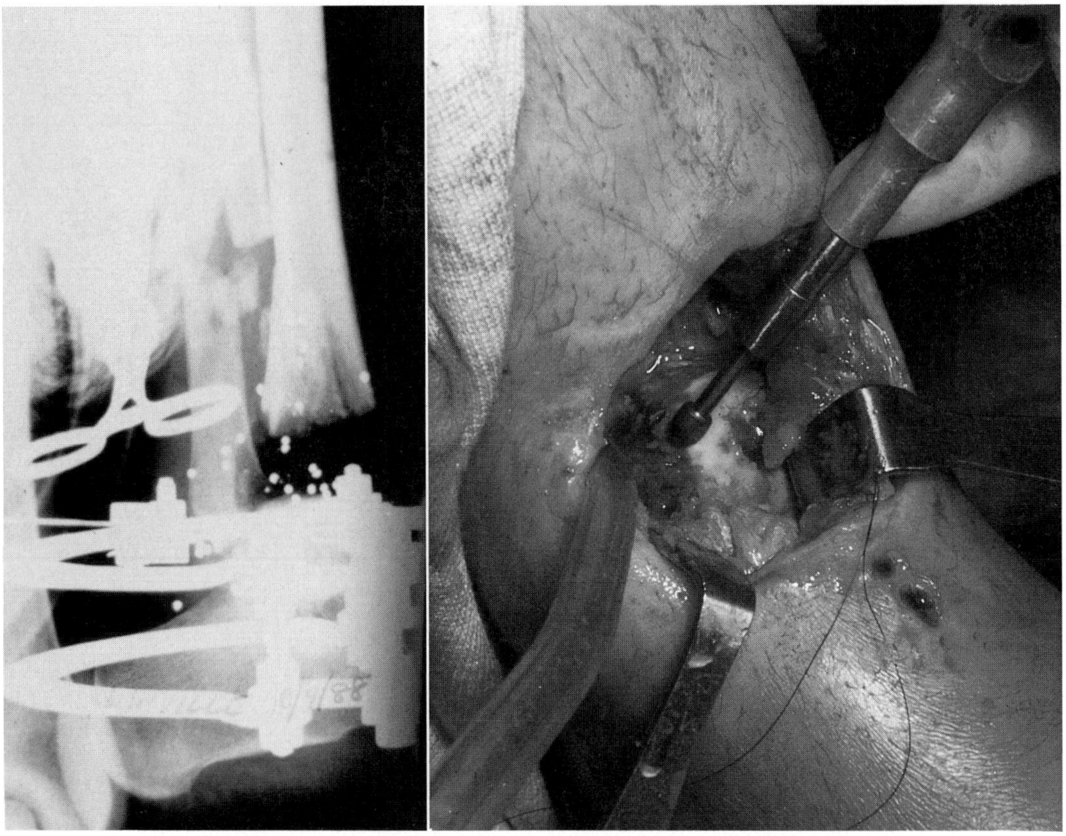

Figure 6 *A,* Intraoperative radiograph of a 21-year-old man injured in a hunting accident. His ankle joint has 6 cm of the distal tibia and talar dome absent. *B,* Necrotic, infected bone and cartilage were debrided with a rongeur and curette. The Midas Rex was used to debride the remaining bone to viable, bleeding ("paprika sign") bone. Culture-directed, intravenous antibiotics were given for 4 weeks. *C,* Intraoperative radiograph showing the tibia collapsed to the talus for ankle fusion and the proximal tibia frame and corticotomy for bone lengthening. *D,* This 6 week postoperative radiograph shows the completed collapse and compression of the tibia into the talus. Also shown is the early bone regenerate of the proximal tibia. *E,* This 4 month postoperative radiograph shows the proximal regenerate of 8 cm of bone; 6 cm was lost in the injury and 2 cm was lost as the tibia was compressed into the talus to obtain ankle fusion. *F,* This 17 month postoperative radiograph shows a solid ankle fusion and a mature proximal tibia regenerate.

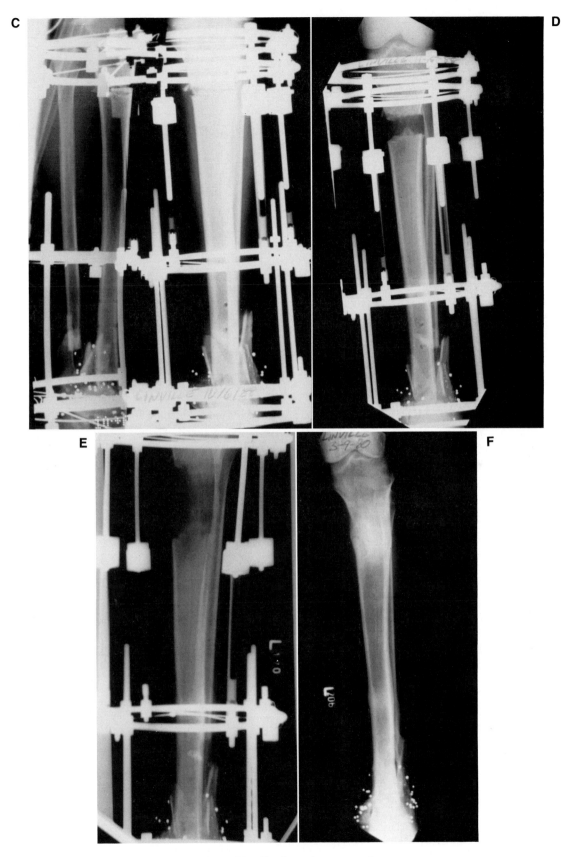

Figure 6, cont'd. For legend see opposite page.

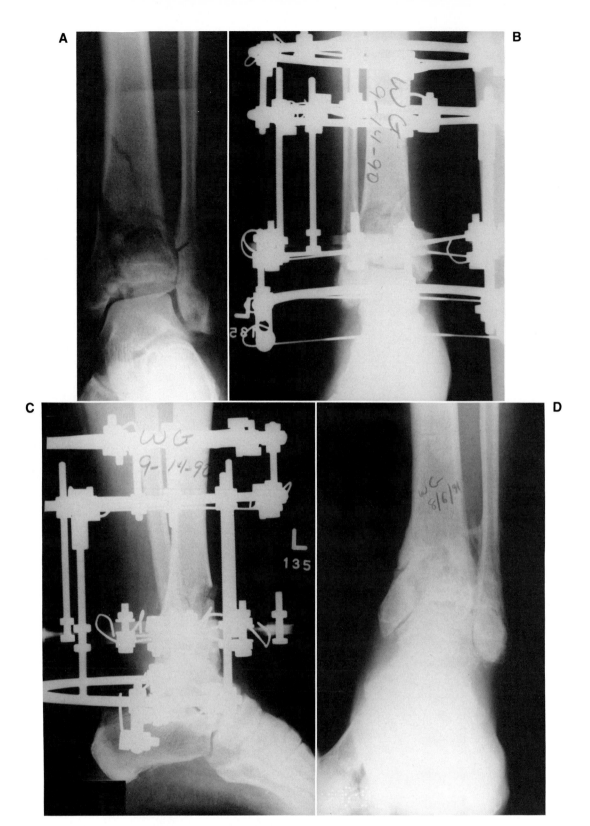

Figure 7 *A,* A preoperative radiograph of a 58-year-old white male with a distal tibial pilon fracture from a 6 foot fall. *B,* Intraoperative anteroposterior radiograph of the pilon fracture reduced with the Ilizarov frame. The talus and calcaneal half-ring is distracted from the tibial rings to create ligamentotaxis. Note the olive wires medially and laterally. *C,* Intraoperative lateral radiograph. The distal tibia fragments are reduced with medial and lateral olive wires and with arc wires. The arc wires are two wires drilled from the medial to the lateral ankle (one relatively anterior, one posterior), and then they are "arched" together, compressing the anterior and distal tibia bone fragments. *D,* Radiograph taken 11 months after injury, showing traumatic arthritis. The patient has no pain except when he mows his lawn; he does not take arthritis medications.

ment joint range of motion and function of muscles, nerves, and vessels of the entire extremity. Preoperative radiographs such as standing plus range-of-motion films, scanograms, and computed tomographic (CT) scans may be needed to show joint abnormalities such as dislocation, ankylosis, and heterotopic bone. A clearly written evaluation with precisely stated limited goals is helpful at the initial visit, for preoperative and immediate postoperative assessment, at discharge, and for each follow-up visit.

Postoperatively, all patients require close monitoring, appropriate casts, splints, and physical therapy. Casts are applied for 6 weeks to allow fibrous tissue growth for soft tissue deformities and for 6 to 15 weeks to allow bone consolidation for fusions and regenerates. Further splints, casts, and surgery may be necessary to maintain the corrected position or prevent recurrence as the child grows.

DISCUSSION

Severe foot and ankle problems of the soft tissue and bone are correctable with the Ilizarov technique. Severe "complex" deformities with varus, valgus, and bone, joint, or muscle abnormalities are correctable, but require a more complex frame. Further, these complex deformities may be difficult to maintain in the corrected position without postcorrection surgery. Treatment of severe foot and ankle bone deformities and injuries also is possible with this technique. Limited goals may be appropriate for patients with severe deformities. The surgeon should formulate a clear preoperative plan and prepare for problems that may be encountered during treatment and maintenance of the correction. Even with its limitations, the Ilizarov technique is helpful for many severe deformities and injuries that previously were unsolved problems.

Acknowledgments. The authors thank Diane M. Anger and Billy R. Ledbetter for their preparation of this manuscript and Lee Rose for his art work.